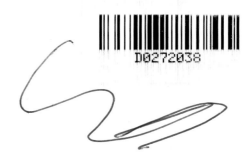

D0272038

Living with
JACKO
FROM TOUCHLINE TO LIFELINE

Alison
and
Peter Jackson

Written with

Andrew Collomosse

GREAT NORTHERN

Great Northern Books
PO Box 213, Ilkley, LS29 9WS
www.greatnorthernbooks.co.uk

Every effort has been made to acknowledge correctly and contact the copyright holders of material in this book. Great Northern Books apologises for any unintentional errors or omissions, which should be notified to the publisher.

ISBN: 978-0-9576399-3-5

Design and layout: David Burrill

Printed and bound by CPI Group (UK) Ltd, Croydon, CR0 4YY

CIP Data
A catalogue for this book is available from the British Library

To our wonderful children,
Charlotte and Oliver

Contents

Acknowledgements

In many ways, *Living with Jacko* has been a labour of love for both of us but it would not have been possible without all the people who have helped and encouraged us along the way. And, in some cases, much more than that. Special thanks, therefore, to Dr Karen Dyker, consultant clinical oncologist at St James's Hospital, Leeds, and all the radiotherapy staff at the hospital. And also to Dominic Martin-Hirsch, consultant ear, nose and throat surgeon with the Calderdale and Huddersfield NHS Trust, and the Macmillan nurses and speech therapy unit at Calderdale and Huddersfield.

We'd like to thank Great Northern Books for publishing our story and Rosemary Conley, Harry Redknapp and Gabby Logan for their kind forewords. We have sourced many of the pictures from our own collection but thanks to the Yorkshire Post, Huddersfield Examiner, Bradford Telegraph & Argus, Halifax Courier and Lincolnshire Echo for their pictures. A thank you for pictures, too, to Barry Wilkinson of Picture House, Ilkley, David Wright, Ian Dobson and Julian Brannigan in the North-East, Rosemary Conley Diet and Fitness, Appleyard Jaguar and Caremark. A big thank you to Richard Coomber for his diligent work in editing *Living with Jacko*, to Malcolm Lorimer for his knowledge of all things Bradford City and to Lynne Greenwood for her editorial advice. And to Andrew Collomosse, who came up with the original idea and has been with us throughout the journey. And finally, on a personal note from Peter, a special thank you to all the thousands of people who backed him and believed in him as a player and manager.

Andrew Collomosse is a freelance sports writer, based in Hebden Bridge, West Yorkshire. He has previously collaborated on the autobiographies of footballers Nat Lofthouse, Jimmy Armfield, Neil Redfearn, Tom Cowan and Peter Swan and cricketers Richard Blakey and Ian Austin. In 2010 he wrote *Magnificent Seven*, the story of Yorkshire's successful side of the 1960s.

Forewords

Harry Redknapp

You won't find too many former football managers working hands on as carers…but when I heard that's what Peter Jackson is doing, it didn't totally surprise me. He's a good sort and he'll do well at it. He'll give it everything and go at it 100 per cent. Just like he did as a player and manager.

I first saw Peter when he was a young player at Bradford City. I was manager at Bournemouth and he struck me straight away as a strong character and a leader. The kind of player you would always want to have on your side and I would have loved to sign him.

But he was a lad who could play at a higher level so it was no surprise when he went to Newcastle in 1986. I thought he would have played in the top flight for a bit longer really but by the time I took over at West Ham in 1994, Peter was 33 and approaching the end of his career.

He always looked likely to go into management because he was a man who was ready to lead from the front. I kept an eye on how he was doing and he knew I was at the other end of a phone if he needed anything. That's important in this game because virtually all managers have worked in the lower divisions and we know how tough it can be. He still knows he can call me any time.

Harry Redknapp has managed Bournemouth, West Ham, Portsmouth, Southampton, Spurs and QPR and played for West Ham, Bournemouth and Seattle Sounders

Rosemary Conley

Alison was one of our shining lights. I knew as soon as I met Alison that she would be a perfect ambassador for Rosemary Conley Diet & Fitness Clubs. With her background in nursing I knew Alison would have a caring personality, which is one of the basic needs of our franchisees.

While being overweight shouldn't be compared with suffering an illness, I was always careful in appointing franchisees who would be sympathetic and empathetic to the members who came to us. They were people who needed help to lose weight and become fitter and would be lacking in confidence. They would need nurturing. Alison delivered on all those fronts and the members loved her for it.

Alison was so successful that she expanded her original territory and took on a number of employees to be instructors in her ever-expanding franchise. She was able to create a wonderful combination of being an excellent weight-loss and fitness instructor but at the same time was a highly efficient businesswoman. Alison always looked amazing and was an inspiration to us at Head Office and to her class members.

We were sad to lose Alison after five years when she sold on her franchise. Happy memories!

Rosemary Conley is the founder and president of the Rosemary Conley Diet and Fitness Clubs. She was awarded the CBE in 2004

Gabby Logan

I met Alison and Peter when my dad, Terry Yorath, worked with Peter at Huddersfield Town. They were always a fun and loving couple and I was really sad to hear about Peter's illness. But the way they have come through this is testament to their strength, both as individuals and as a family.

Gabby Logan is a television presenter and Chancellor of Leeds Trinity University

Prologue –
a time and place for us

Peter Jackson

Born: April 6, 1961, Bradford, West Yorkshire.
Professional Footballer with Bradford City, Newcastle United, Huddersfield Town, Chester, Halifax Town. Football Manager at Huddersfield Town, twice, Lincoln City and Bradford City. Football Agent.
Director, Caremark Calderdale, a Halifax-based company providing domiciliary care and support for elderly and disabled people and the terminally ill.

Alison Jackson (née Whiteley)

Born: February 10, 1958, Halifax, West Yorkshire
Cadet Nurse, Student Nurse, Staff Nurse Oncology Ward, Ward Sister, BUPA Nurse, Medical Representative, Franchise Owner for Rosemary Conley Fitness Programme, Store Manager for Clarins Perfume, Cabin Crew for JMC Airline, part of the Thomas Cook Group, Corporate Sales Manager for Appleyard Jaguar, Bradford, Recruitment Consultant for MGMS International Recruiting.
Managing Director, Caremark Calderdale

Alison Whiteley and Peter Jackson met in the Time And Place Nightclub, Bradford, in the early hours of Wednesday, September 3, 1980. Earlier that night, Peter had been playing at centre-half for Bradford City against Liverpool at Anfield in the Football League Cup. Alison, a staff nurse on the oncology ward at Bradford Royal Infirmary, was having a night out with friends.

Peter. The season before we'd finished fifth in the old Fourth Division. Liverpool had been league champions for the second year in a row. We beat them 1-0 in the first leg at Valley Parade on August 27. It was a fantastic night, the first time I'd seen Valley Parade so full in all my years' going there and watching City as a kid and then playing for them after signing professional in 1979. There were 16,232 crammed in. We went over to Anfield the following Tuesday. I'd watched Liverpool on the telly in European Cup finals, FA Cup finals and loads of massive games and now we were going to play them in front of the Kop, defending a 1-0 lead. We got beat 4-0.

For some bizarre reason – otherwise known as Bobby Campbell, our Northern Ireland striker who'd scored the goal in the first leg – we didn't go for a drink in the Anfield players' lounge after the match. Instead, he took us to this pub behind the Kop. We could have gone and had a look at the trophy room or drunk in the same lounge as Kenny Dalglish, Ian Rush, Graeme Souness and the rest…but no, we all followed Campbell because he was the big man around the club. Imagine visiting players going into the local boozer after a match at Anfield today? I don't remember whether or not Bobby actually knew that pub from past experience. I certainly don't recall it being anything special!

Anyway we had a drink or two before getting on the bus for the journey back home. We didn't reach Bradford until around half past midnight and headed straight for the Time And Place nightclub. It was in a cellar underneath the Midland Hotel, next door to Forster Square station. We all went as a team; not to celebrate being beaten 4-0 but because over the two legs we'd done OK against one of the best teams in Europe.

There were only two clubs in Bradford in those days and Time And Place was very Seventies, straight out of Saturday Night Fever. Men even used to wear white suits like John Travolta. I was never much of a dancer – Alison has always been a better mover – and always felt really self-conscious. I used to think people would be watching me and just used to bob about.

We were all wearing our club blazers and like the rest of the boys, I reckoned I looked pretty smart…even if the blazers did have an image of a bantam, the club's symbol, on the breast pocket. People probably thought we had something to do with Bernard Matthews' poultry business. Bootiful, you might say!

City fans were coming up to us, asking, "How've you gone on?"

"Got beat 4-0."

"What was it like playing against Dalglish and Rush?"

"Got beat 4-0."

We were checking out the girls and after a while, Alison walked by and I asked if she fancied a dance. She didn't know me from Adam but I vaguely knew her because she was in the same class at school as Gerard, one of my two elder brothers. Anthony is the oldest, then Gerard and then me. I could have had the pick of the whole nightclub, of course; all I had to do in those days was click my fingers and the girls would come running! Or that's how I remember it. Alison might have a different take on that. Either way, she said no.

Alison. I didn't go to Time And Place regularly but went along that night with a few of my nursing friends after work. I was going out with a boy – I can't remember his name – who was a big Bradford City fan and we'd arranged to meet at the nightclub after he got back from Liverpool. He'd gone with a group of lads and I suppose they must have broken down or something because he still hadn't turned up after midnight. I thought, "Well, I'm not hanging around waiting for you."

As I was walking past the bar, a spotty young lad with curly hair asked me if I wanted to dance. He was wearing this funny blazer and I remember thinking he must have been a member of the Brighouse and Rastrick Brass Band or maybe the St John Ambulance.

I hadn't noticed him before and I just said no. I didn't really give him another thought but by the time it got to half past one, I started thinking – as you did in those days – "How am I going to get home? I wonder if that lad is still around." He was still there with the rest of his brass band so I strolled past the bar again and this time when he asked me to dance, I said OK.

Peter always says I must have spotted the playboy in him and thought there'd be a sports car waiting outside. In fact it was a Fiat 127. Yellow. And about as big as our settee. Finding out he was a footballer didn't do anything for me. I had three brothers and a dad who were all football crazy and supported Halifax Town. But I had no interest whatsoever. When he dropped me off, he took my phone number and said he'd bring me some tickets for the match against Bournemouth on the Saturday. I never went to the match but he rang me afterwards to ask if I'd enjoyed it. I said, "Yes, it was fabulous, thanks," even though I didn't even know whether they'd won or lost. Then he asked me out for a drink the following week. He arrived smelling strongly of toothpaste.

Peter. I lived in Keighley, about 15 miles from Alison's home in Shelf, which is between Halifax and Bradford, and I stopped and cleaned my teeth twice on the journey. I was that bothered about not having bad breath. We went to a pub in Elland, the Bridge. I can't think why. Neither of us had been before. In those days, people didn't really go out for a meal. If they did it would most likely be chicken and chips in the basket. An Italian or anything like that was way out of my price bracket, more like a couple of drinks and a bag of crisps at the Bridge Inn in Elland. With a game of pool thrown in. How to impress a girl on your first date!

I had to explain the rules to Alison, how to hold the cue and so on. I'd been incredibly tense and nervous all day and when I leaned over the table to play my first shot I couldn't help farting. Or that's what I thought. Instead, I suddenly realised I'd got more than I bargained for and had to go dashing off to the gents, which luckily was right there beside me. It took me what seemed like an age to make myself respectable again.

Alison. So I'm standing there by the pool table, thinking, "I'm on a first date in a revolting pub playing pool with a young lad who happened to give me a lift home from a night club…and he's disappeared into the gents for half an hour. Sweet personality or not, how long have I got? When can we go home?" I honestly wondered if he'd done a runner on me but couldn't work out how he could have escaped from the gents without me noticing. The night ended quite quickly after he came back. He didn't tell me about what had actually happened for another three years.

Peter. I thought I'd blown it, I honestly did. But I called her again a few days later and we arranged to go out the following week.

Alison. Tuesday night at the Acapulco nightclub in Halifax…we really knew how to hit the high spots. It opened in 1962 and believe it or not, it's still there today, claiming to be the UK's oldest nightclub. It was really dark and seedy and I can't think what made us go there. But the night went really, really well from the start. We danced, talked a lot, laughed a lot and had loads to drink.

Late on, when we were sitting on a sofa in the corner, we decided we'd get engaged. Peter had a little brown wallet in his back pocket that contained a tiny diary. He said, "Right, so when will we get engaged?" We plumped for December 13. Then he said, "And we'll get married when?" We picked out June 6 the following year. He tore out the page and we both signed our initials underneath the dates.

It was probably done half in jest and half on a whim because nobody can really fall in love that quickly, can they? And maybe the drink played its part, too. But I knew already what a lovely personality Peter had and that he was the kind of person who would never let me down. And everything grew from there.

I suppose there would have been loads of opportunities for either of us to get out of it if things weren't working out but we were just besotted with each other and spent virtually all our time together from then on. He proposed nine days of meeting me, we were married within nine months and there was never a moment's hesitation for either of us.

Peter. Alison's dad Brian was really formal about some things…like getting engaged. Brenda, her mum, knew what we were planning but not Brian. And when Alison told her mum, she also asked how we should approach it. Her mum said that we would have to do it properly, that I'd have to go and ask her dad one-to-one. I went round to her house for tea and we had spaghetti Bolognese. Then Alison and her mum disappeared; I suppose they said they were going to wash up. I said, "Brian, can I ask you something?"

"What's that, Peter?"

I thought, "Christ, how am I going to get through this?"

"I want to get engaged to Alison. Do you mind welcoming me into your family?"

"Is it not a bit too soon?"

"No, we both feel it's the right time." And he just said, yes, of course.

I had no real life experience at the time, just football. And I still say asking Alison's dad if we could get engaged is the most nerve-racking thing I have ever done.

Alison. We always kept that little piece of paper we tore out of Peter's diary at the Acapulco and 25 years later, our daughter Charlotte had it framed and gave it to us as a silver wedding present. And yes, we did get engaged on December 13, the day after City had played at Southend in a Friday night match, and had a party for family and some of the City players at Silks wine bar in Bradford.

Then we were married on June 6 at All Saints Church, Shelf. Peter always says he doesn't know if we were romantic or just plain daft but we damn well did it anyway!

Peter. And the rest is history...

1. Tuf shoes, long floaty hair and QE2

For six years, Peter Jackson and Alison Whiteley were childhood neighbours in the village of Shelf, midway between Halifax and Bradford. "I went to the same secondary modern as Peter's elder brothers, Anthony and Gerard," recalls Alison. "But at that stage I didn't know Peter. By the time he was old enough to go to secondary school, his family had moved to Keighley. And our paths didn't cross again for over ten years."

Alison's Story

There was about ten feet of snow outside when I was born on February 10, 1958. Dad should have taken mum to hospital but the weather put a stop to that. And even though he called the midwife, she couldn't make it to our house in time. So he had no choice but to deliver me himself. He was a practical man, a chief chartered engineer who was part of the team who designed the drill that bored through the Channel tunnel in the late 80s and early 90s. But even so, delivering babies was not the sort of thing dads expected to do in those days – or today, for that matter!

I was their second child, born three years after my sister, Elizabeth, and followed by my three brothers, Paul, Mark and Jonathan. Mark lives in Harrogate now and Paul in Glasgow but three of us still live not far from our old family home and we see a lot of one another. All our children are close, too.

Mum and dad gave me a perfect, happy childhood. I've always thought that if you can do that for your children and leave them with the kind of good memories I have then you can't do any more. And I like to think both our kids, Charlotte, who was born in August, 1983, and Oliver, who was born three and a half years later, had the same kind of happy childhood.

At first, mum and dad lived in a small three-bedroomed house, number two, Moor End Gardens in Pellon, an area of Halifax. Me and Lizzy shared a room with bunk beds, Paul and Mark had twin beds and when Jonathan was born, he slept in a cot in mum and dad's room. We moved soon afterwards. There was no central heating so we had open fires in the winter and there was a paraffin heater, a creamy-brown contraption that burnt with a blue flame and smelt strongly of paraffin, on the landing during the night.

The road was more like an avenue and there were about ten families living there. I used to play out with kids of the same age. There was a big field at the back where we'd play in the summer and a wall where we used to sit and talk. In school holidays, we'd sometimes be out at seven o'clock in the morning and not come back until bedtime, apart from meals. In the street, in the field. Everybody lived in each other's houses.

In my mind's eye, I remember a massive garden, a big coal bunker at the back of the house and a garage with a swing seat suspended from the roof. But it all seemed so different and so much smaller when I went back a few years ago. I was driving a BMW at the time and it was nearly too wide to get up the avenue; yes, the same avenue I remember as being really grand. I parked outside our old house and I was just having a look when this man drove up. He'd been to the supermarket and wanted to turn into the drive of number two. I had to move forward out of his way. He must have wondered what I was doing because when he'd parked, he came over and said, "Can I help you?"

I replied, "Yes, this is where I was born. I was just driving past so I thought I'd come and see if it's still the same."

He said, "Well come in and have a look. I know exactly who you are. We bought this house off your mum and dad, Brenda and Brian Whiteley. Come on in."

His wife made me a cup of tea and they said it was OK for me to have a look upstairs. It had hardly changed at all. It was really, really weird to go back but also a special moment because I'd lived there for nine happy years.

I suppose, looking back, we must have been quite well off because we always had a car when a lot of families did not. Mum never worked; mums weren't really supposed to work in those days. Dad did a lot of mechanical drawings for the railways and travelled around the world, which was a big thing. Hawaii, China, places that were really remote at that time but where people now go on holiday. So it was mum who really brought up the five kids. And it was the kind of home where, when my dad walked in from work, we all had to be washed and scrubbed and sit quietly until he'd had his tea and read the paper. A lot of families were like that in the early Sixties.

We used to have our family holidays in farmhouses in places like Tenby and Saundersfoot on the Welsh coast with my mum and dad's best friends, Mavis and Eddie Walton. They had three kids, Susan, Jackie and Kevin. Bucket and spade holidays for two weeks every year. We never went abroad but the sun always seemed to shine. Childhood memories again! We never really bothered with suntan lotion – if we did it was probably about factor one – and came home as brown as berries.

When I was nine we moved to a brand new four-bedroomed house in Shelf, between Halifax and Bradford. Dad had just got a new job in Leeds and Shelf was more convenient for travelling. That was when I met my best friend, Christine Patterson. We're still best friends today and nothing's changed, except she's Deegan and I'm Jackson now. On my first day at my new school, Shelf County Primary, she was the first girl who came up to me and started talking. I sat next to her in class and she showed me around. We got on famously well from the start and even now we still play games and do silly things together.

It was a difficult time for me. We'd uprooted home and I had to switch schools just before I sat my 11-Plus exam. I failed and instead of going to Brighouse Girls Grammar School like Lizzy, I went to Queensbury Secondary Modern – not that it did me any harm at all.

It was there that I first came into contact with the Jackson brothers. They also lived in Shelf and Anthony and Gerard both went to the secondary modern. Anthony was a prefect, the one who whacked you at the top of the steps and served your school dinners. We were frightened to death of him. Gerard was in my class but at that stage I didn't know their younger brother, Peter.

There was a good group of local girls from Shelf who went to the same school and we became friends. When we were 14 or 15 we used to go out to the discos in Halifax, which seemed terribly grown up, although we always had to be in by ten. I met my first boyfriend Stephen when I was 15. He was older than me and my dad didn't know about him. Mum did and wasn't too happy about him being older but he was a nice guy.

On our first date, he took me for a drink in a pub. I'd never been in a pub in my life and when he asked me what I wanted to drink I'd absolutely no idea what to say. I looked across the shelf behind the bar and said the first name I recognised. Martini. It seemed like a grown-up thing to drink He asked me if I wanted anything in it. "Like what?" I thought. But I said, "No, I'll have it neat." I've never tasted anything as disgusting in my life!

I always used to fight with Lizzy. I'd nick her clothes when she was out and wear them myself. She used to say to me the next day, "You've been into my wardrobe, haven't you?"

"Never."

When I was 14, she had this fantastic grey and pink patchwork smock. Really trendy at the time. I was going to the school Christmas party and begged her to let me borrow it. No chance! So the minute she walked out of the front door I went to her wardrobe and took it anyway. I wore it at the party along with a pair of manky old Tuf shoes, regulation school footwear that my mum insisted I had to wear all the time. Yes, even at the school Christmas party. I hated them.

When the party ended at around seven o'clock, four of us set off home. We had to change buses halfway and me, Christine and the two other girls were racing to catch the second bus. I followed Christine across the road, right in front of a car accelerating away from the roundabout at a junction called Stone Chair. It scooped me up and threw me into the air. The car drove off and the driver was never found. I must have done about three somersaults before I landed in the middle of the road. It was pitch black, freezing cold and sleeting.

I was unconscious for a while and woke up to find about 50 coats on top of me. All the people on the buses had got off and were trying to help. I must have been in complete shock because I remember sitting bolt upright and saying to Christine, "Where's my shoes?"

She looked a bit baffled but spotted one of them and said, "One of them's here, I can't find the other."

"Right, well just throw it as far away as you can!" She chucked it over a wall into the car park of the Stone Chair variety club. Then I lay down again in agony. I'd fractured my pelvis in two places. Christine ran to her house and they called my mum and dad, who came flying down a few minutes later. The first thing mum said? "Where's your shoes?"

I was in hospital for three weeks and they let me go home on Christmas Eve, which was probably a bit early. I was on crutches and everyone made a big fuss of me. I loved that! Lizzy's smock was a goner, of course, as it was ripped to shreds in the accident and covered in blood. And the missing Tuf shoe? Mum went on a search and found it in the variety club car park! Can't win 'em all, I suppose, but because of my injuries, I was allowed to wear a brand new pair of Levi jeans at school for the rest of the winter.

Christine and I did all sorts of cheeky things and discovered some hilarious ways to acquire boyfriends. There was a music magazine called Sounds and people put in adverts for guitars, amplifiers, sound systems or whatever. Not us. We put in an ad saying, "Two gorgeous girls seek two hunky guys," and gave my home address, 15, Greenacres, Shelf.

We got absolutely loads of replies, maybe a hundred. From all sorts, even people in prison who'd written on toilet paper. Mum was horrified. "What have you done this time? You just cannot do things like this." That's what she thought. We chose what we thought was the most promising letter and arranged to meet these two 'really trendy and hip' (their description!) boys outside C&A in Bradford at two o'clock on a Saturday afternoon. We said we'd be carrying a T Rex album.

It was a lovely sunny day but things took a turn for the worse when we spotted our two 'hunky guys'. They were revolting, absolute nerds. One was wearing really odd clothes and the other a vest. We hid the T Rex album and walked straight past them. They were still there an hour later when we went back to have another look.

Did we learn our lesson? No. Soon afterwards, on a family picnic to Ilkley with mum and dad and my three brothers, we put our telephone numbers in a plastic bag and hid it under a rock at the Cow and Calf on Ilkley Moor. It was found by two Jewish boys from Roundhay in Leeds. One of their fathers owned a jewellery business in the city.

To keep our parents happy, we'd always been in the Girl Guides and then the Rangers and as it happened there was going to be a Rangers party on the Saturday night. When the boys from Roundhay rang, we asked them if they'd like to come. They said they'd pick us up at seven.

Our mums agreed to let us go to the party with them but we had to be in by ten o'clock and not a second later. They picked us up at the top of our road in this beaten up car. It was full of fumes, a really pungent smell, and we thought, "They must smoke strong cigarettes." That's how clueless we were because they'd obviously been smoking joints or something. But we'd no idea.

We climbed in, set off and then they told us we were going to Manchester for the night, never mind the Rangers party. We said we had to be back by ten, no later. They said that would be OK. We'd no idea how long the journey would take and it wasn't until we saw a sign to Nottingham that we realised we were nowhere near Manchester; in fact we were on the M1 and on our way to London.

There was nothing we could do except sit tight and start thinking about what to do when we finally got back home. When we arrived we parked outside these great big houses and one of the boys said, "You two just sit in the car and don't move. We're delivering some jeans." They walked round to the boot and disappeared into one of the houses with all these pairs of jeans.

There was no way we could have moved, even if we'd wanted to. Where could we have gone? It was already well past ten o'clock and we were praying that Mum and Dad would have gone to bed early and wouldn't miss us. I said to Christine, "Look what time it is. When we get back home we are dead." We'd hardly had time to think how we might play it when the two boys came racing out of the house and leaped into the car, shouting, "Come on we're off. The police are on to us." God knows what they were really up to. We raced out of London and headed back up the M1.

They stopped at a service station for a sleep halfway back but we didn't dare get out of the car and ring home. Instead we hatched this plan to creep in quietly, ruffle the beds and then pretend we'd woken up at crack of dawn and gone for an early morning walk. We finally arrived back in Shelf at five o'clock in the morning.

As it happened my sister had been working in Torquay for the summer and was coming back that day to a welcome home party. There was no welcome home for us! As the car pulled up, four adult faces appeared at the window: my mum and dad and Christine's parents. Dad had rung the police at midnight and then called Christine's mum and dad. I thought, "Oh my God!"

We told the two boys they'd have to come in and explain that the car had broken down and we hadn't wanted to ring and wake them up. But they never had a chance to say a word as dad, ranting and raving, chased them down the drive and out into the road. They leaped in the car, raced off at the speed of light and we never saw them again. Christine was dragged off home and we were completely grounded for a month. Bang went our chances of going to a Rolling Stones concert in Manchester soon afterwards and we ended up selling the tickets to Christine's cousin, Terry. Mind you, we made a profit on them. Happy days!

Believe it or not, we felt we'd been really badly done to. In our eyes, we'd done nothing wrong. It wasn't our fault the two boys had decided to go to London, was it? Everything was probably more innocent in those days and I suppose if Charlotte had done the same thing when she was 15, I would have been absolutely petrified. I would have tried to stay calm, for Peter's sake, and when she returned home the first emotion would have been relief...then I would have pretended to be furious. So I suppose not a lot has changed in 38 years!

And looking back, I suppose our parents didn't know the half of it. In those early teenage years, we were quite wild children really. We started going to gigs at Bradford University. We were heavily into music, bands like Deep Purple and Black Sabbath, real rocky bands. We thought we were really chic with our cheesecloth blouses, smocks and long floaty hair. We never did anything bad or malicious and never got into serious trouble. But we were two cheeky little girls who always seemed to get away with things. Just!

Mum and Dad were very keen for all the family to do well at school and Dad put pressure on us. He used to sit down and scrutinise our reports and would say to me, "You must do better at this, Alison. You must try harder at that." I suppose Lizzy paved the way for me. As the oldest, she always had to toe the line and be in on time. She went to the grammar school and was destined to go on to bigger things whereas Alison was going to float by on her looks and her personality.

I did OK at school. I was in the A stream and got good grades at my O levels. But nothing was ever really expected of me academically. Of the five of us, Mark and I have always been the cheeky personalities and sometimes got away with murder. The other three stuck by the book more and concentrated hard at school. Like me, Mark went to the secondary modern, left school after his O levels and has had a successful career in car sales. The others all went to grammar school and took their A levels. Like Mark, Lizzy and Jonathan work in the motor trade and Paul is a property developer.

When Christine and I left school at 16, we decided we weren't quite ready for more studying and thought we'd have a few weeks off. Nothing like the gap year they have today when they go and travel the world. Instead, we had six weeks working as chambermaids and waitresses at the St Nicholas Hotel in Scarborough. We lasted three weeks before we were sacked. We used to go out every night, hit the clubs, roll back in the early hours of the morning, do our duties and then roll out again the next night.

When we came home, it was decision time. Christine had already decided she was going to be a nurse and is now a Clinical Nurse Specialist in Children and Adolescent Mental Health. She has worked in the National Health Service for 37 years. The official plan for me was to go to college in Bradford to train as a chef. I'd signed on for the course before I left school and Mum and Dad had bought a complete set of knives, which cost a couple of hundred pounds. I had aprons, all the gear I needed and everything was organised. Then on the Sunday night before I was due to start, I said to my mum, "I'm not going tomorrow."

"What do you mean?"

"Don't tell my dad but I'm just not remotely interested. I don't want to be a chef." Lizzy would have got a real bollocking if she'd behaved like that and I did think dad would go absolutely ballistic when he found out. But because it was me, it was a case of sit down and let's talk. Mum was just so matter of fact about it. "Right, luvvie. It's your life, what do you want to do?"

I said, "I'm going to be a nurse."

"OK." She must have pacified my dad because within a few days I'd had an interview at Bradford Royal Infirmary and enrolled as a cadet nurse. My parents took me over to Field House, where all the cadets lived, and I look back on my three-year training course as a student nurse as the happiest years of my young adult life.

It was hands on nursing, you had fun on the wards and in those days there was time to nurse patients. The training went in cycles: two weeks in nursing school and then three months on a ward. It didn't seem like hard work, probably because I enjoyed it so much, although it was something I took very seriously. I worked at it really hard and after three years, took my State Registered Nurse exam and passed.

I was 21 when I qualified and immediately became a Staff Nurse on the oncology ward. It had been my last placement as a student. We all did three months on medical, three months on surgical, three months on mental, three months on obstetrics and so on. That gave you a flavour of every single ward so that when you qualified, you were in a position to say, this is what I want to do. Oncology was very challenging for a 21-year-old but it was something I was passionate about. I'd really enjoyed my three months on the ward and that's where I wanted to be.

Nowadays cancer treatment has a good success rate but that wasn't the case in the early 80s. It was about giving people a dignified, pain-free death. The oncology ward I worked on was a long room with smaller wards off the side. Patients came in for treatment on the long ward and were transferred into the side wards to die. Cancer was always black and white to me. You were diagnosed with it and you died from it. That was the only side of oncology nursing I'd seen, a side that involved bad news at the end.

It must have affected my approach to people being ill because I always used to say to the kids when they were poorly, "For goodness' sake, the minute you're diagnosed with cancer, you've got something to worry about. If you're not going to die, shut up, get to school and get on with it." I even said the same sort of thing to Peter when he was moping around after being sacked by Huddersfield Town for the first time in 1999 and the story ended up in the national Press.

So when Peter was diagnosed with lip cancer in 2007 and then throat cancer the following year, I had to do some serious brainwashing. If I'd carried on thinking about cancer as I had 30 years earlier, I would have believed Peter was going to die. I knew treatments had improved enormously and I also knew I wanted to nurse him myself. So I had to change my mindset.

But I still thought, "How am I going to square this with the kids?" Cancer had always been doom and gloom and making things as pleasant as possible for people who were going to die. Now here was my husband, and their dad, diagnosed with a serious cancer.

Peter's Story

Rita, Sue and Bob Too!, the 1987 cult film about two Yorkshire lasses having a fling with a married man, was shot in Buttershaw, the Bradford estate where our family lived when I was born. So it was Leslie, Joan, Anthony, Gerard…and Peter, too, when I completed up the line-up of the Jackson five at St Luke's Hospital on April 6, 1961. I don't remember anything about our time in Buttershaw because we moved to Shelf when I was two. We stayed there for six years and then it was back into Bradford again, this time to Heaton, just a mile or so up the road from Valley Parade.

My dad had a demolition company called Jackson Moran, one of the first in Bradford. He was a hard worker, did well with his business and in 1968, when I was only seven, we went on a family holiday to Italy. Not too many people travelled abroad in those days so it was a really big deal. None of the other kids at my school, Lilycroft Primary, had been abroad.

Then when I was ten we went on a Mediterranean cruise. Not just any old cruise, this was on the QE2. Imagine it! Alison still goes mad when I talk about it. She was one of five kids and remembers family holidays to English resorts…and there was me swanning around on the QE2! I went with my mum and dad and my auntie Cathy, who lived in Settle in the Yorkshire Dales. And believe it or not, the captain was called Peter Jackson! I still have the picture of us shaking hands.

I don't remember whether there were any of the rich and famous on board but that was what the QE2 was all about so there probably were. I wasn't interested. I was just happy running around the boat. I made quite a few friends on board and started taking an early interest in girls. One night I decided I'd take myself off to the cinema. I was supposed to be in bed at ten and when my auntie Cathy went to check the cabin at half eleven to see if I was OK, she thought I must have fallen overboard. The first I knew about the panic going on outside the cinema was a tannoy announcement asking for Peter Jackson to report back to his cabin…and they weren't talking about the captain! I picked up a bit of a bollocking for that.

We had some good holidays and went all over Europe because my dad always said he and mum worked hard and deserved a nice break every year. From 1972, when we moved to a smallholding in the village of Riddlesden, on the outskirts of Keighley, they would leave Anthony, Gerard and me at home to look after the place. Anthony would have been 19 when we moved and Gerard is three years younger than him. The move to Keighley came after dad sold out to Ogdens of Otley, a big demolition company. Looking back, he should have kept his own business and if he had, he might easily have become a very wealthy man.

Keighley is where I really grew up and a lot of people think I was born and raised there. But although Alistair Campbell, Labour's Head of Communications under Tony Blair, and actress Mollie Sugden, from *Are You Being Served?*, feature on the list of Keighley's finest, I'm a Bradford lad. In fact at first it was hard moving from Lilycroft school, where I had a lot of friends, to a new school, Swire Smith Middle School, in a new town. From a school where I knew everybody to one where I knew nobody and I was only 11.

We didn't actually move into the new house until after the start of the summer term so I had to travel from Bradford to Keighley and back every day. Many a day, me and mum set off and I was so nervous I'd be sick in the car and we'd have to turn back. I felt so lonely and isolated and it wasn't an easy time. But things slotted into place when we started to play football regularly. I was quite good even then and at that age, if you're good at football, everything else fits in around you. Before you know what's happening, you're king of the school. It still took a while and a bit of adjusting but I eventually made a lot of friends there and afterwards when I moved on to Greenhead High School.

We lived in a big white house on top of a hill overlooking the Aire valley. I still go back sometimes and on a clear day the views are marvellous, looking out over Keighley and Oakworth and then right the way over to Haworth and the moors beyond. I loved life on the farm after living in the city. We only had 16 acres…but they were my 16 acres! I knew every tree, every wall, every blade of grass, every hut, every stable, every animal, every bird's nest. In fact I collected birds' eggs until I was 17, which shows how worldly wise I was! My mates from school used to come up and we'd camp out in the summer and then play football all day. I never had a proper set of goalposts like kids have today so we used sticks instead. Or even jackets or jumpers. But it was magical on that farm.

I even had my own horse, Prince Pendle Flyer. My dad bought it for me in Bacup. I thought it would be an old horse and we'd feed him, saddle him up, jump on his back and trot round the field. But the Prince was a different kettle of horse and a bit lively to put it mildly. It wasn't even broken in. My dad and I did our best and we managed to get a saddle on it…but even that took a couple of months. Eventually we hired a couple of girls who knew what they were doing to break it in and look after it. They rode it as well.

I did all the jobs on the farm and I often think I'd love to do something like that in the future, go back to basics. I helped with the haymaking, with rearing cows and with the chickens, ducks and geese. Not to mention the turkeys at Christmas. We used to feed them up and then a butcher would come and slaughter them. It was a bit barbaric really. We grew them up from being little chicks and then hit them on the head with a hammer before drawing and plucking them. We never sold any, either, just gave them all to family and friends. I can't remember my dad ever really selling anything.

Maybe he was a bit too generous sometimes but his youngest son had far more of the entrepreneurial spirit! There was a long drive leading up to the farm and every weekend my mum would send me out with a crate of eggs, some egg boxes and a handful of small change. I had this sign, Eggs for Sale, written in big letters on the side of a shoebox. I put a brick inside to stop it blowing away. I haven't got a clue how much I charged for a dozen. The traffic flow wasn't exactly great and what there was consisted mainly of farmers from higher up the hill. They probably had about 58 hens of their own so they were hardly likely to need too many eggs. I'd stand there all day waiting for motorists on the road to stop and I can honestly say I never sold a single bloody egg! So my first dream of becoming a millionaire was over almost before it started.

That was when I hit on Plan B: to become a goat herder. One morning in the school holidays, me and my mate Andrew Northrop set off to Bingley auction market on the bus and bought a baby goat. I think we paid a quid for it. I hid it under my jacket and we smuggled it back to Keighley on the bus. We can't have smelt too fragrant. We'd prepared a little pen and when we got home we put the goat in there and started to feed it cow's milk. It died after three days. Nobody told us we should have been feeding it goat's milk!

Time for Plan C and this time I hit the jackpot. With cows. I went to auction and bought my first calf for about twenty-five quid. I fattened it up for the next few months and then sold it for slaughter for around three hundred pounds. I started off with one and in the end, after about four years, I was looking after eight or nine. Selling them off paid for our honeymoon to Ibiza in 1981.

My dad came from a big family in Settle. He had seven sisters and I spent a lot of my time up there in my school holidays, staying with my auntie Cathy or auntie Celia. It was great walking around the fields and I used to get a load of hand-me-downs from all their kids because I was the youngest. One of my cousins was a lad called David Sharrock, who was three years older than me. He lived at Hellifield, between Settle and Skipton, and supported Preston, which was about 20 miles away. Even so, it was probably his nearest club. He had a Preston North End parka that was passed on to me one summer. And when I went back to Greenhead for the autumn term, kids couldn't work out why this lad from Bradford was wearing a PNE parka. I thought it was massively trendy but I came in for a lot of stick about it.

As well as the farm and my summers in the Dales, my big passion as a youngster was Leeds United. I had a season ticket in the paddock from about the age of nine. My dad had a ticket, too. Now that most grounds are all-seater, they don't have paddocks any more but our spot at Elland Road was in the standing area at the front of the West Stand. It was a smashing view. I grew up supporting the great Leeds side of the Don Revie era in the late sixties and early seventies and we used to go all over with them, even as far as Southampton and to matches in London. My first sight of Wembley was at the FA Cup final in 1972 when Allan Clarke scored the winner against Arsenal. And we were in Paris for the European Cup final in 1975, the year after Revie left and when Jimmy Armfield had succeeded Brian Clough after his 44 days as manager. Leeds lost a controversial match to Bayern Munich and we were standing behind the goal where all the crowd trouble started that eventually led to Leeds being banned from Europe for two years.

My weekends were spent playing football for school and watching Leeds United and I kept scrapbooks with cuttings of all Leeds' matches. I also had a paper round at first, delivering the papers on my Chopper bike, and I was in a football programme club as well. I saved up what I earned from the papers and each week I'd send off for a different club programme, Torquay one week, Liverpool the next and so on. Within the space of about two years I collected programmes from all 92 league clubs. Fast forward around 25 years and I'd played at all 92 league grounds as well. Amazing! But gradually, as I started getting noticed as a player, the trips to Elland Road and the programme collecting began to tail off.

I don't really recall how my own football started. I wasn't from a big football background because while my dad was keen, he was never really a player; he said he used to be a goalkeeper. Anthony and Gerard weren't bad players but nothing exceptional. I played for Greenhead School on Saturday and we had a teacher, Mr Jackson, who was great for me. He was a big, ginger-haired man who liked his rugby. But he was keen on football, too. His name is Stuart but I call him Mr Jackson to this day and I'm still frightened to death of him!

When I was about 14, I used to hang around smokers' corner at school, having a sneaky fag. I was already a pretty decent footballer and one day Mr Jackson came round the corner and spotted me. He gave me a right bollocking. "Jackson, you've got a talent for football and you should use that talent. If you want to go down the right road, stop smoking and make the most of what you've got. Don't throw it away." I didn't have another fag for over 30 years...and when I did, I suffered the worst possible consequences.

I also played in the local Sunday League for Bingley Juniors. They were a good side. I was a centre-forward, scored a few goals and soon started getting noticed. The first real step on the ladder was being chosen by

Keighley Boys when I was 15. And then Yorkshire Boys. Yorkshire schools' football wasn't split up into areas like it is today and there was just the one team selected from the various city and town teams. So for a lad from a small place like Keighley, which wasn't really known as a football town, to get a trial for Yorkshire Boys was an achievement in itself. And to be picked for the final squad of 15 or 16 was amazing. I was presented with a badge for being in the squad and the headmaster at Greenhead allowed me to wear it on my blazer, sewn over the top of my school badge.

However it was soon obvious that I was not quite good enough to play up front at that level so I was switched to centre-half and stayed there for the rest of my career. We played against other county sides and the next step up from there was the big one: England Boys, playing against Scotland at Wembley or Hampden. That was everyone's ambition but you had to be some special player. I was never that good. But I did play against one or two of the lads who made it into the England squad and most of them ended up being signed by Manchester United, Arsenal or one of the other big clubs. A few years later a lot of them had disappeared without making a single league appearance whereas the big rough centre-half from Yorkshire was captaining his local league club.

Scouts always came to watch our games and it wasn't long before I was invited for a trial at Sheffield United and then Burnley. United had a really good side, with players like Tony Currie, Alan Woodward and Trevor Hockey, and I spent a week there followed by a week at Burnley. Their chief scout at the time was Harry Potts who, as manager, had led them to the League Championship in 1960, the European Cup quarter-final the following year and the FA Cup final against Spurs in 1962. The main road outside the stadium at Turf Moor is named after him. Kids who'd been invited for schoolboy trials used to stay at his house for a week and he had a visitors' book in the hall. We all had to sign it when we arrived.

Steve Bruce also had a trial there around the same time but wasn't taken on and eventually signed for Gillingham before moving on to Norwich and then hitting it big at Manchester United. Ironically, over 20 years after our trials with Burnley, Steve took over from me as manager at Huddersfield Town after I'd been sacked in 1999.

There were two of us staying with Harry and his wife, me and a mate called Simon Dalby. One evening Harry said he'd take us to the pictures in town. He dropped us off outside the cinema and arranged to pick us up when the film was over. I can't remember the film but it can't have been too riveting because halfway through I went to the toilet…and found a wallet with sixty quid inside. It was a lot of money in the mid-seventies. I'd been given about fifty pence spending money for the week and here was sixty quid! What should I do? I didn't agonise over it for long. I gave my mate twenty, kept forty for myself and all of a sudden I was the richest kid in school! I honestly still feel really guilty about it to this day.

Rich kid or not, it didn't work out for me at Burnley. I signed Associate Schoolboy forms in 1976 but was released after a year and found myself looking for another opportunity. It came in the shape of a three-month trial with Bradford City. They didn't have any money at the time – not a lot changes! – so one of the directors, a guy called Bill Roper, bless him, said he'd pay my wages for those three months and at the end of the trial, I signed apprentice forms. Eighteen months later, I was making my first team debut at Hereford and after another six months I was the club's youngest captain at 18. So things moved pretty quickly.

Catching a bus from Keighley to Bradford every morning, passing my driving test, playing for the reserves, captain of the reserves at 16, first team debut at 17, first professional contract and captain of the first team before I was 19. I had arrived. Having said that, I'm not sure what I would have done if I hadn't made it as a pro. I was average at school; no brainbox but good at sport. I simply never had any ambition to be anything other than a professional footballer and I was so focused that I didn't really look at any other options. It was either football or football.

I was never the best player but I'd always had a good attitude towards training and playing and a good work ethic. I knew that would be half the battle at a professional club. When I arrived I could see some of the other players didn't have the same dedication and I used to think, "How can they be doing this job when they aren't up for it day in, day out?"

Not long after I started playing for the first team regularly, we had a night match at Southend. In those days teams didn't go through an organised warm-up routine out on the field but at about ten past six, soon after we arrived, I got stripped and ran out on to the pitch on my own. There was no one else warming up – it was each player's choice.

Sitting in the dugout, eating a pie, were Bobby Campbell and John Hawley, two of the senior players. They had a bit of a laugh about me warming up on my own and gave me some stick. "Bloody hell, Jacko, if you're that keen, you'll go well in the game, you'll have a good career." Three years later, I got my big move to Newcastle. I never lost my single-minded approach and I'm convinced it was one of the main reasons why I went on to play over 600 league games for four clubs.

There was a dark side to my progress, though. My mum lived just long enough to see me start playing in the first team before she died from breast cancer. She was 47. I lost her when I was 18 so she never saw me push on from those early games. It was a terrible time and I took it really badly. I was so upset at first that one day I broke down in front of George Mulhall, my manager, during pre-season. He understood what I was going through and told me to take a few days off and to come back when I was ready. But that was never going to work. It meant I would have to be back home all day in a house full of memories and I was back training after a couple of days. I suppose nowadays a young player in that situation would be given counselling.

It was awful to see this beautiful lady deteriorate so much in such a short space of time and leave my dad, my brothers and me on our own at home. Our world just went bang. Since then the three of us have all had some success in our chosen careers and it just seems so tragic that she hasn't been there to enjoy it with us or see her six grandchildren. She died in Cookridge Hospital in Leeds before I met Alison so she never knew her either. Not long after she died, my dad received an offer for the farm that he couldn't refuse, sold up and moved down into the valley, in a little bungalow in Bingley. He never married again.

Joan Veronica Teresa Alice Carroll. She was Irish and her dad, Tony, lived nearby as well. A big fella, about 6ft 4in. He was a rep for a firm who manufactured prosthetic limbs and when I was a kid in Bradford, he sometimes took me to school or gave me a lift home. He drove a little three-wheeler car and the back was full of false arms and legs. I was never that keen on him picking me up!

Her brother, Ronnie, lived up the road from us in Manningham and was a chief inspector with the Bradford police. He always took an interest in my career, too, and when I was appointed manager of Huddersfield for the first time in 1997, he came along to watch my first match in charge against Charlton. It was the last time I saw him alive. He went home that night and dropped dead. Terrible.

All my family were involved as I was making my way up the ladder, though, and I discovered how much when my brother Anthony was moving house not so long ago. He found some old scrapbooks in the loft. There were cuttings in there going all the way back to the start of my career, with headlines like "Jackson signs for Burnley" and "Jackson joins Bantams." Old stories, old headlines from long, long ago. But sometimes it seems like only yesterday.

2. Don't let on that Dad's a footballer

Alison and Peter were married at the Church of St Michael and All Angels at Shelf, on June 6, 1981. "We'd decided we couldn't afford a honeymoon," says Alison, "even though Peter was the captain of Bradford City. That must seem strange to people who think that even in those days, footballers earned a lot of money. But then at the reception, he told me he'd booked ten days at Portinatx in Ibiza as a surprise. Couples didn't usually live together before the wedding then so it was a case of Peter carrying me over the threshold when we arrived home. He had to climb up three steps to the front door. Fortunately he didn't drop me."

Alison's Story

I learned early in our marriage that a wife is second best to football. It is a player's whole life. They are all boys together, it's their vocation and a professional sportsman is 100 per cent absorbed by his sport. If he has a happy marriage running alongside it, that's a bonus. But the worst thing anyone could ever say to me is, "You must have had a great life. Your husband's been a footballer and football manager, earned lots of money and all you've had to do is sit back and powder your nose." Wrong. I have worked for a living, either full-time or part-time, since we were married. I wouldn't have wanted it any other way. When the kids were tiny, I wanted to be there for them as a mum but even during those few years, I could never have imagined living the life of a Footballer's Wife, sitting at home waiting for Peter.

When he was still playing, he'd often come home after a game and I wouldn't even know the result. I wouldn't have a clue. He'd walk in the house and I'd say, "Hello, love, did you win? What do you want for tea?" Football was never really talked about. We never sat down and dissected matches, talked about how Peter had performed, who'd played well, what the manager thought. And I think that was a good thing. It gave Peter a chance to just chill into the family home and it's obviously worked because we're still together over 30 years later.

From the start, I said I would have my own life and my independence and get on with it. I've always thought that the worst thing you can possibly do in life is rely on somebody else. You have to stand on your own two feet and that has been my attitude all along. I also get bored very easily. I'll start a job, try to get to the very top and when I get there, I'm ready to take on another challenge. I've done it all my life. If I can't get any higher, I say,

"Right, bored now, step back and start right at the bottom again."

It probably dates back to my time as a student nurse when I walked on to a ward knowing nothing and left three months later with an understanding of that subject. I was then prepared for the next challenge and ready to start all over again. In my career, though, it hasn't been three months but three years. That's usually been the timespan before I've started looking for something else. And throughout our marriage, our two lives have run parallel. Peter has had his job and I have had mine.

But I soon discovered after marrying Peter that a person's approach to you does change when they find out you're married to a footballer. Even in our early days before most people had heard of Peter, I would be introduced as "Alison, she's married to Peter Jackson, who plays for Bradford City." It was something I just learned to live with. I'd never really bothered about football before we were married. I can remember as a very young child going to watch Halifax Town a couple of times with my dad and granddad and standing there thinking, "What's all this about? I'm bored, time to go home." Once, when Peter dropped some tickets off for a Bradford City match soon after we started going out together, I said to my dad, "Look dad, I don't want to go, will you have them instead?"

I went to a few of Peter's matches, just to show a bit of interest, but I was never really bothered. And football didn't really start to play a much bigger part in my life after we got engaged in 1980. Instead we were more interested in saving up enough for a deposit on a little two-bed bungalow. I wasn't on much money as a staff nurse at Bradford Royal Infirmary but we scraped enough between us to raise a deposit. I think the house cost £14,000.

Our wedding was very traditional, at 11 o'clock on a beautiful sunny morning. I remember everyone else going off to the church and leaving me at home with my dad. The last thing he said before we left the house was, "You look lovely." Then he opened the door and this little dog from across the avenue came running up the drive and jumped straight up the front of my dress. I was horrified but fortunately there was no major damage. I had five bridesmaids, my sister Lizzy, Gerard's wife Sharon, and three of my nursing colleagues. Strangely, my best school friend Christine Patterson wasn't one of them. She had been doing her training as a psychiatric nurse and we weren't in regular touch at the time. She was at the wedding, though, along with one or two of Peter's team-mates.

It was a lovely service but when we came out of the church, it was pouring down. The weather had changed completely. There were a lot of people outside but it was all a bit of a blur for me. And for Peter, too. He'd driven over from Keighley with his dad and brothers, all wearing top hats and morning suits, and he always says he must have looked like a fish up a tree. Strangely, one thing he can remember is that when we came out of church, he spotted Maureen Long, who lived in Shelf and four years earlier had survived an attack by Peter Sutcliffe, the Yorkshire Ripper. She was sitting on the wall outside the church. Obviously a lot of people knew who she was but she didn't know either of us. Peter had always been fascinated by the story of the Ripper, who was from Bradford, and it did seem a bit odd that she should be there.

We were just so excited. That's how it should be, isn't it? And we woke up really early the next morning, all thrilled about going off on our honeymoon. The suitcases were packed and we still had loads of time to kill so we went off for a long walk until the taxi arrived. When we came back from Ibiza, there was a big hole in the fence at the back of the garden and it looked as if someone had broken through. Peter rang 999 and said, "Can you help us. While we've been away, someone's cut a hole in the fence and might have been trying to break in." We didn't know he should have been ringing the local police station, not the emergency service, and the chap at the other end gave him a real bollocking.

That first home was at 24, Devon Way, Bailiffe Bridge, in Brighouse. It was brilliant. You never forget your first little house. There was a kitchen, lounge and two bedrooms but we turned the second one into a dining room. We were real homemakers. We had a new kitchen, a new bathroom, a wedding present from Peter's dad, and we decorated everywhere. Wicker furniture was all the fashion and Les Chapman, who played for City, knew someone who sold it and got us some on the cheap. And like any couple, it was such a thrill to be moving into our own home with our own pots and pans, spending our first Christmas there. Living there meant we were a proper couple and we were so proud. Nearly 20 years later when Peter was manager of Huddersfield Town, he received a letter from a little lad wanting his autograph. He lived at 24, Devon Way! We couldn't believe it and Peter went round and delivered it personally.

Soon after we were married, I became a ward sister, the youngest in Bradford at the age of 21, on the medical ward at St Luke's Hospital. I must have interviewed well! I was earning more than Peter at the time. I'd often be working shifts while Peter would usually be home from training at around half past one. So he had a lot more time than I had to tackle the jobs around the house. I had to take two buses to work then he'd come and pick me up afterwards because we only had the one car…he'd moved up from a Fiat 127 to a Ford Escort by then. We didn't become a two-car family until Peter was given a sponsored car by the club, a red Escort. That's when we bought a red Ford Fiesta for me and we had consecutive number plates, ending in 102 and 103.

We didn't have a massive social life. We tried to go out on a Saturday night, usually for a drink with family or friends. Either that or a takeaway, which was a treat, or sometimes an M&S meal, which was an even bigger treat. We couldn't afford anything else. And if we did go out for a meal, we had to plan well in advance and save up. And for a long time there were no extravagant foreign holidays. We scrimped and saved to have enough to go away. Terry Gray, one of the Bradford City players, had a caravan at Primrose Valley near Scarborough and we once spent a week there. I think he charged us 25 quid.

A bit later, when we had enough for a holiday abroad, we always grabbed the brochures as soon as they came out. We'd get as many as we could and sift through them until we found the cheapest family holiday in Spain. We'd be just about the first people to book. We went with Lizzy and her kids and they were really great times. We'd buy our holiday clothes out of the Grattan catalogue and when we arrived we'd sort out the cheapest all-in menus: ten pesetas or whatever for starter, main course and dessert, with some wine thrown in.

As time went by we used to say to the kids, "Whatever you do, don't let on Dad's a footballer." All of a sudden everything changed if word got out, how people talked to him, how they approached us as a couple. All they wanted to talk about was football. So we used to go to amazing lengths to avoid saying what he did for a living and when we made friends with other people in the hotel, he'd just be Peter. We never really told an outright lie but we became experts at changing the subject when the topic of jobs cropped up. We were just Peter and Alison from Bradford. It became our holiday mission to remain anonymous, although I'm sure some people ended up thinking we were a bit dodgy!

These days we can look back and say we've travelled all over the world and seen some really magical places. But we still look back and say those first holidays were as good as anything we've ever been on. The memories are just as good as they are from our round the world tour over twenty years later.

When we discovered I was pregnant in December, 1982, we decided to move to Brownberry Grove in Shelf, a three-bed semi at the end of a cul-de-sac. We moved in just after Christmas and I gave up work about twelve weeks before Charlotte was born. Peter's season had just finished and he said, "Right, you take it easy and relax. I'll do a bit of work to earn some cash to make up for what you were earning." And he went to work for his brother Anthony's demolition business. That would be absolutely unheard of for a footballer nowadays days but Anthony had always told him that if he needed some extra money he could go and help him. So off he went and while the rest of the players enjoyed their break, Peter was slaving away on site.

Before his first day he rang Anthony and said, "Make sure you look after me. I want a seat up front, not stuck in the back of the van." The van picked him up at half past six in the morning to set off for Manchester and he was chucked straight into the back. Ten men were already in there, some drinking, some smoking Capstan Full Strength cigarettes. He felt ill before he even got to work. But he stuck it out…and again the next day and the next. And Anthony saw he was OK money-wise. Needless to say, nobody at the club knew about it.

He was treated like any of the other workers and, of course, health and safety wasn't like it is today. There was no rigmarole to go through before he was taken on. He just turned up in the morning and got stuck in. He used to come home absolutely knackered and black bright. He managed a couple of weeks before saying enough was enough. And when he finally packed in, he said, "Remind me that if there's ever a time when I'm not involved in football, I won't be working in the demolition business!" It was good for him, though, because he'd left school and gone straight into the little world of football, which in many ways isn't part of the real world. It's a sheltered existence and two weeks on the demolition site gave him an insight into what life was really like. And from that day, he got his head down even more at football.

When Charlotte was born on August 28, 1983, we were delighted she was a little girl. Delighted and relieved because we'd done out the nursery in pink and bought loads of pink clothes. If it hadn't been a girl we would have been horrified. But I was absolutely certain it would be. How did I know? There were no scans but I just knew my little girl was going to have blue eyes and blonde hair and be absolutely gorgeous…and that we'd call her Charlotte. And she was! When Oliver was born in January, 1987, I wasn't anything like so certain that he would be a boy but I wasn't too bothered somehow. I thought it would be nice to have one of each but for some reason it didn't seem to matter so much either way the second time.

I always knew that I wouldn't be going back to nursing straight after Charlotte was born. I don't remember whether or not there was maternity leave in those days but there was never any chance of me taking it because I wanted to bring up Charlotte in the kind of background in which I'd been brought up, where mum stayed at home, looked after the kids and gave them the best start she could. I knew that if I went back part-time I would eventually have been persuaded to do a few more hours here and there and before long I'd be back working nearly full-time.

Peter wasn't earning much as a Fourth Division footballer, even though he was club captain, and for a while with just the one salary we were really strapped for cash. We'd sometimes go round to my mum for tea or we'd 'borrow' a few of her sausages for our own meal. She'd give us washing powder and things like that. But basically we just had to make do and mend. It didn't bother us. There was no question of sitting around waiting for hand-outs or benefits. I've always believed that if you don't have enough money, you should get off your backside and earn some.

We never used credit cards – I don't think either of us even had one – so we paid with the cash we had in our pocket. We never owed anyone a penny, apart from the mortgage. We never bought anything on HP. We decided that if we didn't have the money, we wouldn't spend it. A lot of people think footballers' wives have a cushy number. That once they marry a footballer, their lives are glossy and lovely and they don't have to lift a finger. It wasn't like that for us in the early years.

So I decided to find as much part-time work as I could. While I was pregnant I'd worked as an Avon Lady selling cosmetics and then my first job after Charlotte was born was with Tupperware, first as an agent and then a manager. We still have stacks of it in the loft. I became an area manager for Tupperware after a while and a few years later, when I was working full-time for a drugs company, I had two company cars, a blue Ford for the drugs company, where I was a medical rep, and a white Fiat for Tupperware!

Another part-time job was as a manager for Naturally Yours Cosmetics, with a team of ten girls, and I also ran jewellery parties. I used to go to a wholesaler in Leeds, buy loads of jewellery and then hold house parties where women could come along and buy. Maybe the best example of my entrepreneurial skills, however, was my Mars Bar Diet. One evening I went into the Prince of Orange pub in Shelf and asked if I could run a diet class one night a week, the Mars Bar diet. The landlord agreed so I put up a few posters in the neighbourhood and when I turned up for the first class, they were queuing outside the door! I created the diet myself and allowed them 700 calories a day...plus a Mars bar, to be eaten at any time. Some of them used to cut it up into little slices. For years, I kept bumping into girls who'd been on my diet.

Peter joined in with some of the schemes, too, like my baskets of dried flowers, which were very fashionable at that time. They were really good, if I do say so myself. As it happened, the lady next door had a flower shop so we used to pretend that she made the baskets up in her spare time and we were selling them on for her. Peter took one into work one day and loads of the players and staff were interested in buying them as presents for their wives or girlfriends. We ended up with so many orders that we joked that we'd set up our own cottage industry. We could hardly keep up. It reached the point where there was barely room in the car boot for Peter's kit bag because of all the dried flowers. One day, Terry Yorath, the former Leeds United player who was first team coach at the time, took Peter to one side after training on a Friday and ordered four baskets. I spent the whole weekend putting them together. To this day, they all think the baskets came from our next door neighbour.

Peter also had a brainwave that we could earn some extra money by taking any spare junk and bric-a-brac to car boot sales. It seemed to be a good idea at the time but I only did one and it frightened me to death. As soon as we opened the door, people were pushing us out of the way and reaching into the car, trying to grab things before we'd even set up the table. So Peter became the main man. He enjoyed it, except when people recognised him and said, "You're Peter Jackson from City aren't you? What the bloody hell are you doing at a car boot sale?"

But that only happened once or twice and he was never ashamed to admit that he was doing it because we needed the money. Even so, I can't imagine the captain of Bradford City doing it now unless it was for charity. There was a sale at Brighouse, another at Thornbury roundabout between Leeds and Bradford and another in the car park at Tesco at Buttershaw on the outskirts of the city. He took along a pasting board and a set of legs and chucked all the junk into the boot. He used to drive a hard bargain. And when he ran out of our own stuff, he put the word around at the club that a sale was coming up and players would turn up on the Friday armed with bags of stuff. Kids' clothes were always a good seller. Come to think about it, we've a load of old clothes now that we never wear so maybe Peter could have another go...or maybe charity shops are a better bet.

Of course times changed after Peter's big money move to Newcastle in 1986. All of a sudden, we had to get used to people coming up to us in the street, wanting to talk football or asking for an autograph. We'd be in a restaurant, either on our own or with friends, and they would just wander over to our table and start a conversation. It was difficult to handle at first but after a while we realised that was just how the Newcastle fans were. They were totally fanatical and it never occurred to them that they were imposing or that Peter might not want to interrupt a meal to talk about football.

Being recognised everywhere was strange but something we had to get used to. For Peter it became part of the job and to a lesser extent, it has been the same ever since. It's something we've learned to accept but we will always look back fondly on those early years when times were tough. And such a lot of fun!

Peter's Story

By the time Alison and I were married, I'd been playing first team football for Bradford City for just over two years. I'd signed apprentice terms in November, 1977, after my three-month trial funded by director Bill Roper, but in those days, life as an apprentice professional was a different world from what kids experience today. Today, any youngster signed by a professional club as an academy scholar can expect to play football, football and more football, to be trained and coached properly, to be taught how to look after himself and be offered the chance to complete his education. We didn't have any of that.

The most important thing for us wasn't training, playing football or being coached. Education? You're joking. These days the YTS lads can't even pick up the goal nets after training in case they damage their back but for us it was hard labour from day one. There were three of us. Me, Barry Gallagher, a forward who played around 100 games for the club, and Ray Ellington. Tibor Szabo, who played a handful of first team games in the late seventies, was the head apprentice. He was a year older than the three of us and we had to report to him. He never really did the same work as us but ticked off the various jobs we had to do as we finished them.

We were just general dogsbodies whose main function was to clean the dressing rooms, sweep the stands and terraces, clean the pros' boots, prepare their training gear and matchday kit, take divots out of the pitch. Sometimes we went down to City's Canal Road training ground at Apperley Bridge on the outskirts of the city. But what did I do on my first two visits? I spent the whole time behind the goals running around collecting balls from the pros' shooting practice.

I soon dropped into a daily routine. Every morning I caught the ten to seven bus from Keighley and arrived at Valley Parade at eight o'clock. Sometimes I'd work right through to six in the evening and I wasn't allowed to leave until the work was finished. If the first team were playing a night match, we had to sort out all the dirty kit afterwards and then clean the dressing rooms before we could go home. And if the jobs weren't done right, we'd collect a wallop for our pains and be told to do it again. That was normal and everyone accepted it without question because they'd all been through the same treadmill themselves, either at Valley Parade or elsewhere.

The pay-off came at Christmas when the senior pros gave us a tip. Fantastic! We lived for that. And if the club were feeling generous or they'd had a decent season, there might be a bonus at the end of the season as well. To be fair, we did play a bit of football. We used to train on the car park every Tuesday and Thursday night – our only real coaching. And, of course, we played for the junior team in the Lancashire League; don't ask me why Lancashire and not Yorkshire. It was a fantastic learning curve because as well as playing similar clubs to us, we were up against the big hitters, too. We used to play against the A or B teams from all the top Lancashire sides, including Everton, Liverpool and the two Manchester clubs so there were some pretty decent players around. I was made captain when I was 16.

It was in a youth team game, against Chester in 1978, that I collected my first yellow card. Every professional remembers his first booking and I've still got the paperwork from the FA telling me when, where and why. And I went on to collect my fair share of bookings over the next 20 seasons. As a centre-half, they came with the territory and I was sent off about eight times as well. But that first booking sticks in the memory for a special reason.

Chester's centre-forward looked a bit useful and we'd been having a bit of a dig at one another from the start. Eventually we squared up, exchanged a few pleasantries and when the fuss had died down, the referee called us over and asked for our names. "Peter Jackson," I growled. The ref wrote it down. "And you?" he asked the Chester player. "Ian Rush." Two years later, on December 13, 1980, I was watching ITV's World of Sport on a Saturday afternoon – we'd played at Southend the previous night – when a familiar face flashed up on the screen. Presenter Dickie Davies announced, "Ian Rush will make his Liverpool debut at Ipswich this afternoon." Rush had moved from Chester to Anfield for £300,000 the previous April.

Soon I was playing for the reserves in the old Central League as well and was appointed second team captain when I was 16, too. The reserve team was an even better experience because I found myself playing against seasoned pros as well as young kids like myself who were trying to make their way. There would also be trialists and young players who had just been given a one-year contract to see if they would make it. I don't remember too many who did and there was a very big turnover of players everywhere.

But the combination of old pros, eager youngsters and trialists desperate to make a go of it meant the football had a pretty competitive edge. And we were up against good sides including both Manchester and Liverpool clubs and the big Lancashire and North East sides as well as Yorkshire rivals Huddersfield, Leeds and the Sheffield clubs. My first Central League game was against Sunderland at Roker Park.

I learned fast and on March, 24, 1979, I made my first team debut against Hereford United at Edgar Street. I was 17 and still an apprentice but I was ready for the challenge. I didn't really expect it to happen so quickly but I was determined to make the most of it. I'd always wanted to make my debut before I was 18 and from the start, I'd set myself targets: playing for the juniors, being made captain, playing for the reserves and being made captain there. Then playing for the first team.

And I'm convinced that all the hard work I'd done over the years put me on a sound footing. I firmly believe young footballers today have it far too easy. There was never any chance of me doing a bit of training and then jumping into the car, driving home and putting my feet up…not least because I didn't have a car and I had my apprentice duties to attend to. It was hard graft but I was going to make it count.

I suppose there might have been more glamorous places than Edgar Street to play the first of my 771 first team appearances in all competitions but that didn't matter to me. It was an incredible day and I was so excited, so proud to be making my debut. Some kids play their first league match at 16 but they are usually the exceptional ones, so to be chosen as a 17-year-old, and still an apprentice, felt really special. I remember waking up at home – we didn't travel overnight even though Hereford is 130 miles away – and I was already feeling sick and nervous. That feeling stayed with me all the way down to Hereford and right until the start of the game. There was nothing at stake but I was on my way…and how was I to know I'd go on to play at every league ground?

I was chosen because John Middleton, one of the regular centre-backs, was injured. And the side included four ex-Leeds United players, Paul Reaney, Mick Bates, David McNiven and Rod Johnson. Before joining City, Reaney and Bates were members of Don Revie's squad that I'd supported so fanatically as a kid so you can imagine how it felt to be lining up alongside them for my league debut. Also in the side was Terry Dolan, who'd played for Huddersfield in the old First Division and ten years later was appointed manager of Bradford City when Trevor Cherry left the club. In 1988, Terry took City to within a whisker of the top flight and also managed Rochdale, Hull City and York City. He was my reserve team coach when I was in charge at Huddersfield for the first time between 1997 and 1999.

And alongside me in defence was Steve Baines, another former Huddersfield player, who eventually achieved football rarity status: an ex-pro who crossed the great divide and became a league referee. There was only a small crowd and we were beaten 3-1. But I remember making my first pass, kicking my first clearance out of the ground, knocking my first backpass to the keeper. I did OK. And how could I know that Hereford would be destined to play another key role in my career 32 years later during my time as City's interim manager in 2011?

We were struggling at the wrong end of League Two when I succeeded Peter Taylor on a temporary basis at the end of February, with just a single priority: keep the club in the league. Failure might easily have meant extinction because the club had major financial problems but we achieved our target with one game left...with a 1-1 draw at Hereford. So my career had come full circle. I made my debut as a player at Edgar Street and saved the club there as manager.

George Mulhall was the manager who gave me my chance and that was special, too. I always had a lot of time and respect for George, although I was frightened of him at first because he could be a hard man. But he was the one who spotted something in me as a kid and had taken some time out to coach me. Sometimes in an afternoon, he'd hang a ball from a steel girder above the groundsman's entrance at the old Bradford End for me to practice my heading. George and Bernard Ellison, who was in charge of the City juniors at the same time, were my early mentors and I still bump into Bernard every now and then. He always says he was the man who set me on the road to fame! Until recently he was involved with the club as a scout.

And not only did George hand me my league debut, I played my final competitive match for him 18 years later. I'd left Chester, my last league club, at the end of the 1996-97 season and George immediately offered me a chance at Halifax Town in the Conference. He wanted me to be his captain. But when the chance came along three months later to take over as manager at Huddersfield, he didn't stand in my way. I owe him a lot.

On my 18th birthday, a week after my debut, I turned professional and was given my first senior contract. It was about a month before the end of the season, traditionally the time when the retained list was announced. And I soon learned that new contract time was an unnerving experience for all the professionals, young or old. Every year, on the Monday after the last match of the season, all the pros would line up outside the manager's door to find out if they'd been retained. It was like a conveyor belt and they'd all be a bit twitchy. There wouldn't be too much of the usual dressing room banter. After a player went in, there would be an anxious wait before the door opened and he reappeared. Someone would ask, "What have you got?" and the replies would vary from a year, two years or in some cases even three. And, of course, there were the ones who'd been released.

There was no room for argument or negotiation, no agent to talk on your behalf. The manager would say, "You've got a year on a hundred and twenty quid a week," and that would be it. Take it or leave it. You were grateful for anything you could get, to be honest, and even if you reckoned you were worth an extra ten quid, you'd settle for five if that was all that was going. So I was lucky, to say the least, that my first pro contract was for three years. If I'm totally honest, though, the length of that deal wasn't because I was an outstanding player; more that I was young and if I progressed quickly, I'd be an asset they might be able to sell and make a bit of money on because I was still under contract.

I made eight more appearances that season and another 12 the following year, when City finished fifth in the old Division Four. I played in the last eleven games and then started to play regularly from the start of the 1980-81 campaign. During the season, George Mulhall made me captain, the club's youngest skipper. It was a tremendous honour. After George left in March, 1981, Roy McFarland came in as player-manager. Roy, who'd made nearly 500 appearances for Derby and won 27 England caps, was one of the great centre-halves and obviously he was going to be first-choice. That meant I was going to be in the mix to play alongside him.

Even at 34, he was one of the best centre-halves I have seen. He was a top-class all-round player and was usually the first pick in five-a-sides in training…and not just because he was the manager! I learned a lot from Roy. I appeared in the first 21 matches after he took over but then for a while my form dipped and I only started nine of the last 25 games as we finished second and won promotion to the old Division Three.

Maybe that was just par for the course in a young player or maybe because I was aware that there were rumours of clubs watching 'Peter Jackson, Bradford City's up-and-coming centre-half.' Big clubs like Liverpool, Manchester United, Tottenham were all reported to be checking me out and I admit I started to feel a bit of pressure. And by the time I lost my place, Roy had taken the captaincy off me and given it to Billy Ingham, the former Burnley midfield player. It was a big disappointment and I was upset about it at the time. But with hindsight, the captaincy was a lot of responsibility and perhaps too much for a young player who was also learning his game. It was probably the right thing for Roy to do. Would I have an 18-year-old as captain? Probably not.

Roy left in November, 1982, returning to Derby as part of a new managerial set-up under Peter Taylor, Brian Clough's right hand man at Derby and Nottingham Forest. He was replaced by Trevor Cherry, the former Leeds and England defender who had also captained Huddersfield Town early in his career. Like Roy, Trevor had played nearly 500 times in the top flight and won 28 England caps. He came in as player-manager and was ever-present in the back four for 28 matches after making his debut at the end of December. I played alongside him in central defence for most of his first two seasons in charge.

And it was from that point that my career really kicked on, mainly because Trevor appointed Terry Yorath as his number two. Terry became my mentor. He set everything going again after my career had stood still for a while and he pushed me forward. Terry gave me my confidence back. His man management and coaching were excellent, his knowledge of the game was first rate and it reached the point where if I needed advice about anything, I would turn first to Terry. So much so that when I was going to sign for Newcastle in 1986, I rang him up at half past six in the morning to ask him what sort of money and contract I should be asking for. I'm not sure he appreciated the timing!

Cherry inherited a good young squad, a lot of whom were local lads, people like me, Stuart McCall, Ces Podd and later Don Goodman. Then there were players who came in from outside like Eric McManus, the goalkeeper, Chris Withe, Garry Haire, John Hawley, Bobby Campbell, Dave Evans and John Hendrie. Together it was a pretty potent mix. Like most young sides, we had a tremendous spirit and we simply never knew when we were beaten. Our philosophy was that even if we were two-nil down with three minutes left, we could still win 3-2. It didn't happen, of course, but with that kind of spirit running right through the squad, there weren't too many occasions when we were two goals down anyway.

We were a good side and good people. When we went out, we all went together. It was all for one and one for all. We couldn't afford big days out, like an afternoon at the Races, but most Tuesday afternoons we had a session at the Belle Vue pub, across the main road from Valley Parade, and got over it on our Wednesday off.

When we played away from home one of us would always be responsible for making sure there was a crate of beer on board to drink on the way home, usually we were celebrating but sometimes we had to settle for drowning our sorrows. You won't see a drop of alcohol near a coach these days. Over a season we'd put all the players' fines into a kitty and then put it towards a trip to Magaluf or somewhere equally exotic! We were a small, tight squad of maybe 15 players, who enjoyed training, enjoyed playing, enjoyed winning and hated losing together and above all, enjoyed one another's company. Most of us are still in touch.

The club had major financial problems at the time and in 1983, went into administration with its future in the balance for a while. But the off-the-field difficulties were never allowed to affect our development on the field and as a unit. And if you ask any of that squad to name their happiest time as a player, there's a good chance they will say Bradford City. Valley Parade really was a happy Valley for us all and by the start of the 1984-85 season, when the club was on an even keel once more and Trevor had made me captain again, we were ready for a serious promotion challenge. How could anyone have foreseen the triumph and tragedy that lay ahead?

3. Just a melted blob of yellow plastic

In 1980, at the age of 19, Peter became the youngest captain in Bradford City's history. Before their game against Lincoln City at Valley Parade on May 11, 1985, he was presented with the Third Division Championship Trophy. Just before half-time, the 77-year-old wooden main stand caught fire and in one of sport's worst tragedies, 56 people lost their lives. "We were a young team and we grew up overnight," says Peter. "As captain I had to co-ordinate the aftermath: players attending functions, hospital visits. And funerals, of course. It was humbling. It still is. Twenty-five years afterwards, I was in M&S in Halifax when this lady came up to me and said: 'I've always wanted to thank you for what you did for me on the day of the fire.' I must admit, I filled up."

Alison's story

Charlotte was only 18 months old and we imagined at the time that she would have no memories of the fire. But it affected her almost straight away. Before the fire, she had always been a good sleeper. She had a regular bedtime and would go down at half past seven without any trouble. But almost from the day of the fire, until she was nearly five years old, she would never, ever sleep in her own room.

We'd put her into her cot and straight away she would cry and scream and try to clamber out. We'd take her downstairs for a few minutes then put her back in her cot and the same thing would happen all over again. And again and again and again. We persevered because that was the thinking at the time. But she just would not have it. When she progressed to her own little bed, she'd simply climb out and creep quietly downstairs. We'd suddenly be aware that she was in the room.

For months and months, I had to lie down on the floor beside her and eventually she would nod off. But as soon as I moved a centimetre, she'd be awake again. In the end, we put her mattress at the side of our own double bed and she'd sleep fine with Peter and me alongside her.

When she was three she started going to playschool and one of the first things she was asked to do was paint a picture showing what her mummy or daddy did. She painted a big orange triangle, the shape of a bonfire and behind it a man in a striped shirt. The teacher asked what it was and she replied, "That's daddy and that's the fire." And we'd thought a little baby wouldn't have any memories of that dreadful day. Thankfully, she doesn't recall anything now.

It should have been one of the happiest days of our lives. Instead, it was one of the worst. Before every match Peter had a set routine that began with steak and chips for tea the night before. The dieticians wouldn't like that these days, would they? Then he had to go to bed at the same time every week, before 10pm. Yet however much he tried to make the game against Lincoln just like any other match, it was never going to be that. This was the day Bradford City would be receiving the Division Three Championship trophy and Peter was the captain. I remember him leaving for the match far earlier than usual because he was so excited and so keen to get down to Valley Parade.

My mum called during the morning to see how we all were and said dad was getting ready to go to the match as well, again far earlier than he needed to. My brothers were all going, too. So was Peter's dad and his brothers. And, of course, me and Charlotte. It was going to be a big family occasion. Dad picked us up at around 12.30pm, normally it would have been an hour later. We parked up as usual in the Polar Ford dealership on the main road, where my brother Mark worked. And we realised straight away that there was a fantastic atmosphere all around the stadium.

Because Charlotte was so small, I'd decided beforehand not to sit in the stand and instead went into the players' lounge at the city end of the ground. It's still in the same spot today. There were a couple more wives in there with their babies and we were all so thrilled when the team came out about half an hour before the kick-off and Peter was presented with the trophy. The players did a lap of honour and I just remember looking at all the happy faces of the fans and being so proud of Peter.

When the match kicked off, I sat in the left hand corner of the bar, keeping one eye on the football and one eye on Charlotte. I couldn't actually see right into the stand to my left because there was a big wall in the way but a few minutes before half-time, I was aware that there was a bit of a hoo-ha at the far end of the ground. One or two fans were spilling on to the pitch.

Football hooliganism was still a big problem at the time and I thought somebody had started fighting or causing trouble. I couldn't understand why anyone would want to do that on such a happy day. Almost immediately the game stopped and the players all seemed to be looking into the stand at something I couldn't see. Then all of a sudden the doors at the back of the bar were pushed open and people who had been in the stand started pushing their way into the room and heading for the exit at the far side of the bar.

My instinct was to grab hold of Charlotte and fight my way through the crowd and out of the doors at the back. But so many people were coming into the bar that way that it was impossible. I knew something was happening out in the stand but I was helpless to do anything about it. All I could do was pick up my baby in my arms and try to stop us being pushed too far into a corner and getting crushed. It had all happened in a few seconds and I still had no idea what was going on.

There was no noise, either inside the room or outside in the stand. No real panic. No shouting or crying out. It was eerie. Through the open door I could hear a windy, whirring noise, a kind of whoosh. Charlotte and I were being squeezed right into the corner away from the exit and I was getting really, really frightened. We were facing the pitch and there was nowhere for us to go.

I didn't cry for help or anything but I was starting to really panic when a pair of arms were wrapped around us both and we were dragged bodily through the crowd of people in the room and out of the exit door. It was Peter, still in his kit. Looking back, I think some of the fans stepped aside to let him pull us through. Obviously they now knew what was happening outside, recognised him and could see he was trying to rescue his wife and baby.

We squeezed through the door. Outside there was a wall and a flight of stairs leading down to the players' tunnel area. By the time we escaped, the heat was overpowering and the room was already filling with smoke. People were pushing and scrambling to get down the stairs and on to the pitch. There was a ten-foot drop from the wall down to ground level and Peter jumped over.

I passed Charlotte down to him and he shouted, "Jump, just jump. I'll catch you. Jump!" So I jumped. I was wearing a brand new pair of leather pants and for a split second, I thought, "Bloody hell, I bet I've scuffed my new pants." Peter was holding Charlotte in one arm so he eased me down to the ground with his other hand. Then we ran out of the ground and on to the cobbled street outside the stadium.

Peter knew exactly what was happening because he'd seen the fire starting from the pitch and he knew he had to get us as far away as possible as quickly as he could. As we ran away, I looked back and for the first time saw the smoke billowing out of the stand. I thought, "God, dad's in there, so are Paul, Mark and Jonathan. And Peter's family." For the first time I was terrified. Peter led us halfway up the street and then we stopped beside a wall. He told me to wait there with Charlotte and said he was going back into the ground to see what he could do. I said, "No, you can't go back in there. What can you hope to do?"

He said, "I've got to go back in." I pleaded with him not to do it. By this time there were people who'd escaped from the stand wandering around with their burned clothes stuck to their backs. The clothes had melted in the heat. They were in a daze, in total shock and had no idea that they were badly burned. It was horrific. The fire engines and ambulances started to arrive and everyone seemed to be rushing around in all directions.

There were loads of people wandering aimlessly about asking where their loved ones were. I was asking the same question. I knew Peter was safe but what about my dad and brothers, what about Peter's dad and brothers? It was obvious even then that people must have died in the fire. Peter said he'd go and try and find out where they all were and I begged him not to try and go back into the stand. But he couldn't have done so even if he'd tried.

The houses in the street were occupied almost entirely by Asian families and they had all come out on to the street with blankets, cups of tea and glasses of water, asking people if they wanted to come inside to use the phone – there were no mobiles then. Eventually, after what seemed like an age but was only a few minutes, my dad found us. Peter had spotted him and told him where Charlotte and I were and he told us my brothers were all OK, too.

One of the residents asked if I'd like to ring anyone to say we were safe and I said, "Yes, I just want to phone my mum." She'd said she was going to listen to the match on the radio so I knew she'd know what had happened and would be worried to death.

I said, "Mum, I can't talk for long, I'm using someone else's phone. But Charlotte, me, Peter and dad are safe. So are Paul, Mark and Jonathan." That's all she wanted to hear. I rang off. She said later that it had been the worst thing that had ever happened to her because she felt so helpless. She was just sat at home listening to the radio when she heard that the fire had started. Then the flames burned through the radio cable at the ground and the line was cut off. So she'd no idea what had happened after that. She always said my phone call was the most important she had ever had in her life. Something she would never forget.

Word eventually filtered through to Peter that all the players had to meet up at the pub at the top of the road, the Belle Vue, and he told me that's where he was going. It was a pretty seedy place as I recall but they had to find somewhere to do a head count. I told him that Charlotte and I would be OK, that we'd go back home with my dad and the important thing for him was to make sure his dad and brothers were safe as well. Thankfully they were. And so we left. As we were driving home, I couldn't help wondering if it had all really happened. It just seemed so unreal, the kind of thing you see on the telly and think how terrible; the kind of thing that happens to other people.

I don't think I was in shock, more a sort of daze. Dad dropped us off at home and then all I wanted was for Peter to be home soon as well and to know everyone was safe. I don't remember what time Peter eventually arrived but I seem to think it wasn't as long as I'd expected. Like me, he was still in a daze about it and he hadn't been in long when a great big outside broadcast van pulled up outside the house, accompanied by a couple of motorcycle outriders.

I don't remember whether it was the BBC or ITV or who the commentator was. But Peter was asked if he'd go outside and talk about what had happened. He nodded and went out. He still had his kit on. They wanted to talk to me as well, and afterwards I made tea and biscuits for everyone while my mum kept an eye on Charlotte until the television people had gone. The film of the fire was on all the news bulletins and we just sat there watching it over again and feeling numb. Eventually, I put Charlotte to bed and I went, too. Peter stayed up all night, stunned.

It was a day I could never, ever forget. First the silence, the whooshing sound and then the noise as the rescue started. The burned people and the crushing. The smell is still as vivid as it was all those years ago. For a long time afterwards, if I went to a ground where the stand had old wooden floors, I was petrified. I used to think that if it had happened once it could happen again but of course the Valley Parade fire meant that wooden stands are now a thing of the past. I've never been a nervous person at all but those wooden floors filled me with terror. And to this day, whenever I go into a stadium, a cinema or any big public building, the first thing I look for is the fire escape and my quickest route to it. And if I'm ever in any kind of crush, I wonder straight away how I'm going to escape. I've been there before, you see.

Peter went back to Valley Parade the following week and had a look in the bar at where Charlotte and I had been before he forced his way in. He walked over to where we were standing when he spotted us and on the floor was a melted blob of yellow plastic. It was Charlotte's little Tippy Tuppy feeder. Just a melted blob of yellow plastic.

Would we have died if Peter had not come in? Who knows. To the best of my knowledge the flames never reached there and I don't think anyone died in the room. But clearly the heat and smoke were overpowering and anyone who had not been able to escape would have perished.

How did it affect me? Once the immediate aftermath had settled down, I was able to draw a line under it and move on. I don't honestly think there have been any other long-term effects. The day itself remains an absolutely horrendous memory and something I will never be able to erase from my mind. And I think anyone who was there would say the same thing. Of course it would have been very different if one of my family or Peter's relatives had been killed or burned and I know I would never have got over the trauma.

In the aftermath, I had to be there for Peter as he attended funerals and organised the players' hospital visits and fundraising evenings for the survivors and the relatives of the dead. We were both on autopilot at the time but I saw a light at the end of a long tunnel and aimed for it. I just thank God we all still had a life ahead of us.

Peter's Story

During my two years as an apprentice at Bradford City, one of the jobs we had to do after every match was clear the main stand of all the litter left by spectators. It was an old, dilapidated wooden stand that was built in 1908 and had long since seen better days. There were holes in the floor, under the rows of seats and on the stairways. And when we were clearing up, we'd just brush everything down those holes.

For years, generations of apprentices had done exactly the same thing so you can imagine how much rubbish had piled up down there under that old wooden stand. It was a tinderbox. All it needed was a stray cigarette down one of those holes and whoosh.

The stand had already been condemned as we prepared for our final match of the 1984-85 season against Lincoln City on May 11. In fact the demolition teams were going to move in two days later and knock it down once and for all. Tragically, however, that last match, when we would be presented with the Division Three Championship trophy in front of a full house, would prove to be one game too many for the old stand.

I can't remember being as excited about a football match. I'd hardly slept a wink all night. I was a local lad and I was going to be the first Bradford City captain to lift a championship trophy for 56 years. Imagine that! It was a really big honour for me, almost like winning the FA Cup. My dad and brothers were going to be there; so were Ali, her dad and her brothers. And little Charlotte, too. It was the kind of day every footballer dreams of and it was going to happen to me. I had shredded wheat, bacon and eggs and toast for my breakfast as usual…and then I couldn't settle all morning.

I usually got to the ground at about half past twelve, which was earlier than most of the other players. But I was even earlier this time. It was a sunny, windy day and there was a real party atmosphere as the fans started to arrive, with lots of supporters in fancy dress. And a party atmosphere in the dressing room, too. I've talked earlier about the fantastic spirit right through the club and particularly in the team and it really shone through that day.

Valley Parade was nothing like the top-class stadium it is now. There was a small, covered standing enclosure at the city end of the ground, an open Spion Kop at the opposite end and another small, low terraced stand on the Midland Road side. And then there was the main stand with its rows of seats, some wood and some plastic, behind an old-fashioned standing paddock area.

About half an hour before the kick-off we lined up and walked down the tunnel and out on to the pitch. A huge roar greeted us and we walked to the centre of the pitch and unfurled a banner, reading 'Thank You Fans!' I put the same picture in my office at Valley Parade when I became the manager in 2011. Then I was presented with the trophy and we did a lap of honour. Usually, a trophy ceremony used to take place after the game, followed by the lap of honour, but for some reason they decided to do it the other way round this time. I never found out why.

It was a nothing game for both sides and while it would be unfair to say we were going through the motions a bit, it wasn't particularly intensive.

With five minutes to go before half-time the score was still 0-0.

The first sign that something might be wrong was a puff of smoke at the kop end of the main stand. It grew bigger very quickly indeed and in no time at all the strong wind was blowing the smoke down the stand towards the City End. A few spectators were spilling from the front of the stand into the paddock and then on to the pitch and already I could see flames, also fanned by the strong wind, starting to run along the tarred roof of the stand.

Yet from the pitch we could also see that the people underneath obviously had no idea what was happening on the roof nor, for that matter, in the empty spaces below the stand where the blaze had actually started. They were more concerned about the smoke billowing around them. I knew straight away that this was big trouble. So did all the players. The referee stopped the game and called us together near one of the floodlights and not far from the burning stand.

By now hundreds of people were piling on to the pitch and I remember particularly one young boy who was struggling to clamber over the wall. He was a little coloured lad, no more than six or seven, I suppose. And instinctively I grabbed hold of him and hauled him on to the pitch. It was all done in an instant yet 26 years later, after I'd been given the manager's job on an interim basis, a chap came up to me and said, "You won't remember me, Peter, but you pulled me over the wall on the day of the fire."

As soon as I realised how serious the fire was going to be, my only priority was my family and above all, Alison and Charlotte. I knew they would be in the players' lounge so I just dashed off the pitch and forced my way into the bar. I could see them down at the front so I pushed my way through to them, grabbed hold of Alison and hauled her and Charlotte out of the room. I jumped over a wall on to the side of the pitch, Alison handed down Charlotte and then she jumped, too. We ran out of the stadium and the thing I remember most was the eerie silence outside in the street. There was no screaming, no pandemonium, as you might expect. Just the silence, a whirring noise and the smell of burning.

Once I knew Ali and Charlotte were safe I had to find out if my dad and brothers and Alison's relatives were OK as well. I found her dad and told him where she and Charlotte were. Then as I set off to find my own family I was told that all the players had been asked to report to the Belle Vue pub at the top of the street for a head count.

As I walked into the bar, still in my kit, I saw that ITV's World of Sport was on the television. People in the pub were watching quietly and almost as soon as I arrived, Dickie Davies, the presenter, said there was a news flash from Bradford City. He reported that there had been a fire at the stadium and the match had been stopped. And I remember him adding, "But at this stage there are no reports of any fatalities." Instinctively, I knew he was wrong. I'd seen how quickly the fire had spread through the stand and how intense the flames were. I'd seen some people escaping on to the pitch but knew with absolute certainty that others would have been trapped in the stand. And I knew no one could have survived for long in there.

Almost immediately, live pictures were transmitted with a commentary from John Helm, ITV's man in Yorkshire. It was hard to accept that the horrific pictures on the screen were of events happening 200 yards away and that I'd been out there on the pitch a few minutes earlier.

I don't remember how long I was in the Belle Vue with the other players for the head count but as soon as we knew everyone was OK, I decided to go back to the dressing room and find my false teeth – I'd had two of my front teeth knocked out in a match when I was 16 – and my car keys. There was a fireman on duty near the entrance to the dressing rooms and office block, which had not been affected by the fire, and at first he said we weren't allowed in there. But eventually I persuaded him to let me rescue my teeth, my club blazer and a pair of shoes.

I left the dressing room and walked up to one of the offices that overlooked the ground and saw body bags out there on the pitch. There were a lot, although the official line was still that there weren't many fatalities. I knew different.

By this time I also knew that my dad, Anthony and Gerard were OK. One of the lads said he'd seen them but as there were no mobile phones, it wasn't until I could ring them at home later that I could be sure. All my family and Alison's family had been in A block, at the far end of the stand from where the fire started but even so my brother Gerard was almost caught up in it. He was at the back of the stand and said later it was like a wind tunnel carrying smoke and flames through the stand. He said people were trampling over one another as they rushed for the exits but he managed to find a way out just in time.

My dad was one of the survivors who escaped on to the pitch and one of the first people he saw was Stuart McCall's dad, Andy, who was badly burned. Dad stayed around to help him until the ambulance people arrived.

I climbed into the car and for some reason didn't follow my normal route home, via the city centre. Instead, and don't ask me why, I chose a route that took me past Bradford Royal Infirmary. Maybe it was a subconscious thing. As I approached the hospital, I could see people sitting on the walls outside with bandages on their hands and faces. I simply had to stop and see for myself what was happening inside. Apart from the shoes and blazer, I was still wearing my City strip. I walked into the accident and emergency unit and I just could not believe the number of people in there with burns. It was horrendous, it really was. The smell of the hospital, the smell of burnt flesh.

The staff were doing a fantastic job but they were simply overrun by the number of casualties. I felt the least I could do was try to console some of the victims as best I could. And it was just so moving because there were people lying there with major burns who only wanted to talk to me about Bradford City. They wanted to congratulate me on what a wonderful season we'd had.

They said how great it would be to play against teams like Leeds, Huddersfield, Sheffield United and Sunderland next season and how they wouldn't miss those games for anything. This was from people with sixty or seventy per cent burns. Tragically some of them didn't make it to the start of the new season but survivors still come up to me to this day and remember how they talked to me in the hospital after the fire.

I've no idea how long I stayed but when I got home, the television crews were there with reporters wanting to talk to me. I was just a little-known footballer caught up in an enormous tragedy but minutes later pictures of me were being beamed around the country and beyond. When everyone had gone and Charlotte and Alison were in bed, I stayed downstairs in the lounge. I spent the night on the sofa, still wearing my kit, dumbfounded. Every television channel was showing footage of the fire over and over again and I just sat and watched. Transfixed, numb.

I may have slept, maybe not. Then the following morning, the screens were full of the story again and all the newspapers were carrying reports on their front and back pages and inside. It would have been impossible to get away from it all, even if I'd wanted to. Which I didn't. On the Monday the players got together to talk about what we should do next. The full horror of the tragedy was known by this time and we knew that we would have to attend funerals and visit victims in hospital.

I suppose that if something so awful happened today, the players would receive counselling. They would be given some kind of advice about how to approach visiting people in hospital with sixty or seventy per cent burns. Or how to talk to relatives of the dead when they attended the funerals. We were, after all, a very young side and obviously none of us had ever been through anything remotely like this before. But there was no help, no advice. All we could do was just get on with those awful tasks in the only way we knew. As a team.

I have to say the players were fantastic. As captain it was down to me to draw up a rota for some players to attend every funeral. Trevor Cherry, the manager, and his coaching staff and club officials had their own arrangement. There was another rota for visits to the burns unit and another for fund-raising events in aid of the injured and the bereaved families. Two months after the disaster players from both sides attended a memorial service at Valley Parade and we all gave up our summer to do what we could.

The Bradford players had been due to go to Spain on the Wednesday after the match for an end-of-season trip but obviously that was cancelled, although some of the Lincoln players did go ahead with their own trip to Mallorca. And they had a major scare when their plane landed at Leeds Bradford airport at the end of the return journey, overshot the runway and the passengers had to leave by the escape shoots.

Incredibly, there was a suggestion that the Football League wanted to replay what was in effect an abandoned game. I even had a call from Gordon Taylor, then the chairman of the Professional Footballers Association, asking how the players felt about that. I told him in no uncertain terms that there was no way the Bradford City players would even consider it. The idea was dropped almost as quickly as it had been raised.

I will never forget May 11, 1985. It was a day that started happily and quietly but in the end a day that, in the space of a few minutes, changed the face of football and the safety of football grounds. It was a day that affected me for a very long time. It affected us all. And people all over the country can remember exactly where they were on the day of the Bradford City fire.

Eventually, as a group of players, we had to prepare for the new season. Obviously all our home games would have to be played away from home while Valley Parade was rebuilt, at Leeds, Huddersfield and, for the most part, Odsal Stadium, home of what was then Bradford Northern Rugby League club, now Bradford Bulls. Our first 'home' game, four matches into the season, was against Stoke at Elland Road. I'd been there many times as a supporter and had also played in a West Riding Cup game for Bradford. But I don't recall any kind of special feeling because I was in the home dressing room at Elland Road. It was an important game for Bradford City, our first 'home' match since the tragedy and we needed to win it for our supporters. And we did, beating a good Stoke side 3-1.

Our next two games were played at Huddersfield's old Leeds Road ground, the first an away match against Town, the next a 'home' game against Hull City. In the away dressing room one week, in the home dressing room the next. How bizarre is that? Town beat us 2-0 but we won 4-2 against Hull. Seven of our first nine matches were officially away from home and it wasn't until November 2 that we played out first league game at Odsal. In all we played eleven league matches there, with six at Huddersfield and four at Leeds, and we started with a 1-0 win against Crystal Palace.

We won the next three on the bounce and in the end won six of the matches we played at Odsal. There should have been more but there were a lot of mid-winter postponements and sometimes it wasn't fit for a rearranged game, which was then switched to Leeds or Huddersfield. Odsal is an impressive stadium these days but had not been fully redeveloped at the time. It was a vast bowl that in 1954 had staged a Rugby League Cup final replay between Halifax and Warrington in front of an official attendance of 102,569. But people say the crowd was much bigger, more like 120,000, because a load of fans had got in without paying. So you can imagine what an enormous ground it was and how a crowd of 10,000 or so would look lost in there.

And as well as being Bradford Northern's HQ, it doubled up as the home of the Bradford Dukes speedway team, with a cinder track running all round the pitch. The corners of the pitch stuck out into the track and had to be removed if there was a speedway meeting and then replaced for football and rugby matches. They were just wooden boards with turf fixed on top so often a player would scuff the wood as he took a corner.

At first, we had to change in portakabins right at the top of the ground and then walk down a flight of steps on to the pitch through the crowd. It was a hell of a climb back up for the losers. Eventually, proper dressing rooms were installed under the main stand as part of the stadium's redevelopment.

Despite its drawbacks, however, we didn't mind playing at Odsal. The pitch wasn't the best, the facilities were a bit primitive, the floodlights weren't really up to standard and it was hellish cold in winter. So cold that the fans used to call it Ice Station Zebra. So if we thought it was tough, what was it like for visiting sides? Particularly against a side as committed as we were. After the fire, we stuck together like never before and that togetherness ran right through the club. Not just the players, manager and coaches but the supporters, the office staff, the directors, everyone.

We all knew what a fitting memorial it would be if we could not only survive at the higher level but also perform well. And we did. Given all the circumstances, to finish 13th in what is now the Championship was a tremendous performance by those players.

Lincoln City, our opponents on the day of the tragedy, did not play at Valley Parade again until Boxing Day, 2007. I was manager of Lincoln, Stuart McCall, my team-mate on that awful occasion 22 years earlier, was in charge of Bradford City. It was an emotional day.

4. Talk of the Toon

On October, 23, 1986, Peter left Bradford City and headed north to Newcastle United for £250,000, equalling Newcastle's record transfer fee. New dressing room, same old banter. But for Alison, the move was a complete culture shock. "I felt as if I was in a foreign country, I really did. Everything felt totally alien and that's when the enormity of what we'd done really hit me."

Alison's Story

When I married Peter I knew that transfers were part and parcel of the job. I accepted that at any time I might have to drop everything and move to another part of the country, almost certainly somewhere I'd never been before. Even so, when Peter moved from Bradford City to Newcastle on October 23, 1986, the transfer came completely out of the blue.

There had been no speculation about Newcastle in the media and while Peter had been linked with one or two other clubs in the past, things had gone quiet. There was nothing to suggest that he wouldn't be spending another season with Bradford City, who, later that year, would be moving back to Valley Parade for the first time since the fire.

We'd left the house at Devon Way about 18 months earlier and settled into a new home, a little two-bedroom cottage, built in 1874, in Witchfield Hill, Shelf. We'd snapped it up as soon as it went on the market but once I was pregnant with Oliver, we knew that long-term it wouldn't be big enough for four of us. But for the time being we were really settled. It was a lovely little place to bring up Charlotte, I could take her to playschool and toddlers club with my sister, Lizzy, and we were surrounded by friends and family.

For a while, we'd been receiving joke calls from friends, usually other footballers, pretending to be working for big clubs. The phone would ring and a voice would say, "This is Joe Bloggs or whoever from Everton, is Peter Jackson there, please?" I'd put the phone down and dash through to Peter to tell him Everton were on the phone. Then the true identity of the prankster would be revealed and Peter would go mental.

So when the voice at the end of the line said, "This is Willie McFaul, manager of Newcastle United, is Peter Jackson there?" I replied in what must have sounded like a bored tone, "Yeah, yeah, hang on a minute." Then I called out, "Peter, it's a guy called Willie McFaul. Says he's from Newcastle United." And then as I handed over the phone, I whispered, "It sounds like somebody taking the piss again…" Needless to say, I'd never heard of Willie McFaul.

But this was no joke, this was the real thing. And Willie McFaul was saying the clubs had agreed a fee and would Peter drive up and meet the Newcastle physio at the Scotch Corner hotel on the A1 at 11.30 the following morning for a medical. If that was OK, he'd then drive up to Newcastle to discuss personal terms and, if all went well, join Newcastle United.

Peter said he'd be bringing his wife along, too. That's what some players did in those days because agents were few and far between and Peter didn't have one. It was nice to be involved although I've never played any part in any of Peter's transfers or managerial appointments since. These days, some footballers' wives seem to influence their husband in his choice and in some cases players turn down big offers because their wives don't fancy living in a certain place. That would never have happened with us. The following morning, we left Charlotte at home with my mum and drove up to Scotch Corner. Peter passed the medical at Catterick Army Camp and then off we went, destination Newcastle.

When we arrived at the stadium, it was pandemonium, with reporters, photographers, TV cameras everywhere. Newcastle had paid £250,000 for Peter, equalling their previous transfer record, so he was big news. After he'd agreed terms with Willie McFaul, we walked into the reception area and he was taken down a corridor to the right, to be interviewed and photographed by the football press. I was taken down a corridor to the left for an interview with the news and features journalists. I remember looking around, feeling vulnerable and pregnant, and I looked back for Peter. He turned round at the same time and mouthed, "Be careful what you say." Ever so deliberately.

I was interviewed and grilled on all sorts of subjects. For example, I was asked, "Do you go out a lot?"

"Not really."

"Do you enjoy going to the races?"

"Well, yes, sometimes."

"Does your husband gamble?"

"Yes, we both do when we're at the races."

"How much does he bet?"

And it went on and on. I was – and still am – outgoing, chatty and honest and normally I'd talk away quite naturally. I'd have said, "Yes, we put money on the horses," thinking of our little £3 bet on a day out when they would have been thinking more like £300. They kept trying to catch me out so they could get down to the nitty gritty about their new big signing's marriage. It was the first time I'd had any sort of grilling from the Press but thanks to Peter's warning, I managed not to fall into any traps and was diplomatic with my answers.

Afterwards I called my mum and said, "We're in Newcastle, we're staying overnight in a hotel and we'll be going into a club flat at the end of the week. Then we'll be moving up to Newcastle full-time. So can you put the house up for sale for us and arrange for Pickford's to come and put the furniture in store?" And that was it. We never went back to the little cottage that had been our dream home.

As it happened, there was a guy called Peter Flescher on the City board and obviously he'd known about Peter's move. As soon as he heard we were putting the house up for sale, he was on the phone wanting to buy it. So we never actually put it on the market and made about 20 grand profit after 18 months.

Our apartment was brand new and in a street called Strawberry Place, right in the city centre and next to a nightclub. Peter, me and Charlotte, who had stayed with my mum and dad while we were in the hotel, moved in. It was a really plush apartment, owned by the club, and I think there was another new player staying in the block as well. At around half past nine on our first morning, Peter announced, "Right, I'm going training," and off he went. Leaving me, Charlotte and the pushchair in a strange apartment in a strange city.

I thought, "Peter's going to be out training every day so it's no good me sitting and moping around. I'm going to have to talk to people, to make friends, to get to know my way about." I knew we'd have to go out…but where to? And would we be able to find our way back? I actually toyed with the idea of tying a ball of string to the door handle and pulling it behind me into the city centre so that at least we'd know how to get back. But where to find a ball of string that long?

I'd never been to Newcastle in my life and here I was having to find my way around with a little three-year-old. It was scary, it really was. I locked the door behind us, took the lift to the ground floor and out of the front door of the block. First decision: left or right? I turned right, then took a first left. Just in front of me was a little café. We went in and sat down. The waitress came across and I ordered a cup of coffee for myself and a soft drink for Charlotte. She just looked at me and didn't answer. So I ordered again. Same reaction.

And then it dawned on me that she couldn't understand a word I was saying. When she spoke to me, it was in the strongest Geordie accent I've ever heard in my life and I couldn't understand her either. I thought, "How am I going to be able to live in a place where I can't understand what people are saying?" Peter was going to be fine. He had his football, his team-mates and the dressing room banter. That's the same everywhere for the players and while they're at the club or the training ground, nothing else exists. I knew Peter would adapt straight away.

But as Charlotte and I sat in that little café I realised that I would also have to adapt and fast. I thought, "Well, we're here now so we'd better get on with it." And that's what we did. But living in the flat wasn't easy and I can't really remember what I did on a day-to-day basis.

We used to go back down to Yorkshire and stay with my mum and dad every weekend, driving down after home matches. Sometimes, if Peter was playing away from home, I'd go down on my own with Charlotte or mum and dad would come and stay with us. At first I still saw Yorkshire as my base and it helped me cope with the other five days of the week living in a flat in Newcastle.

Straight away we started house hunting. Peter asked some of the other players where the best areas were and we began looking in Jesmond and South Gosforth. We discovered some new houses were being built just behind the Freeman's Hospital in South Gosforth and chose a four-bedroomed detached.

The house wasn't quite ready so we put down a deposit and then actually moved in on Christmas Eve of all days. Mum and dad came up and helped with the move because Peter had to train as normal. I was first over the threshold, followed by Charlotte, mum and dad, and the first thing I said was, "Where's the Christmas tree?" Even before, "Put the kettle on!" It was Christmas Eve and we just had to have a tree with baubles to make it Christmassy for Charlotte. So dad went off to buy a tree, a proper one, and some lights and trimmings and by the time Peter arrived back from training, the tree was up and running. No curtains, no pictures, no lightshades…but at least we had a tree!

Newcastle was a different world. Bradford was a homely football club where everyone knew everyone else and on match days, the mums would take their kiddies along and have their own little room. Now it was up to me to make my own life and unlike Bradford, I went to every home match at first. I felt it was important for me to meet all the other wives. A lot of them had young children around Charlotte's age so we would all mix at matches.

But it wasn't until we moved into our new home that I really started to make proper friends. Our neighbours, Gordon and Gary, were a lovely couple in their sixties and they went out of their way to make us feel at home. Their son Trevor and his wife Jackie lived about three miles away and we were introduced straight away. They became fantastic friends for the two years we were there. They had two children, around the same ages as Charlotte and Oliver, and me and Jackie did everything together. They've split up now but I still speak to her via Facebook.

We also made good friends with Neil McDonald, one of Peter's team-mates, and his wife Lynn, who was a dental nurse. Like Peter, Neil went into coaching and management after he stopped playing and had a spell as Peter's number two while he was manager of Lincoln. And we also made friends with a couple across the road, Anne and Bob, whose daughter Sue was around the same age as me and became a friend, too. So I had three really good girlie friends and also mixed with the other wives at the club.

Charlotte soon settled into her first school, Gosforth Junior and Infants, and then Oliver was born in the Victoria Hospital in Gosforth on January 22. I went into labour at about six o'clock in the morning and woke up Peter.

He said, "You'll be all right, love. It's the second one. It will be ages yet," rolled over and went back to sleep. At half past eight, I managed to convince him it was going to be a lot quicker. So we phoned my mum and she got on a train from Bradford. Then we phoned Lynn McDonald, who said she could come straight over and look after Charlotte. She arrived at about nine o'clock.

We set off to the hospital in the car and were given a rousing send-off by the builders who were working on the other houses on the estate. They were all Newcastle supporters and knew before we moved in that Peter had bought the house. The first time we went for a look to see how it was coming along, they had scrawled, "Good luck on Saturday, Jacko!" on the plastered walls.

They kept an eye on me while I was pregnant and as Peter drove me away, they were all cheering and waving and wishing me luck. I did my best to smile back through gritted teeth. Peter stopped on the way for a sandwich and a newspaper and we reached the hospital soon after ten. Oliver was born at twenty past eleven, exactly the same time as Charlotte, although she was born at night. But even so, it was uncanny. Peter was with me at the birth but left soon afterwards to collect mum and Charlotte, who was wearing odd socks when she arrived because Peter had got her ready for the visit. The funny things you remember! Oliver and I went home the following day. Oliver was a perfect, beautiful blond-haired, blue-eyed boy. Peter and I were very proud parents as we brought him home to a rousing cheer from the builders. Family now complete!

The next day was Friday and when he arrived home from training, Peter looked round the kitchen and said, "We seem to be running out of food."

"OK," I replied, "you'll have to go to the supermarket." Mum would have gone on her own but she didn't drive.

Peter said, "I can't go to the supermarket on a Friday. I've got a match tomorrow." I ask you! I thought, "Right…," stood up, got dressed, put my coat on and headed for the door. Mum was going mad. I nearly passed out on my way to the door but I was making my statement: "This says it all. Men, football, mollycoddled, selfish." Peter got the message and reluctantly set off for the supermarket.

I joined a gym almost straight after Oliver was born. It had its own nursery and I used to take Oliver along to the nursery and then spend just about all day working out in the gym to lose the baby fat. In the end, fitness and losing weight became an obsession. All the other wives were slim and beautiful and well dressed and I was desperate to be like them. We were at a big club, our life had changed overnight and I felt I had to be part of the glitter. For the only time in my life I became what people now regard as a Footballer's Wife.

My first priority was to trim down from my usual size ten or 12 to a size eight, so I could fit into the expected role model and be like the other wives. That involved almost starving myself, taking in only 400 calories a day, even counting how many peas I ate. Sometimes I used sachets of powdered diet food. I wouldn't even lick a stamp because the gum might contain calories that I couldn't count.

A strict diet like this and working out all the time was a dangerous combination. When I went home my mum would be shocked and say, "Alison, you look awful." I'd look at my size eight figure in the mirror and reply, "No I don't, I look fantastic." But when I see photographs of myself from the Newcastle days, I know she was right. I did look awful, just like a stick. I must have been quite close to anorexia.

The Metro Centre had just opened at Gateshead and like the rest of the wives, I used to go shopping there and spend loads of money on clothes and handbags. There were lots of invitations for players and their wives to attend all sorts of functions – Peter once judged a beauty contest! – and we nearly always said yes.

I don't think Peter really noticed my new shape or the long, blonde swishing hair. He's never really been bothered whether I've been a size eight or a size 14 and always says I look lovely whatever. If he spotted I was surviving on sachets of diet food every night rather than tucking into a decent meal, he never said anything or maybe he didn't think anything of it.

I was trying to conform to the image expected of a footballer's wife, seeing pictures of myself in the local papers, having people ask for my autograph. I was impressionable and wanted to be a footballer's wife for Peter, rather than myself. People wanted to know Peter and I wanted them to see him with a perfect wife on his arm, the kind of wife a player was expected to have, with two gorgeous little children alongside them. We earned nowhere near the money top players can earn today, of course, but I can see where today's wives and girlfriends are coming from. If I felt under pressure then, because of all the media attention, they must be under more pressure now to play the part, look the part and conform to the image expected of them. The players are the icons and always have been; the wives or girlfriends on their arm feel they have to play a role.

I don't think for a minute that they are all stupid and just in it for the money. And a lot of them have been with their partner for a long time, often before he was famous. But they will be very aware that some players, when they have become household names, have dropped a long-time girlfriend like a sack of spuds and taken up with a model, a pop star or whatever. They don't want to suffer the same fate and feel the only way they can avoid that is by becoming a Footballer's Wife.

They get a lot of stick for having expensive designer clothes and a lifestyle to match but isn't that what the public expects? They can't just walk about in a Primark coat…not that I have anything against Primark coats. But imagine the criticism they would receive if they did. They are under constant scrutiny. If they have a spot or a pimple on their face or a bunion on their foot, it will be spotted by a camera lens.

And it always fascinates me how all the top players seem to have beautiful partners or girlfriends. Let's face it, some of the players are pretty ugly but there's no shortage of girls ready to drape themselves on their arm. In many ways I do feel for the long-time girlfriends or wives who suddenly find themselves in the spotlight and having to live up to an image they never really aspired to.

Even when we were in Newcastle over 25 years ago, it wasn't just the players people would recognise, it was their wives as well. If you were involved with Newcastle United, you became a celebrity, public property almost. Once, when Oliver was tiny, I decided not to go to the match and opted instead for the Metro Centre. I dropped Peter off at St James' Park and watched him make his way up to the main entrance with the crowd all over him, people taking photos and asking for his autograph.

I was so absorbed that I didn't realise the car was also surrounded by fans and they started knocking on the window and asking me for my autograph. They were pushing pictures of me and Peter and pieces of paper through the window and shouting: "Will you sign this Mrs Jackson?"

I was thinking, "Shit, what do I write? 'Best wishes, Mrs Jackson,' or 'Kind regards, Alison.'" Peter could see what was happening and mouthed, "What are you doing?" I was tempted to say, "I don't know." But one thing I did know was that I wouldn't be doing it again! It was bizarre, unreal.

Often, when we went out socially, either to a club or a restaurant, we were pestered by women making advances to Peter, just wanting me to rise to the bait. I managed to play the supportive wife all the time but sometimes it wasn't easy. But Peter was always the perfect husband and he'd say to them, "Look I'm with my wife. Is that OK?" And we'd move on. I never had any suspicions about him on that score.

And for the first time in our marriage we had money, real money. I didn't have a car when we moved to Newcastle so I borrowed Willie McFaul's wife's car, a red Fiesta. She was great, although I always knew her as Mrs McFaul…we would never call a manager's wife by her Christian name. Peter had a sponsored car and I soon bought a car of my own, another Fiesta.

We absolutely loved the life. We made good friends, had a great social life and for the first time we could afford an expensive holiday. As soon as Peter's first season ended in May, when Oliver was three months old, we went straight off to Alcudia in Majorca for four weeks. We stayed in a fabulous hotel. Doors started to open for us and we were mixing with a lot of different people, who I suppose wanted some of the reflected glamour from being in the company of a Newcastle United footballer. We knew it might be short-lived, because that's the way it is in football, and we enjoyed it while it lasted. Nice cars, nice clothes, nice holidays.

Then all of a sudden it ended as quickly as it had begun. Peter was dropped after the first match of the 1988-89 season and took his bat and ball home. Peter does take things very personally. On the outside, he's a tough, strong-willed character but inside he takes things very much to heart. I don't. I just say, that's life, shut up and get on with it. No point moaning. But Peter does get hurt.

This time he didn't think about it properly and when Bradford City came in for him soon afterwards, we went back. I said he should buckle down and get back into the Newcastle team but when his mind's set he won't listen. He just said, "No, we're going back to Bradford." He didn't even wait around to see who else might be interested. And we turned our back on what had been a fabulous lifestyle for two years. I think he will admit it was the wrong decision to go back to his previous club as a player; it was different 23 years later, when he returned as manager. But as a player, he under-performed and was very disappointed about it.

It was a massive culture shock. In Newcastle, people were much more fashion conscious, the nightlife was tremendous, we lived near to the city centre with great shopping. And Peter was playing for a top club. Isn't it everybody's dream to play for a club like Newcastle United? He'd been voted Player of the Year in his first season and the fans loved him. They still do. They adore him. Whenever he goes back, he's given a tremendous reception and when he was diagnosed with cancer in 2008, we received tons of emails, cards and messages from people up there.

After such a glamorous lifestyle, Yorkshire seemed really old-fashioned, although obviously it was good to be back among my family. We had nowhere to live and for the first five months, while we were waiting for our new house in Brighouse to be finished, stayed at the Banksfield Hotel in Bingley. We had adjoining rooms, Oliver and Charlotte in one and Peter and me in the other, with connecting doors.

The hotel staff were great, especially to the kids. We soon found a school for Charlotte and every day, when she came 'home' from school, they let her sit behind the reception in her little uniform. Oliver just about had the freedom of the corridor outside our room and used to whiz up and down on his little cycle, wearing his home-knit polo neck jumper and Rupert Bear pants. Businessmen using the hotel overnight had to jump for their lives sometimes.

The cleaners used to take our laundry home to wash. They'd say, "Don't be using the hotel laundry, love, I'll look after them for you." They'd babysit for us as well. Peter was still a big name at Bradford, of course, and everybody thought we were living the glamorous footballer's life in a hotel. But in many ways it was a nightmare, particularly having to spend Christmas morning there and not in a home of our own. Whenever I hear people moaning and groaning about all the preparation they have to do for Christmas at home, I look back to our Christmas in a hotel in 1988 and think they don't know how lucky they are. We went to my mum's for Christmas dinner but opening the presents just wasn't the same.

We used to go along to Brighouse nearly every week and look first at the foundations and then at the building work as the house took shape. I was able to imagine what a lovely home it was going to be and Peter could picture how he would create his garden. He's very proud of it now. Eventually we really settled in. Back home to our roots, our parents, our families and our old friends. And Newcastle seemed like another world.

Peter's Story

It was half past ten at night, a week or so after I'd joined Newcastle. Charlotte was tucked up in bed in our city centre apartment and Alison and I were thinking of turning in as well. Then the doorbell rang. I turned to Alison. "Who the hell can that be at this time of night?" When I opened the door, I was confronted by the sight of Paul Gascoigne and his buddy, Jimmy 'Five Bellies' Gardner. They were pretending to have a fight and laughing their heads off. I thought for a minute that they wanted to come in and make a night of it but it turned out they'd been out on the town and run out of money. They needed some cash for a taxi home and knew I was staying in one of the club flats. I gave them a fiver and off they went, still laughing.

Gazza was only 19 at the time and I'd known him for just a few days. But I'd taken to him straight away. He was a lovely kid, a real character. How could we know that in a few years, he'd be probably the most famous sports personality in the country? In fact, after his tears at the World Cup in Italy in 1990, he became one of the most familiar faces in the world. I cannot knock him. I never could and I never will. As his former England manager Bobby Robson once said, he was as daft as a brush. But everybody loved him. We couldn't help it. Gazza was one of those people who could make everyone around him feel good. That's a rare quality.

He really did have time for everybody. And he was so generous. Even before he really made it big, sponsors were falling over themselves to give him kit and clothes…and he used to give nearly all of it away. Once he was given a top-of-the-range Berghaus winter jacket and as we were leaving training, he turned to one of the autograph hunters and said, "Here, you might as well have this. I don't need it." The jacket must have been worth a couple of hundred quid even then. In fact, I had one as well and I've still got it over 25 years on.

Once I bumped into Gazza at Miami Airport after he had joined Italian club Lazio in 1992. Or more like I bumped into a crowd of people who were milling around someone famous, asking for his autograph and taking his picture. They must have been ten deep. I'd no idea who it was and I had Oliver with me, who was more interested in getting Donald Duck's autograph than this mystery personality. Anyway, I went to take a closer look and there was Gazza, signing bits of paper and posing for pictures.

It had been a while since we'd last played together and I thought, "Should

I bother introducing myself? Will he even recognise me?" He took the decision out of my hands because he suddenly looked up and spotted me. He beamed that huge smile and boomed out, "Why-aye Peter, what you doin' here? I've got me mam with us and you were always her favourite player… she's still got your picture on the wall!"

Gazza had been on holiday in Florida, too, with his usual entourage of about twenty people. But even though he was one of the most famous footballers in the world, he was genuinely pleased to see an old team-mate. We did our best to have a chat but it was impossible with all the people around.

It must have been ten years before I saw him again, at a boxing dinner in Bradford. We were both on the top table and a couple of minutes before the guest speaker was about to start, I happened to ask Gazza how Five Bellies was getting on. "Ask him yourself," he replied, fished out his mobile, dialled a number and said, "Jimmy, I've got someone who wants to speak to you." He handed over the phone just as the master of ceremonies was announcing the guest speaker. All I could do was tell Jimmy I'd call him back.

Gazza was a lovely character but some of the people around him did not give him the right guidance. He had loads of hangers-on when he was at the top but they all disappeared when he started having problems. That's the way sport or celebrity is. And football management, for that matter. If you're in, everybody wants a piece of you; if you're out, nobody wants to know. But the one person who has always stood by Gazza is Jimmy, the man branded as a hanger-on when Gazza was mixing with the rich and the famous. But where were the rich and famous when Paul was struggling and needed some help? Nowhere. And where was Jimmy? Right there alongside Gazza as usual. They were friends as boy and man and were really close. And they stayed that way through thick and thin. I had a lot of time for them both.

My move to Newcastle happened in a whirlwind. We'd been to a funeral earlier in the day and soon after we arrived home Trevor Cherry rang to say Bradford had accepted a bid for me from Newcastle and their manager Willie McFaul would be calling. I was stunned. I would have been happy to stay at Bradford and that's certainly what my dad wanted. He'd always said that after the fire, I should stick around and see the club into the old First Division. He and my brothers used to go to every home game so they would all have been happy for me to stay. Charlotte was three and little Ollie was on the way so Alison's mum and dad wanted to be around her as well. In fact, Alison's dad was desperate for us to stay in Yorkshire because he was a big cricket man and had decided that Ollie was going to play for Yorkshire…they could only field homegrown players in those days.

Alison answered the phone when Willie rang and he told me a fee had been agreed with Bradford and asked me to meet their physio, Derek Wright, at Scotch Corner the following morning, a Thursday, for a medical at

Catterick Camp army base. Then I was to drive to Newcastle to agree terms, sign the contract and do a Press conference. Alison and I tried to take everything into consideration and decided we just couldn't turn the move down. It was my first chance to make it into the big-time and who knows when another might have come along?

I gave Terry Yorath, my mentor at Valley Parade, a 6.30am alarm call on the Thursday morning to ask how much I should be looking for. I would have been on around £200 a week at Bradford and Terry said I should be looking to double or even treble that at a top-flight club. In the end, I think Willie and I agreed on around £500 a week plus appearance money. That was a lot in those days. I'd no idea at that stage what the fee was and asked Willie. He said they'd equalled Newcastle's club record fee of £250,000, for midfield player John Trewick from West Brom six years earlier. I just couldn't believe it. I was in shock. A massive club with great traditions like Newcastle paying a record fee for me?

The Press conference was huge, with around 40 reporters, cameramen, radio and television journalists. Apart from all the interviews I'd done in the aftermath of the Valley Parade tragedy, I'd only really been used to chatting to one man, David Markham from the Bradford Telegraph & Argus, or sometimes a few of the regional and national press after matches. I'd never experienced anything like this. I was wearing a yellow M&S jumper, not exactly groundbreaking fashion, and wondering what people who were used to seeing top-flight players in all the best gear, would make of it. To be honest, I was blown away. Everything had happened in the space of 24 hours since that call from Willie McFaul.

Willie was a genuine bloke and I came to like him a lot. He showed faith in me as a centre-back in the days when football was a man's game and you had to be tough to survive at any level, particularly in the top flight. When I look back at film of some of the tackles in the eighties, it was pretty x-rated stuff. No one would get away with it now but back then defenders had a licence to go in hard and everyone just accepted it as part of the game. It was survival of the strongest and you had to stand up and be counted. But nowadays some of those tackles would mean a five or six-match ban. The strikers weren't blameless either, particularly with people like Billy Whitehurst around.

In fact, big Billy might just have been one of the reasons I joined Newcastle. Bradford City were drawn against them in the second round of the League Cup and Billy missed the first leg at our temporary home at Odsal, which we won 2-0. I was relieved he wasn't around, to be honest, but I was under no illusions about what to expect at St James' Park in the second leg. Newcastle won a corner early on and Billy came straight over to me and said, "Come near me at this corner and I'll smash you."

The ball came over, I went for it, won the header and sure enough, he caught me. But I knew that I'd had to stand up for myself straight away and if I'd ducked out of that header, Whitehurst and everyone else on the field and in the dugout would have spotted it. He would have trampled all over me for the rest of the match. Instead, I gave as good as I got, we lost 1-0 but went into the third round and two weeks later I signed for Newcastle. And the day that I signed, Billy moved on to Oxford…and Alison and I ended up living in his club flat!

My first game was against Aston Villa away two days later before I'd really had time to get to know my new team-mates. But one name everyone was talking about was Gascoigne. He was just starting his second full season in the first team but already people were hailing him as a genius. And he was. Gazza was in the squad that travelled to Villa Park and he and Paul Stephenson, another of the younger players, arrived with their overnight stuff and boots in carrier bags. Before the next away game at Leicester, I gave him a suit holder.

I had an OK debut, nothing more. I was very nervous beforehand and finished up needing a couple of stitches in a cut above my left eye after a clash with Gary Thompson, their centre-forward. We lost 2-0 and were bottom of the league. Then it was time for my home debut against Oxford on November 1. I made sure the first challenge was a big one and I sensed straightaway that the fans were going to take to me. I won the Man of the Match award and collected a second soon afterwards.

Whitehurst didn't play for Oxford thank God, but he was waiting for me when we went to their place later in the season. I'd become a bit of a cult figure by that time, Newcastle's big, tough centre-half, so there was plenty of banter flying between us before, during and after the match. Thankfully I escaped in one piece but like a lot of other centre-halves who were around at that time, I will always rate Whitehurst as the most difficult opponent I faced.

Four weeks later, I appeared in my first live television match, against West Ham at home. There were only a handful of matches broadcast live in those days so it was a really big occasion. They were top of the league with an attack that included Frank McAvennie and Tony Cottee, both internationals, and we beat them 4-2.

I raced down the motorway afterwards and went for a drink with my brothers, who'd been watching the match live. They told me how Ron Atkinson, who was working as a pundit – he'd just been replaced as manager of Manchester United by Alex Ferguson - had said, "This young lad Jackson from Bradford is doing really well." Imagine that? Magic! And I really realised I'd made it when I featured on one of those old Panini stickers that kids used to collect!

Even our training sessions were watched by a decent crowd. At Bradford there might have been one or two on a nice day and a few schoolkids in the holidays or at half term. But half-term at Newcastle would see a couple of hundred arrive and the club had to employ stewards to keep them in order.

Funnily enough, though, the facilities at the training ground were nothing particularly special, certainly by today's standards, and I suppose the same could be said about the stadium. They were in the process of knocking it down for redevelopment and the dressing rooms were well past their sell-by date, with all the players using a big old communal bath after the match.

From the middle of my first season, we changed in portakabins, just like the early days at Odsal. They were pretty basic, the kind of thing Sunday League players would use. It wouldn't happen today. The cabins were behind the goal and there was a corridor for us to walk on to the pitch. The home and away cabins were next door to one another and the walls were paper thin. There was sometimes a bit of aggro between the two sets of players on the way back to the cabins after a match but it never blew up into anything serious.

My biggest worry after I signed was that I didn't know any of the other players and there were some pretty big names around like Peter Beardsley, Glenn Roeder, the captain, David McCreery and John Anderson. How would they react to the arrival of the new record signing, a young lad from Bradford most of them had probably never heard of before our two League Cup-ties? I needn't have worried. I was accepted straight away and settled in really well.

Newcastle was, and still is, a football mecca…I think it's illegal to wear another club's shirt around the city! Players were VIPs and it came as a bit of a shock at first to be recognised everywhere. But as time went by, I came to terms with the celebrity status as Alison and I were invited to all sorts of functions and mixed with people from all walks of life who wanted to know us simply because I played for Newcastle.

And then, at the end of my first season, came perhaps the biggest surprise of my career. I'd been invited back to Valley Parade as a guest of honour at the Bradford City Supporters Club Player of the Year presentation and even though it clashed with Newcastle's presentation night, I didn't imagine there would be a problem. But Willie McFaul had other ideas. "Sorry, Peter, you can't miss this one for any reason. The same applies to all the players."

"Come on, Willie. Bradford want me there to present the awards and after everything that happened there, it would really mean a lot."

"No, I want you at ours." End of story and I wasn't too happy, to be honest. After all I'd been through at Valley Parade I desperately wanted to go back and say thank you to everyone. I didn't get particularly dressed up and was looking for an early get-away as soon as the awards were over. When the ceremony began, the announcer said, "In third place, Peter Beardsley." Peter went up on to the stage and collected his award.

"Second is Paul Gascoigne." This time, Gazza went up to huge cheers all round. I started looking around trying to work out who the winner was going to be if it wasn't either of those two. "And the winner is…Peter Jackson." I was absolutely gobsmacked. And to this day, I see winning that award as one of my biggest achievements in the game. Imagine some of the names on that trophy: Jackie Milburn, Malcolm Macdonald, Kevin Keegan, Chris Waddle…and Peter Jackson. I knew the fans liked me because I was committed, wholehearted and got stuck in. But this really was something else.

Playing for Newcastle in the top flight also enabled me to complete my full set of all 92 Football League grounds. I was well on the way after playing with City in the fourth, third and second tiers and had appeared at all the grounds outside the top level. But before going to the North East I thought I'd struggle to play at too many top-flight stadiums. However by the time I left after two seasons, I was a fully-fledged member of the 92 Club. And going to grounds like Old Trafford, Anfield, Goodison Park, Highbury, White Hart Lane and Stamford Bridge was something I'd dreamed about as a kid. Doesn't everyone?

We had some great matches, winning at Arsenal, Tottenham and Chelsea and beating Manchester United at St James' Park. And for a very different reason, I'll never forget our 4-1 defeat at Old Trafford on New Year's Day, 1987. The day I scored two own goals! The first happened when Jesper Olsen got away down the wing, whipped in a cross, I went to head it back towards him but instead the ball glanced of my head and into the top corner. Then in the second-half, when we were 3-1 down, I went up for a cross with Frank Stapleton, got the final touch and it sailed past our keeper Martin Thomas. He didn't have a chance with either. Fortunately, Frank claimed that one and nobody argued…and we used to have a laugh about it when we played together for a while at Huddersfield in 1992.

And for two years, I was playing with and against world-class footballers, again the stuff that dreams are made of. Players like Beardsley, who was an unbelievable talent. He'd started at Carlisle and then moved to Vancouver Whitecaps because no one here really fancied him. But when he came back and joined Newcastle he was a revelation. He wasn't particularly quick but he had this ability to just drift past defenders. It must have been a natural gift because it wasn't as if he worked on his attacking skills too much in training. On the contrary, Peter preferred to spend his time in goal!

The day before my debut at Villa Park, we had the usual five-a-sides in training and Peter couldn't wait to get the gloves on and go in goal. I couldn't believe it. I asked one of the other players what was going on and he said that Peter always played in goal and next week he'd be practising his shot-stopping. Sure enough he did…and he wasn't a bad keeper, either. Peter was a quiet, unassuming lad who kept himself to himself. Not in an arrogant way, that was just his nature. There were enough loud players around in the dressing room with Gazza and Darren Jackson leading the way, but Peter just went about his business quietly. He moved to Liverpool in a big money deal at the end of my first season and his career really took off from there.

Soon after he left, Mirandinha joined us for a new club record £575,000, the first Brazilian to play for an English club. He'd played four times for Brazil, scoring his only goal against England at Wembley, and when he came to the training ground after signing, all the players stayed behind to watch him working out on his own. Hundreds of fans were there, too.

He couldn't speak a word of English and communicated with his hands and his big smile. He started having English lessons more or less straight away but had to have an interpreter in the dressing room. And needless to say, with Gazza acting as his tutor he picked up one or two choice phrases. Soon after he joined us, he invited all the players and their wives or girlfriends to a barbecue at his home. It was the end of August and a stinking hot day, about 28 degrees. But Mirandinha still had the central heating on at full blast and the house was dripping with condensation.

It was exciting to play in the same side as Mirandinha because he was so unpredictable; not necessarily one of the very top players but he had flair. And that's what the fans love up there. Inevitably he became a huge cult figure among supporters. There was real hype about him. He and his wife had sponsored cars, with Mirandinha and Mrs Mirandinha on the side. And everywhere he went, people made a big thing of it. One day, soon after he'd signed, he stopped at a local shop to buy an apple. Later that day there was a banner in the shop window saying, Mirandinha Shops Here. The idea caught on and soon every shop he and his wife went into had a similar sign in the window. And a few more that he'd never been near in his life.

We finished 17th in my first season and eighth the following year. But the FA Cup had always been huge in Newcastle, going right back to the 1950s when they won the competition three times in five years, and in both my seasons, we fancied our chances. We reached the fifth round each time.

In 1987, we lost 1-0 to Spurs at White Hart Lane. It was a penalty, I gave it away and Chris Waddle, a former Newcastle player, scored. Spurs were beaten by Coventry in the final. The following year we lost to Wimbledon, who went on to win the Cup with a 1-0 win over Liverpool, one of the great Wembley shocks. And there was already a bit of 'previous' by the time we faced them at St James' in the fifth round after a league game at Plough Lane a few weeks earlier.

That was the match that produced one of the most famous football pictures of them all: Vinnie Jones grabbing Gazza by the balls. The picture was reproduced all over the world and if you look carefully at some versions, it features a third player. Me. Or should I say, my right thigh. Just think, if I'd been one pace further forward, I'd have had a supporting role in a classic sports pic. So near but so far!

It happened after a goalkick from Dave Beasant, the Wimbledon keeper. But even though I was one of the closest players to the incident, I'd no real idea what had gone on because like everyone else, including the referee, I was watching the ball. I heard Gazza scream in agony, shouting, "He's grabbed my bollocks!" But it was off the ball and we all just got on with the game and nobody thought anything of it until after the match.

That's when things started to kick off between Gazza and Vinnie. A fan had given Gazza a bunch of flowers as he was leaving the team coach and he sent them into the Wimbledon dressing room as a present for the man who'd grabbed his bollocks. Vinnie replied with a toilet brush. But even though Gazza was still going on about the incident on the way home, everybody thought he was exaggerating and it was only when we saw the picture in the papers next day that we realised exactly what had happened. Needless to say there was a load of hype when we were drawn against Wimbledon in the fifth round of the Cup and the papers were full of what Gazza was going to do to Vinnie and vice versa.

We were playing well and there was a genuine feeling that if we could beat Wimbledon we'd go on and win the Cup. But they did us 3-1 at St James'. Gazza had a very quiet game – Jones had him in his pocket – and at that time, Gazza really was the key man for us. If he was on fire, he could destroy any side in the land but he didn't turn it on that day and what proved to be my best chance of winning the FA Cup had gone.

The season petered out a bit after that but after a good pre-season, I was really fired up for the start of the 1988-89 campaign, which opened with an away game at Everton. Two of my former Bradford City team-mates, John Hendrie and Stuart McCall, had both moved into the top division in the summer, John joining me at Newcastle and Stuart moving to Everton. And all three of us were involved at Goodison in front of a crowd of over 40,000. It should have been a great way to start my third season at St James'. Instead, we got beat 4-0 and I never played for the club again.

Willie had signed Andy Thorn from Wimbledon in the summer and he lined up alongside me in central defence. I always needed someone alongside me with a bit of pace but Andy and I were probably two of the slowest centre-backs in the league. We were torn apart by Tony Cottee, who scored a hat-trick on his Everton debut, and Graeme Sharp. I was dropped for the next game against Spurs and soon afterwards Willie told me Bradford City wanted me back and had come in with an offer of £290,000, a club record. I said OK, just like that. Perhaps I should have held out for longer to see if anyone else might come in…Stoke were also interested. Or maybe I should have hung around and waited for another chance at Newcastle. Instead I let my heart rule my head and went back.

City gave me a five-year contract. They'd just missed out on promotion to the top flight under Terry Dolan the previous year and after selling McCall and Hendrie, desperately needed to bring in someone who would give the fans a lift. I was going to be that someone. My signing was billed as The Return of a Legend. The money was good and the move gave Alison and I a chance to be back with our families again. And in those days not a lot of players were given five-year contracts. So there was a security element, too.

However, I knew straight away I had made the wrong decision. On my first day back at the old training ground at Apperley Bridge, I felt flat. Newcastle and the glamour seemed a million miles away. Everything was so familiar when what I really needed was a new challenge. I just never fired. I had enormous respect for Dolan and, of course, for Terry Yorath, who succeeded Dolan early in 1989. Then John Docherty took over from Terry a year later and we just never saw eye to eye at all. He made it clear I wasn't part of his plans and I moved to Huddersfield Town on a free transfer in September, 1990. To be honest, leaving was a relief.

That second spell at Bradford was the only time in my career when I felt I let down a group of fans. I struggled a bit fitness-wise and having to live in a hotel for five months, even with Alison and the kids there as well, didn't help. And did I feel some pressure because I was going back to a place that held so many memories and expectations were so high? I don't know. But it never felt right from day one and I just didn't perform as the club slid from the brink of the top flight into the old Third Division. I returned to Valley Parade as a hero; I suppose I left as a bit of a villain.

5. Changing faces, changing places

For Alison, March 1990 was back-to-work time as she embarked on a career that would feature eight different jobs over the next twenty years. It was all change for Peter, too, with a move to Huddersfield Town and the start of the happiest four years of his playing career. "The club was warm, it was welcoming and it just felt right from the start."

Alison's Story

Most mums would admit they reach a point when they think, "What am I? I'm just a mum." Maybe it happens more if their husbands have high-profile jobs, in my case a professional footballer, and they are always the ones back home looking after the kids. Being a mum is hard work but where's the recognition? Sometimes mums feel they are being taken for granted and I was no different.

For me everything came to a head on Mother's Day, 1990, two years after we left Newcastle. Peter was in his second spell at Bradford City, Charlotte was six and Oliver three. I woke up in the morning and thought, "Right, if I stay here for a little while, Peter and the kids will get up and make me a cup of tea and some toast." Nothing happened.

We always used to take my mum out for Mother's Day lunch but at teatime, I thought he might say, "Right, it's Mother's Day, we've got a little surprise for you." Nothing. Or maybe he'd offer to get the kids ready for bed and then open a nice bottle of wine later on. Nothing. Just head down watching football.

So while we were all sitting round the table in the evening, I announced, "Do you know what? I'm going back to nursing." Decision made. It wasn't something I'd been thinking about for a while, it was completely spur of the moment. And it meant back to building my own life again, back to being recognised as me, back in the workforce. Peter just said, "Right, love, whatever you want."

Next day, I spoke to Pam O'Malley, our next door neighbour, who absolutely loved Charlotte and Oliver, and asked if she could help with childcare. We'd moved into our home at the same time as Pam and her husband Fergie and they still live next door today. They took to the kids straight away. Oliver used to love going into their house because Pam gave him heart-shaped slices of toast…and it always had to be Warburton's bread; at home, he was told to eat what he was given!

When Charlotte was still at infants' school, she decided it was time for Fergie to give up smoking. She'd been taught all about the perils of cigarettes, spotted that Fergie, a big Irish guy who ran his own tarmacking company, was a heavy smoker and decided she should do something about it. Her method was simple and direct: she drew pictures of coffins and posted them through the letterbox with a dire warning about the dangers of smoking. He gave up straight away and hasn't had a cigarette for over twenty years.

So it was a natural choice to tell Pam what I was planning and she was more than happy to help us. And my decision to return to work proved to be a turning point for the family. Before that, Peter had been a bit of an old-fashioned dad, happy to leave me at home to look after the kids while he went to work. But now, for the first time, he would come home from training and then go out and pick up the kids from school after I'd gone to work. It was the first time he'd really been a father to his children and they have loved and adored one another ever since. But if I'd carried on being just a housewife, would he have ever really got to know his own kids? Or would he always have been in his football bubble?

I signed up with the BUPA nursing agency. I must admit there were one or two pangs of guilt about going into the private sector after working in the NHS, which had after all given me my training and funding at the start of my career and where I'd had some fantastic times. We used to really enjoy the camaraderie and the hands-on work whereas now it seems far more time is spent with paperwork and assessments. Yes, the NHS has moved on but in my view, not for the better.

For example, my training combined the academic side with work on the wards. That way I gained practical experience from the start and when I qualified, I had a good idea what the job was about on a day-to-day basis. Now, though, nurses train at university and when they come on to the ward, a lot of them have a completely different attitude. They don't want to empty bedpans, change bedding, bed-bath patients. But those things are an essential part of what nursing is all about: making a patient better through basic nursing care as well as medical care. Technical knowledge can only take a nurse so far and I think the balance has tipped the wrong way.

On the wards, we used to have our own NHS cleaners, rather than contract cleaners, and everything was immaculate. They took real pride in their work and so did we. If the ward sister came on to the ward, everything had to be absolutely 100 per cent. If a consultant was doing his rounds, it had to be 150 per cent. And if the matron was around, nothing less than 200 per cent would be enough. Say if you like that I'm harking back to the days of white starched aprons, Hattie Jacques and the Carry On films. But I think we need to go back to the standards of those times.

I have to say that I have absolutely no complaints about the way Peter was treated when he was receiving his cancer treatment at St James' Hospital in Leeds in 2008. I could not fault it. But I have spoken to friends who have had ageing parents on general wards and had to wash them, dress them, toilet them and feed them because nobody else had time to do it. Yet nurses are completing their training only to find there are no jobs. Not enough nurses on the wards but still no jobs for newly-qualified graduates. It beggars belief. When I qualified, I was asked which ward I would like to work on. I replied the cancer ward and I was there next day. There was no question of not having a job to go to.

However, when I decided to go back to nursing in 1990, I didn't make a conscious choice not to go back into the NHS. It was more a question of finding work that suited our particular situation. I flowed back into nursing through the private sector because I could choose my own working hours and fit my work around Peter's football: in the afternoons after training, in an evening when he didn't have a game or on a Sunday when, in those days, he would never be involved with football. If there were any gaps, our neighbour Pam stepped in and over the next few months, I worked as a staff nurse in the BUPA hospitals at Roundhay, a suburb of Leeds, at Elland, halfway between Halifax and Huddersfield, the Yorkshire Clinic near Bingley and some outside agency work.

A lot of my work at Roundhay involved cardiac nursing, patients having bypasses or valve replacements. A lot of them seemed to be in their thirties and forties, successful young businessmen who'd made a lot of money and, in a way, were now paying the price for leading such stressful lives. They may have been big figures in the business world but when they were lying on a trolley waiting for heart surgery, they were as vulnerable as anyone else. And the question in their eyes was always, "Am I going to be all right?"

As the years have gone by and I've had businesses of my own, I've often thought that if heart problems can strike down rich, successful businessmen like them when they overwork, where do I stand with all the hours I put in? But you just accept the stresses and strains and get on with your life, don't you?

The agency also covered nursing homes and industrial nursing in factories and mills. I found the strict timetable that we had to follow in nursing homes was a bit too regimented but factory work was very different because I wouldn't know what to expect from one shift to the next. There might be anything from cut fingers to eyes affected by chemical fumes, to keeping an eye on people returning to work after suffering back problems to looking after someone waiting for an ambulance after falling from a gantry.

My first shift was at a factory in Heckmondwike, in the heart of what used to be West Yorkshire's heavy woollen district. Sadly most of the mills have long gone now. It was a night shift starting at eight o'clock and I was booked in for a couple of weeks because the regular nurse was on holiday. I clocked on not really knowing what to expect. I had a little television in the clinic and I'd taken along a couple of magazines but I sat for hours and hours without anything to do at all, praying for someone to come in. I was bored silly. Finally, at about four in the morning, a chap turned up complaining of a headache. I gave him a couple of pills, made a note of it in the log and that was it until my shift ended at eight am.

The next night I turned up fearing the worst, this time armed with a pile of magazines. But news must have got around about the new, young nurse because when I arrived there was a queue ten deep of lads wanting an aspirin or complaining of some minor ailment like a stiff neck. I dread to think what my predecessor must have been like but she'd obviously deterred the workforce from seeking medical attention! And in the end, I had two really enjoyable weeks.

It was during a stint at the Yorkshire Clinic that I was first approached about returning to nursing full-time. A lot of the consultants and nursing staff knew me from my days in Bradford and they said I was wasted working part-time, that I should return to work as a staff nurse. It wasn't something I had thought seriously about and I wasn't sure I really wanted to do it. But they were people whose views I respected so I took a step back, thought about it for a while and in the end, decided to go for it; back to working regular hours and a chance to really get my career back on track.

Peter had moved to Huddersfield by this time and we continued to organise the kids' care between us, with Pam O'Malley's help. And I soon slotted back into the routine as a staff nurse, treating medical and surgical patients and working alongside the various visiting consultants on their rounds. Each consultant had his own specific day and the staff nurse accompanying him had to know which rooms his patients were in and point him in the right direction. So I had to be on my toes.

I managed to avoid too many mishaps…with one major exception that involved Mr Clayton, a gynaecologist who had a reputation for being a bit of a stickler, to put it mildly. On one occasion, I showed Mr Clayton into a room I believed was occupied by a gynaecology patient when, in fact, the lady concerned was waiting to have a wisdom tooth removed.

Displaying his best bedside manner, he sat on the patient's bed and said soothingly, "Now Mrs Jones, today will just be a routine operation, a straightforward hysterectomy with no complications and I wouldn't imagine you'll be in here for more than a few days."

Mrs Jones sat bolt upright at the news and said, "But I thought I was just having a wisdom tooth out." Mr Clayton turned to me and his expression said it all. I thought, "You're going to be in dead trouble for this, girl," and it was time to start thinking on my feet. So I put on my best smile and said, "OK, we've obviously come to the wrong room…but if ever you do happen to need a hysterectomy, Mrs Jones, Mr Clayton will be the perfect consultant for you."

He added, "And good luck with your wisdom tooth…" but I was certain that he would go absolutely mental as soon as we stepped outside. But in reality, he appreciated that it was a simple human error with no disastrous consequences and just laughed it off.

I had no plans to move away from nursing so soon after going back full-time but occasionally medical reps would come round, giving out their pens and coasters to the nursing staff and offering ski-ing trips in the Alps to the consultants, which doesn't happen any more! For all my working life, I'd been wearing a uniform and I started to look at the reps and think, "Wouldn't it be nice to strut around in a suit, carrying a briefcase and a mobile phone and driving a company car?"

Then one day at the end of 1992, I spotted an advert in the Nursing Journal from a company called RP Drugs. They were looking for a northern rep, operating mainly along the M62 corridor between Liverpool and Hull. I decided to give it a go. I was interviewed, got the job and a couple of weeks later set off to their HQ in Farnham in Surrey for three weeks' training, coming back home at the weekends. There were about ten of us on the course, all women, and it was very intense. But by the end of the three weeks, I had the suit, the briefcase, the mobile and the company car...oh, and the pens and coasters, too!

The company manufactured liquid medication and I used to call on GPs, nursing homes and hospital pharmacies. My patch also included two prisons, the high-security jail in Wakefield and Armley prison in Leeds. In the prison population, a lot of inmates pretend to take tablets but spit them out later, sometimes to sell or swap with other prisoners. So liquid medication is seen as a much more foolproof option. Those visits really opened my eyes. Thankfully, I'd never been in any way close to anybody who had been sent to prison and I found going there a petrifying experience, particularly my first couple of visits to Wakefield.

On my first call, I parked nearby and had to walk past a huge security wall that looked like a mountain from the pavement. I thought, "Hell, how am I even going to get into this place, never mind find the pharmacy? Anyway, walk tall, Alison!" Eventually I came upon a glass door, which was the main entrance. The glass looked two or three inches thick and was no doubt bullet proof but someone had obviously whacked it with something solid recently because the glass was splintered on the outside.

As luck would have it, I arrived at the start of official visiting time and there was a long queue of relatives waiting to go in. I thought, "Do I stand in the queue or do I use the suit and briefcase to pull rank and march to the front?" I marched to the front. I knocked on the door and told the prison officer on duty that I was from RP Drugs and had an appointment with the pharmacist.

The staff searched through my briefcase and told me to go through the security checkpoint, where I was frisked. I felt like a prisoner arriving for the first time and I was very conscious that I was a female in a male prison, a place where women would not normally be seen. An officer escorted me to the pharmacy, which involved walking round a third floor balcony from where I could look down and see some of the prisoners taking their exercise at ground level. They heard my high heels, looked up and started shouting and wolf whistling. It was a case of eyes front, head down and follow the officer. The pharmacist was an older guy and asked me if I was OK. "Yes, I'm fine, just fine!" I lied and eventually, once the security men knew who I was, visits became a little easier. Wakefield has housed some notorious criminals over the years but I worked on the basis of the less you know the better, and never asked anyone who was in there at the time. But they all looked pretty scary to me.

At first, the job was very hard work. Sales is all about selling yourself and building up a rapport with clients on your early visits. So I spent a lot of hours alone in my company car on the M62. I was dealing with people who didn't really have time to see me and were keen to get on with their own work and I found myself talking about our new products to a lot of pharmacists' backs. And it was notoriously hard to build a relationship with GPs because they tended to be suspicious of travelling sales people.

I stuck at it and eventually built up a portfolio of key accounts. But after a while I discovered that having established a rapport between myself and my clients, there was no real need to make personal calls every time. So eventually, I did more and more work from home on the telephone rather than meeting people face to face, one of the main things that had attracted me to the job in the first place. I'd been looking for comradeship in my work but after nearly three years, I found that it was a lonely job and perhaps by that stage, a bit too easy. The challenge had gone and it was time to start looking for something new. How could I know I'd find it by visiting a psychic fair in Bradford?

Peter's Story

I was only 13 when I went to Leeds Road, Huddersfield Town's old ground, for the first time. January 18, 1975. My mate, Mick Wood, lived in Bingley, down the road from our home in Keighley and he was a very big Town fan. His grandma lived at Fartown, where Huddersfield Rugby League club played. Mick used to watch all Town's home matches and asked if I fancied going along to see them play Preston North End. Bobby Charlton was Preston's player-manager at the time and he was the big attraction.

It was a real adventure. We caught the bus to Huddersfield from Keighley, went to his grandma's for dinner and then set off to Leeds Road. Mick gave me a brand new Town scarf to wear and we stood behind the goal on the open end…where the away supporters stood after segregation came in. Halfway through the first-half, I was jabbed in the back by this big lad, who growled, "Give us your scarf, kid!" I took one look at him, decided this was no time for heroics and handed over my scarf. To round off a grim afternoon,

Town lost 1-0.

Fifteen years later, in September, 1990, I found myself back at Leeds Road, this time on official business. Town had started the season badly and Eoin Hand, their manager, was looking for a centre-back. George Mulhall, my old manager at Bradford City, was on the staff at Huddersfield and recommended me. I met Eoin at a hotel near the M62 and the following day drove to the ground to agree terms. As soon as I reached the stadium I felt at home.

I went through the main entrance and the first thing I saw was the nameplate from the locomotive that had been named to commemorate Town's three successive Championships in the Twenties. I wandered along the corridor and out through the tunnel on to the perimeter track around the pitch. I looked across the old ground with its huge terrace on the opposite side and thought, "This is for me." Alison had gone back to work by this time and with the ground just fifteen minutes from home, I was never going to be far away from the kids. In no time at all, it seemed I knew every inch of the ground, outside and under the old main stand.

These days, just about every club has a separate training ground and apart from match days, the players barely see the stadium. At Huddersfield, we usually trained a mile or so away at the Leeds Road Playing Fields and the stadium was the focal point of the club all week. Underneath the stand, a corridor ran the length of the building; left to the dressing rooms, boot room, medical room, joiner's room and laundry, right towards the tunnel, the offices, manager's office, the board room, players' canteen and a small bar for 100 Club members on match days.

Everything revolved around the canteen. We'd grab a cup of tea in there before training and afterwards, we'd have a shower and then head off for lunch together. There was a big old table and we'd sit there for ages. The senior players would have their meal first, good, wholesome food like a jacket potato, and then the kids would come in later. Whereas at Newcastle and Bradford, the players all dispersed after training, at Huddersfield, we stayed together, talking, arguing, laughing, messing about and above all, building a real sense of togetherness. There was a wonderful atmosphere in that canteen, there really was.

My first port of call in the mornings was Nellie Thompson: the laundry manageress, to give her a fancy title. What a character! I'd heard all about Nellie when I was at Bradford from Bobby Campbell and Les Chapman, who'd played at Town before me. So I can't say I hadn't been warned when she came and sat next to me in the dressing room on my first morning. She slapped me on the knee and said, "Now Peter lad, let's look at your cock then!"

Nellie was a big woman with white hair; a widow, a lovely lady. She looked a bit like Supergran. She used to say I was her favourite and every day, without fail, she'd have a cup of tea or coffee waiting for me when I arrived. Her laundry was opposite the home dressing room and she used to sit in a big old chair – it must have been there for 40 years - surrounded by giant washing machines, tumble dryers and piles of kit for the players to pick up when they arrived. I'm sure Nellie never had a day off sick in her life, even after she had a bad fall in the laundry and damaged her ankle. She hobbled for the rest of her days but never complained. And she never had a bad word for anybody.

She used to babysit for us and I'd often pop down to her house and tidy her garden. I had a sponsored car and took her to the supermarket every Friday afternoon. She'd say, "You make me feel like a princess, Peter, when we pull up in your sponsored car." Nellie died in 1993, while Alison and I were away on holiday in the States. We didn't find out until we arrived home and by then it was too late to go to the funeral. I was devastated. I'll never forget Nellie, God bless her. You don't see characters like her at football clubs these days.

Fred Elms, the joiner and odd job man, had been there for years, too. He'd arrived at Leeds Road in 1950 with the contractors hired to rebuild the main stand after it was destroyed in a fire…and never left! The groundsman was Ray Chapple and woe betide anyone who ran on to his pitch during the week. Sometimes after training, one of the lads would say, "Ray's not around today, let's go and have a kick-about on the pitch." But we'd hardly get over the touchline before he'd appear from nowhere and shout, "Get off the pitch!"

At Huddersfield there were loads of characters like that, people no one outside the club knew about who were all little cogs in a big wheel and played a part in making it such a happy place. The club probably lost a bit of identity with the move across the road to the McAlpine Stadium in 1994. Some of the old timers stayed for a while but eventually they moved on

Paul Fletcher was the chief exec and masterminded the move to the McAlpine. He later played the same role at Bolton before becoming commercial director at the new Wembley Stadium and then chief executive at Coventry during their move to the Ricoh Arena. My first chairman was Graham Leslie, who ran Galpharm Pharmaceuticals, based in Brighouse and at one time Town's stadium sponsor. Soon after Graham left, Terry Fisher took over. Terry, a travel agent, was only 30, two years younger then me!

The dressing room was full of people who became good friends. Like Iwan Roberts, the Wales striker who finished up playing over 750 matches for seven clubs, and Iffy Onuora, another striker who was an economics graduate from Bradford University. In 2008 when I was diagnosed with throat cancer while managing at Lincoln, I needed someone to take over while I was having treatment, someone I could trust totally. Iffy was that man.

Straight away, I became a new player. The worries and pressures I'd felt since returning to Valley Parade seemed to evaporate overnight. I really did feel as if a weight had been lifted from my shoulders. In saying that I'm not being critical of Bradford City but I'd struggled there and now I felt I could pick up my career again.

Town were 23rd in the table after losing their first two league matches and had been beaten in both legs of the Rumbelows Cup first round by Bolton Wanderers. They were also our opponents on my debut at Leeds Road. Town lacked a leader and Eoin made me captain straight away. We won 4-0 and I sensed that everyone at the club, particularly the fans, had taken to me. The following week we drew 0-0 at Fulham even though I gave away a penalty, which Steve Hardwick, our keeper, saved.

I have never worked harder on my fitness than I did at Huddersfield. I'd had fitness problems at Bradford and as I was approaching 30, I knew I needed to be as fit as possible. I used to drop the kids off at school and head straight to the ground. After my cuppa with Nellie, I'd be in the gym just after nine o'clock and work in there until 10 when most of the other players started to arrive for a 10.30 start. Then after training and a bite of lunch, I'd go back out in the afternoon and work on my own before going to pick up the kids. I used to run up and down that enormous terrace for what seemed like hours. Either that or round the running track. Sometimes I'd go in on my days off as well and I can honestly say I was never fitter at any time in my career.

The reward was playing some of my best football. I built a good relationship with Graham Mitchell, the other centre back, and the full-backs, Simon Trevitt and Simon Charlton, who later played in the Premier League for Southampton, were both top players. That back four was as good as any I played with. In midfield we had Chris Marsden, who'd come in on a free from Sheffield United, but went on to play in the top flight with Coventry, Wolves and Southampton. Chris had a lot of injury problems but he was a talented playmaker and linked well in the middle with Kieran O'Regan. And there were plenty of goals up front with Iwan, Iffy and Phil Starbuck.

Phil was a born-again Christian and instead of a number on his training kit like the rest of us, he had the word Rev! Initially he came in on loan from Nottingham Forest before signing full-time. He scored 36 goals in 120 league starts and formed a good partnership with Iwan. I'm surprised he didn't go on and do really well but instead, he seemed to just disappear.

Town were a steady, level-headed club who didn't throw a lot of money around but we had a good side and in my first season, recovered from that poor start to finish eleventh. We knew we were better than that and would be challenging strongly the following year. We showed what we were capable of early on by beating Sunderland, who were a division higher than us, in the Rumbelows Cup second round. We won 2-1 at Leeds Road and 4-0 at Roker Park, Sunderland's old stadium.

As a former Newcastle player, I came in for a lot of stick from the Sunderland supporters but gave one of the best performances of my career. One paper actually gave me ten out of ten in their form report! It was one of those games when everything came together for me and it was the start of one of my best spells as a player.

In fact, not long afterwards, I had a chance to join Birmingham, who were in the same division as Town, for £250,000. Terry Cooper, the former Leeds and England defender, was their manager and he offered me the combined role of player and reserve team coach, not bad for someone who'd been given a free transfer from Bradford City 18 months earlier. The money on offer was quite good, certainly good enough for Alison and I to think long and hard about it. But I was comfortable at Huddersfield, the family was settled and at the age of 32, I didn't really want to uproot when I was doing so well with Town.

We should have gone up automatically. We were as good as anything in the division but Marsden picked up a knee injury and between mid-February to mid-March, we lost six out of eight matches. Eoin was sacked. I was bitterly disappointed to see him go. There was only one manager in my career who I didn't enjoy playing for: John Docherty, who was in charge during my last few months at Bradford. Generally I got on well with the rest and particularly with Eoin. He was a former Republic of Ireland manager, he knew the game and I enjoyed his company on a personal level.

His departure inevitably created one or two tensions in the dressing room. When a manager goes, some players are happy because they have been out of the picture for one reason or another; others worry about who might come in and what their future might be. I always felt that players who were out of the team should look at themselves and ask why. And what could they do to get back in? Instead, too many started slagging off the manager. Perhaps that's easy to say for someone who was usually a first choice but it's something I saw from the other side of the fence when I became a manager.

Ian Ross took over from Eoin, Marsden came back and we picked up again, winning seven of our last eight matches to finish in third place, three points behind Birmingham and four ahead of sixth-placed Peterborough, our opponents in the play-offs. After finishing the season so strongly, we were convinced we would win, even though Marsden was missing again. We were 2-1 up at their place and although they equalised late on, we had two away goals so it was in our hands. The second leg has always been remembered in Huddersfield as Black Thursday. We scored very early on but never really performed on the night. Peterborough deserved to win. The fans reacted badly and there was a bit of crowd trouble afterwards with people invading the pitch and police horses coming on to clear them off. I stood in the tunnel with Iffy and watched it all happen. We were both in tears.

We beat Sunderland in the League Cup again the following year but perhaps suffered a hangover from Black Thursday. At the beginning of March we were in the bottom two but then Mick Buxton, who had led Town to two promotions in his time as manager from 1978 to 1986, returned as Ross's right hand man. We won 12 of our last 16 matches and finished 15th. I had a lot of time for Mick. He was a bit dour but totally straight and honest. He treated everyone, a senior pro like me or a young kid just starting out, exactly the same and earned everyone's respect. I wish I'd played under Mick in his prime.

Ross lost his job at the end of the season and in July, 1993, Town appointed their 15th post-War manager: Neil Warnock. After starting in non-league, it was his fourth job as a league manager and he'd already taken Notts County into the top flight. Neil was a massive personality and he blew in like a whirlwind. As soon as he arrived, he told us there would be a system of fines for players who stepped out of line: turning up late, leaving their kit around, dirty boots and so on. The fine would be twenty or thirty quid and when you think that, say, half a dozen players a week would pick up a fine, the kitty soon began to build up.

Neil told us that he'd collect all the money together and at Christmas, have a champagne party at his home in Holmfirth. By the time we played Bournemouth at home just before Christmas, there was a hell of a lot in the kitty and after the match, we all put our best gear on, hired taxis and headed off to Holmfirth, looking forward to a big night.

There were 15 or 16 players and their wives, all convinced that there would be a few cases of bubbly to go at but instead, there were only eight bottles on the table and a few cans of ale to share between the lot of us. That wasn't going to go far. There was a bit of food as well and all the surfaces, including the top of the telly, were covered in cling film to prevent any stains. We polished off those few bottles in no time and stood around waiting for reinforcements. Nothing. Instead, at five to ten, Neil looked at his watch, told us Match of the Day was on in ten minutes and said, "Right lads, t'champagne's gone, Match of the Day's starting so off you go!" And we all went home. wondering when we'd be spending the rest of the money!

Warnock brought Mick Jones with him as assistant manager and Kevin Blackwell as reserve keeper and player-coach. He ranted, raved and immediately started bringing in his own players, some of whom I'd never heard of from non-league. One of them was Darren Bullock, who arrived from Nuneaton Borough, did really well and stepped up a level without trouble when Town were promoted in 1995; others failed to make it. At first things didn't push on as everyone expected and Warnock came in for a bit of stick from the fans. But gradually he put together the side that was promoted at the end of his second season.

It's no secret that as a player, I never got on particularly with Neil. He would no doubt say the same thing. Yet as managers we have always been good friends, chatted regularly on the phone and been out for a bite of lunch every now and then. He has survived in management for over 30 years and to do that, he must have something special.

Everything was black and white with him. If he liked you, you were OK. If he didn't, he made it clear from the start. If you weren't part of his plans, you were bombed out. But he was canny enough to see how popular I was and straight away appointed me as a reserve team coach, where I worked alongside

Blackwell. I'd done all my badges and was looking to go into the coaching side when I eventually retired so it was a good move for me. And it was a move that demonstrated to the supporters that Neil saw me as an important part of the backroom team as well as a senior player and club captain.

We both knew that I was approaching the end of my career but I believed I was still a big player and even though we were struggling, I started in 30 of the first 35 league matches and scored Town's last FA Cup goal at Leeds Road, in a first round replay against Telford. I also featured in all our matches in the Autoglass Trophy, from the first round against Doncaster in late September to a two-leg northern area final against Carlisle United at the end of March. We won the first leg at Leeds Road 4-1 and then hung on in the second leg, losing 2-0. Town were going to Wembley for the first time since 1938 and I had no reason to suppose I wouldn't be playing there for the first time in my career. To lead out a side at Wembley is every player's dream and for me, it was about to come true.

It was then that the cracks started to show between me and Neil. Thanks to the Autoglass Trophy, the club was on the move. The fans sensed it and started to get behind Neil. The jeers that had at first accompanied his direct style of football turned to cheers as Wembley became a reality. Rightly or wrongly, I started to feel that he had used my appointment as reserve coach to stay in with the fans and now, with things moving in the right direction, he was ready to ditch me. Sure enough, on March 24, two days after we reached the Autoglass Final, Neil signed Pat Scully from Southend. He made his debut against Plymouth at Leeds Road on March 26. I dropped to the bench and never started another match for Huddersfield Town. And that included the Autoglass Final.

In the week before the match, and four weeks after our win at Carlisle, Neil called me into his office. He came straight to the point. "I know you've played in every round but I'm not going to play you at Wembley. You'll be on the bench and I'll bring you on at some stage." Then he added. "But I want you to lead the side out." I could have said no, I suppose. But I still saw it as a massive honour, even though I would have to go straight to the bench after introducing the players to Michael Howard, the Home Secretary and guest of honour, instead of tossing up with the Swansea captain. I must be the only man to lead out a side at Wembley and then sit on the subs' bench for two hours.

However the decision to leave me out made a statement: there is no more Peter Jackson at Huddersfield Town. I couldn't understand it at the time, in fact I thought it was deplorable. But now, having been a manager myself, I ask would I have done the same thing? And the answer is I probably would. There was never a slagging match between Neil and me, either in private or in front of the other players because as club captain, I knew how important it was to keep the dressing room together. We both just knew that when he brought in Pat Scully, it was the end for me and we never really had much contact after that.

Over 30,000 Town supporters went down to Wembley and it was a fantastic occasion for the club and the town. Even though I knew I wouldn't be starting, it was wonderful to be involved in the build-up. We spent a few nights at a hotel near Wakefield that had its own golf course, travelled down to London on the Saturday and walked on the pitch at Wembley. And leading the side out next day, with my family in the stand, was one of the highlights of my career. Not too many players have done that and I was immensely proud. But the afternoon went downhill from there.

Swansea took the lead early on but Town equalised through Richard Logan, another of Neil's imports from non-league, midway through the second-half. Soon afterwards, the fans started chanting for Jacko. I was sat a few yards away from Warnock so he must have heard it, too, but no joy. At full-time, the scores were still level and I thought, "I must be going on now." Still no joy. Half-time in extra-time? No joy again. Finally, with a minute of added time to go and penalties inevitable, Warnock called: "Jacko, do you fancy going on and taking a penalty?"

I thought, "You must be joking!" Imagine going on for a penalty shoot-out, kicking the ball for the first time at Wembley and sending it sailing over the bar. No chance! Anyway, by that stage I'd lost it. I couldn't have gone on, there was no desire any more. As Town's captain and someone who'd played in every round, I should have been involved at some stage. If it had been a play-off final, a do or die match with a lot of money at stake, I would have accepted being consigned to the bench. But it wasn't. It was the Autoglass Trophy Final, a showpiece occasion that, more than anything else, was a day out for the fans.

Town lost the shoot-out. Afterwards I did have doubts about whether to go and pick up my medal because I was so upset about not going on. In the end I did so, as a mark of respect to the competition and the Town fans. But afterwards I walked straight off to the dressing room and couldn't wait to climb aboard the bus and get home. When we arrived back in Huddersfield, there was an official function for the players, with a few drinks and a bite to eat. I just turned up to show my face and then went straight off home. After four seasons and 195 games, my Huddersfield Town career was over.

There was one more disappointment, however. On April 30, 1994, Town played their final game at Leeds Road. There was nothing at stake either for Town or Blackpool, our opponents, and I was desperate to be involved at some point. But I knew deep down that it wasn't going to happen. I was the past, the man who was leaving the club and the stadium where I'd spent so many happy hours. To be sitting in the stand as Town played that last match was very sad. It was the end of an era for Town and for me and the end of the happiest time of my playing career. How could I know that in three years, I would be back at the club as manager?

6. All the fun of the fair

By mid-summer, 1994, it was all-change again. Peter left Huddersfield for Chester and a daily commute of 150 miles. "Even in those days, the M62 was a nightmare. Sometimes the journey would take an hour and a half, sometimes three hours." And the following year, Alison took a career swerve into the world of leotards, lycra and the Rosemary Conley Organisation.

Alison's Story

In 1995, the annual Bradford Psychic Fair was held at the Midland Hotel in the city centre. I'd never been to anything like it before and usually I wouldn't have given a second thought to spending Sunday afternoon there. But Mum was into that kind of thing. She always said she had healing hands and when we were kids, she'd stroke us if we didn't feel well. She never took it any further either then or later but always retained an interest. So when my sister Lizzy and I heard about the fair, we decided it would be nice to take her along.

The organiser started by giving a talk in which she pinpointed one or two people in the audience who she felt might have some spiritual qualities. She didn't pick on any of us. There were tables all round the room where people were looking at palms, gazing into crystal balls, reading Tarot cards and so on. I had always been a bit sceptical, although I did go with an open mind, and in the end, I decided to try the Tarot cards.

I took a seat across the table from the reader. She was just an ordinary middle-aged woman, not a Gypsy Rose Lee or anything like that. Twice, while she was reading the cards, my mum walked past and each time, the reader lost her concentration and had to start all over again. It didn't worry me but she was really upset about it and after the second interruption, she pointed at mum and asked, "Who was that woman who just walked past?"

"Oh it's my mum, she's probably just been to the toilet."

"Well that has never, ever happened to me before. I've never had to break off in the middle of a reading. Your mum must have real spiritual power and she should do something with it." Mum never bothered.

Anyway, it proved to be third time lucky with the cards when we started again and I couldn't believe how accurate she was when she started talking about my work. She said, "I don't know what you are doing now, but whatever it is, it's the wrong job for you. You need to be surrounded by people and I think you are probably finding your work a bit lonely." How could she know that's exactly how I was feeling about my job with RP Drugs? I'm sure I hadn't given anything away in advance.

She went on, "Whatever your next job is going to be, you will decide on it just like that…" and she clicked her fingers. "It will come to you in a flash, something you have never even thought about." Then she added, "And it will happen today." On the way home, we all dissected what our readers had said and I must admit I started to think, "What if she's right? Will something happen today?"

OK, I was a bit bored with my job but the salary was good, I was successful and eventually I would move on to something else in my own time. I had no reason to suppose it would be a spur of the moment decision as she had suggested. When I arrived home, I made myself a cup of tea and picked up the Sunday Times magazine. I was flicking through the pages when I saw an advert placed by the Rosemary Conley Organisation, asking for people to become franchise managers. I thought, "That's it, that's what she means! That's what I'm going to do."

It was something totally different for me. I'd never been into keep fit, running marathons or climbing rocks but I thought, "I can do that. I'll be an instructor." I made the phone call the next day and arranged to go down to the Rosemary Conley offices in Quorn, near Loughborough, for an interview later in the week. It was an intense interview, with Rosemary herself, her financial director and two more business advisers grilling me. They made it clear that first, I had to be the right kind of person to become an instructor: positive, enthusiastic, energetic, a people person. Then second, did I have the business acumen to run a franchise?

I didn't really have any business experience, apart from setting up the Mars Bar diet and running Tupperware and jewellery parties all those years earlier, but I must have done OK because I was invited back for a second interview…and my next career path was set out for me. I handed in my notice at RP Drugs, signed all the paperwork at Quorn and then embarked on another intensive training course, this time courtesy of Rosemary Conley.

Rosemary had built a successful business on the back of her book, The Hip and Thigh Diet, which sold over two million copies. By the late nineties, she was definitely the market leader – people called her the Delia Smith of the diet world. She was a television celebrity and became a millionairess but because she had started out as a housewife, she always said, "Women feel I am one of them."

She was a proper businesswoman who succeeded through sheer hard work and passion and was a role model for all women who wanted to have a successful career. She certainly became that for me and I learned a lot from her. She was a great person to work for and I never felt as though she was just taking my management fee and then afterwards not giving me or my franchise a second thought. I used to go down to Quorn once a month for training updates and she was always there and very hands-on. Her franchisees came to know her well and it was a good relationship on a personal level. But if she had anything that needed saying to us, she would come straight out and say it.

She had a public image to maintain: the kind, caring woman who wants to change people's lives through her diet and exercise regime. And I think she genuinely did feel that way and was doing it for the right reasons. I never thought for a minute that she was false. Yet on the back of that, she was a driven, single-minded businesswoman who knew exactly what she wanted and where she was going in her career.

Rosemary also made a point of meeting our families and sometimes on a Sunday, Peter and I would take the kids down to Quorn for one of her family days. I suppose hundreds and hundreds of franchisees have come and gone since 1995 but I'm pretty sure that if, even now, someone were to mention Alison Jackson to Rosemary, she would remember me as one of her early managers. I don't say that in a big-headed way but as an illustration of the type of person she was: a serious career woman but also a lovely lady.

She lived in a mansion near Melton Mowbray but the business headquarters where her training courses were held was a massive old mansion house, standing in its own grounds in Quorn, a beautiful building with oak-panelled walls and lovely ceilings. There were ten or twelve of us on the course, a manageable number, and we stayed overnight in a hotel nearby, driving into Quorn every morning for our training. It was a delight to be there.

As well as learning how to become a Rosemary Conley instructor, we were taught how to run the business side of the franchise and given training, around the boardroom table, in marketing and advertising. There were visits from top dieticians to teach us all about Rosemary's low fat diets, which in those days worked on the basis of less than four grams of fat per hundred grams of food, combined with a regular exercise regime. So it was quite an easy diet to stick to, which is one of the reasons why it was so popular. We learned about body metabolism and how the exercise regime and the diet must be complementary.

We also started our Royal Society of Arts Exercise to Music qualification. I have always been quite musical so when we were training, I adapted fairly quickly and if, for example, my routine involved dancers joining in on the beat of eight, I could bring them in on time, no problem. But some girls struggled because their sense of rhythm was not too good. Also I was still pretty fit physically so I didn't have any major problems in that area.

In addition to overseeing the entire operation, Rosemary held two classes of her own every week in Loughborough and as part of our training we went along to one of them. We were given the chance to meet some of her ladies and talk to them about how they felt a class should be run. Almost all of them were totally in awe of Rosemary and couldn't believe how much weight they had lost because of the diet. She was an inspiration to everyone.

She used to travel around the country and hold seminars or conferences to which all the ladies in her classes were invited. They were big events at places like the Sheffield Arena. Whenever she was in Yorkshire, her franchisees had to work alongside her during the presentations and we'd take along a group of our ladies to meet her. She always found time to talk to them and if any had brought along a copy of one of her books, she would sign it. Sometimes they took part in her fashion shows, modelling Conley leotards and tights, which were very fashionable in those days

Once we had finished the initial training course, we could still not become instructors until we had the RSA qualification so we had to go away and construct our own individual routine for the exam. Then, of course, we had to practise the routine with a willing student…which is where Peter came in. Although I'm not so sure willing was necessarily the right word in this instance! As soon as we'd packed the kids off to bed, I'd say, "Please, please come and help me out." He was thinking more in terms of a quiet evening in front of the telly but instead, I'd have him doing all the exercises, like V steps, box steps, knee lifts, and then I'd start on my dance routine. He was totally uncoordinated but he had a go, although I don't think he talked too much about it to his team-mates at Chester, the club he joined from Huddersfield in 1994. I just wish I'd taken some photos!

I also roped in my brothers, Paul and Jonathan, and had them dancing around the lounge; groups of friends, too. In fact anyone who could help me perfect the routine, not least in reaching the point where I knew my left hand from my right…not as easy as it sounds because as the instructor is facing the class, her right hand is their left hand and so on. I still sometimes get confused today.

It was practise, practise, practise all the way to the big exam, even when we went on a family holiday to a villa in Carvoeiro on the Algarve in Portugal. We had a maid who came in and cleaned every day and although she couldn't speak a word of English, I cajoled her into dancing the routine beside the pool. I thought if she can follow it without understanding a word, I must be on to a good thing. I passed.

Before I could set up my classes, I had to organise the business side of the operation. Each franchisee paid Rosemary a fixed fee, I think it was £10.50, for staging a class so I had to work out how many classes, and with how many clients, I would need to run each week to start making a profit. And once I knew how many classes there were going to be, I had to find enough venues to hold them: church halls, school halls, hotels throughout the Bradford, Halifax and later Huddersfield areas.

I had leaflets printed and used them to advertise the classes anywhere and everywhere and eventually started with 14 classes. On some of my first evenings, I'd arrive at a venue, unpack all my equipment, put on my outfit – leotard, trainers, a fashionable sweatband on my wrist, no doubt – and then only three or four people would turn up. But I did my best to make sure the class was enjoyable and the following week, those three or four would each bring along a couple of friends and in the end, there would be 30 or 40 in the class.

As the number of classes increased, I had to start recruiting new instructors to cope with the demand. The first was Helen, my brother Paul's wife at the time, and then I recruited Jonathan's wife, Joanne. They both passed their RSA exam and began running classes of their own. Then my third sister-in-law, Mark's wife Jenny, became interested, too, took her RSA exam in Harrogate, and worked for a franchise there. So it was a real family affair. A good friend, Tina Payne, also became an instructor along with Michelle and Lindsey, two members of one of my first classes who had really done well.

Eventually, I had 15 instructors running 55 classes a week while I took more of a back seat on the office and management side. Helen also helped me out in the office, which doubled up as the fifth bedroom of our home in Brighouse. Every Friday, all the girls would come along with their registers and bags of money, which we would have to count right down to the last penny for the company accounts. We'd always have lots of coffee and buns, which Rosemary might not have approved of but we convinced ourselves that they helped us concentrate. And those weekly meetings were important in developing a sense of camaraderie among the instructors and giving them a chance to raise any issues there might have been.

We also staged some big events, including a Rosemary Conley marathon at the McAlpine Stadium, as it was then known, in aid of a breast cancer charity. Peter was manager of Huddersfield Town by that time and he came along with most of his players. Some of the Huddersfield Giants Rugby League players were there, too. So there was a rare combination of big, burly footballers, even bigger and burlier Rugby League players and about 250 women of all shapes and sizes, aged between 18 and 80.

It went on for five or six hours and I changed the instructors every 20 minutes or so. Some people just hopped around as best they could, others really went for it and the professional sportsmen totally entered into the spirit. The ladies were thrilled to bits to be stood next to a Town or Giants player and there was loads of publicity, both in advance and on the day. We raised over £2,000, which was a reasonable amount of money in those days.

Three times a year I took a group of 49 ladies down to Springs Health farm in Leicester. Every week when they came to their class, they would pay £5 towards the cost of the trip. We'd set off on a coach first thing and arrive in Leicester at around nine o'clock. They'd do a session of aerobics then water aerobics, tan sessions, beauty treatments and, of course, eat a low fat healthy lunch. Some people went every year. We'd take a pound off everyone as they boarded the coach and then buy 49 lottery tickets...I think we did 15 trips in all and won just £10 from our total stake of nearly £7500. We bought a couple of bottles of wine with the winnings and drew the lucky winner out of a hat.

One of the great things about the Rosemary Conley diet was that it wasn't about a trained instructor teaching aerobics to a small group of fairly fit dancers, aged around 20 to 30, who started from a pretty high level. This target audience was any age over 18, any fitness level, any weight so I saw all shapes and sizes, especially when they were squeezed into their leotards, T shirts or whatever. In any group there might be 60-year-old ladies weighing 20 stone, who would have to be taught at a very low pace. They would be grouped on the right hand side of the room and in the middle would be ladies who had already lost some weight and were ready to move on to another stage. And on the left would be the intense group, usually younger, slimmer and fitter than their instructor.

One group would be leaping around, another moving more moderately and a third group would be taking it really easy. So to the slow group I'd say, "Right, just a little walk, nothing too strenuous…and you slow down a bit, Edith!" To the middle group, it would be, "Come on you lot, step it up a bit now, you can do better than that!" And to the super-fits, I'd joke, "I'm not even watching you lot, you're far too good for me!" It was important that they all felt I was involved with them, whatever their standard

My mum and Pam O'Malley, our next door neighbour, shared the cashier duties, taking the money as the dancers arrived. And eventually they joined in, too. Mum was a diabetic and also suffered from heart disease. But even though she just diddled around in her little tracksuit, thinking she wasn't doing a lot, it was far, far better than anything she'd done for years and she was fitter than she'd been for a long time. Not long after the classes finished, she became ill and passed away 18 months later, which perhaps proves how important that little bit of exercise was in prolonging her life.

In the end, I only ran four classes myself but they were really enjoyable and we always had such a laugh. At each session we'd weigh all the ladies first, which always produced plenty of joking, and then before the exercises started, I'd give a motivational talk about some specific topic, low fat food, eating healthily, the importance of exercise and so on. There were about 30 different topics in all.

I never believed in being too regimental. At Christmas, I used to say to the ladies, "Go and have a fantastic day, eat whatever you feel like but just be sure to go back to the diet the next day." Or at Easter, "Have an egg for goodness' sake! If you don't you'll only feel deprived." Then in the summer I'd tell them, "Go away for two weeks and enjoy yourself. You've saved up all year for it. Forget about the diet…but the minute you put your key in the front door and turn it when you get home, you're back to healthy eating and your exercise."

I believed that if people decided to live like that, they wouldn't go far wrong. And I liked to think they identified with me, too. I wasn't some super-fit, skinny size eight ordering them about, I was a wife in her mid-thirties with a couple of kids who had a healthy diet but also knew how to enjoy life. People came because as well as losing weight, they enjoyed it. So when, after a year or so, the weight loss began to dwindle they would still come because it was a fun place to be. And to this day, I keep bumping into ladies who came to the classes and they always say, "When are you going to start again?"

I eventually sold the business in 2000, when I was due to re-sign the franchise agreement for another five years. I was a bit concerned about that because even though Rosemary still looked stunning, she was in her mid-fifties and not getting any younger. How much longer would I be able to sell the classes on the strength of her name? And was the bubble of the low-fat and exercise diet eventually going to burst? If so, would it be in less than five years? And one of my instructors, Shelagh Brayshaw, was keen to take over the franchise. Shelagh was from Keighley, Peter's home town, and when she was 16, she'd made the national press by becoming a Bluebell Girl at The Lido nightclub in Paris.

In the end, I decided that maybe the business had peaked and I couldn't imagine it would grow any bigger, if at all. There's always a good time to sell a business and for me, this was it. Was I right? Well the Rosemary Conley Organisation was still going strong ten years later and she was awarded the CBE in 2004, so who knows? But I never had any regrets.

Above all, though, when I had to make the decision, my dad was really ill with prostate cancer and I felt that with all my nursing qualifications, I really should be there to help him and mum. I sold the business to Shelagh about five or six weeks before dad passed away. He was in and out of the Overgate Hospice in Elland during that time so I was able to help my mum support him. It would have been a huge regret to this day if I had not been able to give them the time they needed because of work commitments.

But I will always remember my days with Rosemary Conley as one of the happiest times of my working life, five years that kick-started my career and taught me about the entrepreneurial side of business. I was totally involved and loved a job where, unlike my work as a medical rep, I was meeting and mixing with people all the time. Some of them are still good friends. It was hard work and not every Rosemary Conley franchise manager has been successful by any means. But I like to think I succeeded because people came to the classes knowing they would enjoy their workout with me. It worked both ways.

Peter's Story

Only once in 18 years as a professional did I think, "I've had enough of this." During my first season at Chester City after I'd signed from Huddersfield, initially on loan, in September, 1994.

We hadn't made the best of starts in the league; in fact we were in the bottom four virtually all season and were eventually relegated into the old Division Three. And on November 29, we met Crewe at home in the Auto

Windscreens Shield, the successor to the Autoglass Trophy in which Huddersfield had reached the final earlier that year.

Chester's fiercest rivals were Wrexham and games between those two were always seen by both sets of supporters as the real local derby. But Crewe is only 25 miles down the road from Chester so there was always a little bit extra for the fans when the sides met. There were only 1,890 people in the Deva Stadium that night…and I don't recall many Chester fans seeing out the full 90 minutes. We were awful and lost 6-0. I was marking Ashley Ward, who later played in the top flight with five clubs and cost around £8.5m in transfer fees, and he scored a hat-trick.

Afterwards Mike Pejic, our manager, went absolutely mental. He stormed into the dressing room and shouted, "Right, keep your kit on, we're going running." I thought, "Oh, God, no!" All players want to do after a defeat like that is get in the car, hit the road and forget about it. And in my case, hitting the road meant a 75-mile drive to Brighouse which, even on a quiet night, took the best part of an hour and a half. However, Pejic had other ideas. He ordered us back out on to the pitch and then he ran the bollocks off us. Run, run, run. I've no idea what time we finally finished but I didn't get home until nearly one o'clock in the morning, And if that wasn't bad enough, Pejic had ordered us to report back in at 8.30am.

So I set the alarm for half past five, staggered off to bed and five hours later clambered back into the car and set off on the return journey to Chester. We trained hard until 11 o'clock and then had to sit and watch a video of the match. He seemed to stop the recording on freeze frame to conduct an inquest into just about every incident and I finally drove away from the ground at 5pm. Straight into the height of the rush hour around Manchester.

The traffic was horrendous and I eventually reached home at nearly eight o'clock. I was 33, I'd played the best part of 700 games in all competitions, I was approaching the end of my playing days and for the first and only time in my career, I asked myself, "Is this really worth it?" By the end of training on Friday morning, I'd decided that it definitely was and went on to have three really happy seasons at Chester, a smashing little club.

I first heard about their interest from Neil Warnock, the Huddersfield manager. He'd already told me he wanted me out but when Chester asked if I could go there on loan, I had reservations. But Neil said: "Look, you won't be playing here so you might as well go and get some games in. Then take it from there." I said, "OK, I'll see how it works out." Alison was still working for RP Drugs at the time, although she set up her Rosemary Conley franchise the year after I joined Chester, and we'd already decided we weren't going to move house at that stage of my career. So going to Chester would mean commuting, something I wasn't too sure about. Virtually all the journey was on motorways, the M62 and M56, and quite honestly I didn't fancy making that 150-mile round trip every day on my own.

Then early in my loan spell, Pejic signed Nick Richardson from Cardiff.

Nick was a Halifax lad, the younger brother of Lee Richardson, who I signed for Huddersfield from Oldham three years later. He lived near me so we agreed to share the travelling. Dave Flitcroft and Andy Milner also commuted every day from south Manchester and we arranged to link up with them near Wilmslow and travel on to Chester in one car. That made life a lot easier. I met Nick every morning at Ainley Top, just off the M62 near Huddersfield, at around half past seven in the morning. I drove a BMW 3 Series in those days, with a personalised number plate, 555 PAJ. Nick had a big estate car and when he was driving I'd settle down in the passenger seat and have a kip. He was a few years younger than me but we became good mates and still have a laugh about the Chester days when we meet.

All four of us took along a packed lunch, usually a sandwich made the night before and a bag of crisps, and we took turns to provide the flask of tea. Sometimes in winter we also had a flask of soup for the journey home. And as soon as we finished training, on pitches at Chester Racecourse because the club didn't have its own training ground, we raced back to the stadium, dashed into the shower, rushed to the car and set off as early as we could to make sure we didn't hit the afternoon traffic around Manchester. Three of us would get stuck into our food straight away while the driver had to wait until the front seat passenger had finished and was free to double up as a waiter. There'd be crumbs and crisps all over the place. The glamour of professional football!

There was no way of knowing how long the journey in would take so we had to give ourselves plenty of leeway. Inevitably there were times when we'd arrive ridiculously early and others when we'd stagger in an hour after the rest of the players and pick up a fine for being late. But we had some laughs.

Flitcroft was a real character. There was never a dull moment when he was around, either in the car, on the training ground or in the dressing room. His elder brother, Gary, was a big star with Manchester City, living the dream in the top flight and probably earning ten times as much as Dave. But Dave's attitude, application and desire were spot on and he's taken that same ethos into a successful coaching career with first Rochdale and then Barnsley, where he became manager in January, 2013. They were good days. I was made captain soon after signing full-time, won a couple of Player of the Year awards and made my 600th league appearance while I was there. Cyrille Regis, the former England striker, reached the landmark at around the same time and we were both presented with commemorative medals before a home match. Memorable!

Big Cyrille had arrived a year after me and was coming to the end of a 20-year career that featured five England appearances. He was a true gentleman. I'd played against him a few times and he was always a real handful. But off the pitch, you could not wish to meet a nicer guy. He was cool, calm, sophisticated and had a genuine presence, an aura. When he spoke, people sat up and listened...even nightclub doormen at Christmas!

That was in 1995 when we all decided to go to a nightclub in Wilmslow after our Christmas do. When we arrived there was a long queue waiting to go in but Mark Guterman, the chairman, thought he was the Big I Am around the place and pushed to the front. "Chester City," he said to the doorman.

"So what?" was the reply. So the chairman came back to us and said rather sheepishly, "Sorry lads, he won't let us in." Without saying a word, Cyrille strolled nonchalantly to the front of the queue, said good evening to the doorman, who smiled, said, "Hello, Cyrille," and told his two bouncers, "Right, let 'em in!" Cyrille was even older than me – I gave him three years' start - but he was still an awesome figure on the pitch and scored seven goals in 29 appearances for Chester. I wish I had played with him in his prime. We became quite close while we were there and stayed in touch afterwards when he became an agent. It was an honour to finish my league career with someone like Cyrille.

Of course he wasn't at the club when we were on the receiving end of that hammering from Crewe and after we'd been beaten in six of our next seven league games, Pejic lost his job. We were relegated at the end of the season, by which time Kevin Ratcliffe, the former Everton and Wales defender, had taken over as manager. He'd been working alongside Pejic as player-coach.

I'd known Kevin since our schoolboy days, when he was captain of South Wales and I was captain of Yorkshire. He was a good manager and a good coach and I'm surprised that he didn't go on and do better. After leaving Chester in 1999, he was in charge at Shrewsbury for four years but after beating Everton in the FA Cup third round in January, 2003, they went on a disastrous run and were relegated from the Football League at the end of the season. Kevin eventually moved on to the media side, working as a match summariser for BBC Radio Wales.

But he played a part in making my last seasons as a league player a really enjoyable time. I'd known for a while the end was coming because from the middle of the 1996-97 season, I was carrying a double hernia that I knew would need an operation eventually. But I struggled on for as long as I could. I scored my last league goal against Doncaster at Belle Vue in November. We won 1-0 and I seem to recall it was either a 30-yard volley or a towering far post header. One match report confirms that it was indeed a header, in the 77th minute from a Flitcroft corner, but the word spectacular does not feature in the description of the goal.

My last FA Cup-tie was a second round match against Boston United at the Deva on December 7, 1996. We'd beaten Stalybridge Celtic in the first round and after our 1-0 victory over Boston, we were drawn at Middlesbrough in the third round. Middlesbrough went on to reach the final that year, losing to Chelsea, and their side included big names like Fabrizio Ravanelli, Juninho, Emerson, Craig Hignett and Gianluca Festa. They hammered us 6-0 and sadly, I wasn't involved after being sent off for a second bookable offence in the previous round. Boston had a striker called Leroy Chambers, who'd been at Chester the previous year, and we'd never got on. Predictably there was a bit of niggle from the word go and I was sent off as early as the 36th minute.

But the Jacksons were still represented at The Riverside Stadium with Ollie as the Chester mascot. He was nine at the time and for a while he'd been travelling over with me for home matches. The club used to keep a seat for him in the stand. So he was thrilled to bits to be the mascot at a Premier League ground. The Middlesbrough lads really went out of their way to make him feel at home, posing for pictures with him in the dressing room and on the pitch. We still have them today.

The team travelled up to Middlesbrough on the morning of the match, picking up Ollie and me at Wetherby, and we stopped off at a pub on the A1 for our pre-match meal. After we'd finished eating we had an impromptu game of 'Chicken' on the dart board. It's the game where one of the players holds his hand up on the board while the others take turns to throw a dart. If he moves his hand, he's a chicken! I remember Ollie turning to me at one point with a look of disbelief on his face, as if to say, "Is this really how professional footballers behave before an important FA Cup-tie?"

Meanwhile Chester were going well in the league and reached the Division Three play-offs, losing to Swansea in the semi-final. But I wasn't around to help them. I had to miss the closing stages of the season because of the hernia and made the last of my 651 league appearances against Barnet at the Deva Stadium on March 8, 1997. We won 1-0. I'll always remember little Chester City as a good time in my life. I'm still in touch with people there and when the news broke in 2008 that I had been diagnosed with cancer, a short tribute was read out before a home game, giving details of my stats with the club and elsewhere and wishing me a speedy recovery. For me, that summed up Chester City and I was delighted when Chester FC, as they are known, were promoted to the Conference at the end of the 2012-13 season.

So in the summer of 1997 I was a free agent and at 36, the prospects of finding another league club were not great. I'd completed my coaching badges so I was definitely looking for an opportunity to move on to the coaching side as a first step on the road to my ultimate goal, management. Then Halifax Town came calling.

For me, Halifax has always been The Club That Won't Die because I've almost lost count of the times they've been on the brink of disappearing without trace. They have had so many knock-backs and time and time again, they've been close to collapsing altogether. But somehow they've found a way to survive and even now, after being forced to drop down into the Unibond League after going into liquidation in 2008, they're climbing back up again, now known as FC Halifax Town. They have been promoted three times in four seasons and are now back in the Conference, one level below league football.

The Shaymen will be back in the league eventually, no worries!

For years, the headquarters of the Halifax Building Society, now just The Halifax, was literally a hundred yards away from The Shay, a massive building towering over the main road into the town. The Halifax was a worldwide brand but never once, as far as I know, had they put their hands in their pocket and offered a sponsorship deal to their hometown club. I don't remember The Halifax even having an advert on the perimeter fence around the ground and at one time, Town were sponsored by the Nationwide. That was absolutely criminal.

Halifax have never had any real success, never had any major sponsorship, never had any money. But what they have always had is friendliness in abundance. It's always been an amazing little club and we go back a long way. When I first got married, Halifax often played home matches on a Friday night and I used to go and watch them with Alison's dad and her brothers. To this day people at The Shay welcome me back and whether I'm in work, out of work or whatever, the welcome is just as warm.

Throughout my career, I always kept an eye on how they were doing and it was awful to see them drop out of the Football League for the first time in 1993. Early in 1997, towards the end of my time at Chester, it looked as if they were going to lose their place in the Conference as well. Then George Mulhall, my first manager at Bradford, took over and kept them in the Conference. He rang me early in the close season and offered me a one-year contract. The money was £150 a week, around £350 less than I'd been earning at Chester, but I never had a moment's hesitation.

Because of my coaching and management ambitions, I asked for a clause to be inserted in my contract that if an opportunity came along, I would be released even if it meant Halifax not receiving any compensation. They agreed. And although I only spent a few months at The Shay before becoming manager at Huddersfield at the start of October, I enjoyed every minute.

We used to train on public pitches on Savile Park, a few hundred yards away from The Shay, on Tuesday and Thursday evenings and straight away it felt just like being back at school, playing with my mates. I also used to train by myself on Monday, Wednesday and Friday so once again my fitness levels were higher than most of the others, even though I was the oldest player in the dressing room.

I'd train after taking the kids to school and then I'd usually pick them up again later because Alison was totally involved with her Rosemary Conley franchise. I also did one or two bits of local radio work at midweek matches and a spot of gardening here and there. I've always been a keen gardener and if I heard someone needed some work doing, I'd offer to give them a hand for twenty quid or so in cash. It brought in a bit of money and kept the boredom away.

But Halifax Town was the serious business and straight away, I thought to myself, "This isn't a bad side." Even though they'd nearly been relegated the previous year, there was a tremendous spirit and one or two players, like Geoff Horsfield, a big, strong striker, and Jamie Paterson, a little Scottish midfield player who now lives in Australia, had a bit extra. I looked at both of them when I went to Huddersfield but the asking prices were too high. Horsfield finished that season with 37 goals in 30 games and his agent sent a video down to Kevin Keegan, then manager at Fulham. Kevin snapped him up for £300,000 and he went on to play for ten clubs in 13 years, including Birmingham and West Brom in the top flight.

Horsfield was a real down to earth lad from Barnsley. His dad was a miner and Geoff was always a big fan of Arthur Scargill, the former miners' leader. With Geoff, what you saw was what you got on and off the field. I remember playing Yeovil one night when Graham Roberts, the ex-Spurs and England defender, was their player-manager. They were going well but we beat them 3-2. Horsfield scored a hat-trick and tormented Roberts all night. Roberts was a renowned hard man but Geoff stood up to him and gave as good as he got and more. He really ran riot.

I'd been the first player to arrive in the dressing room at around half past five and Geoff rolled up soon afterwards, straight from the building site. He was eating a McDonalds cheeseburger. When he'd finished it, he chucked the bag in the bin, stripped off, had a shower, put his kit on and went out and scored a hat-trick. Next day he was up at six o'clock and back on site.

One of my first games was a pre-season friendly against Huddersfield, who were then in what is now the Championship. We beat them 3-1 and it could easily have been five or six. Because of a colour clash they were wearing a new change strip of cream and blue, not one of the best strips I've seen. They fielded a strong side but we absolutely ripped them apart and could have won far more easily. There were a lot of Town fans there and they gave me a great reception…certainly a lot better than their own players received as they left the field at the final whistle!

Halifax started the season at 200-1 to win the title and walked it by nine points. There was a rumour that a couple of the directors had put some money on us and if so, they struck lucky because the winnings would have paid for the players' Championship bonus at the end of the season. I wish I'd had a tenner on as well because I sensed after beating Huddersfield that we could be a force. In all, I played in ten games for the Shaymen. We won nine and drew the other so I must be the only player to appear in only ten matches for Halifax and never finish on the losing side! I like to think I played a part in getting the ball rolling for what was a wonderful season for the club and even though I played just a handful of matches, I received a Championship medal. A cherished possession.

Halifax was probably the first and only time in my career when I felt I could play without any fear or pressure, just for the sheer enjoyment of it. I had a great rapport with the fans and everything came together from the word go. Ollie and his mates used to come down and watch and Alison's dad also came to a couple of games, even though he was unwell. He was so proud to see his son-in-law play for the club he loved. I was proud to be there and I would have been happy to go on and play a full season.

Instead, on Friday, October 3, I had a call at home from Malcolm Asquith, the chairman of Huddersfield Town, asking me if I'd be interested in taking over as manager. The call didn't come totally out of the blue. Town were four points adrift at the bottom of Division One, with no wins and just four points from nine matches. Brian Horton, who had been in charge since Neil Warnock's departure in 1995, hadn't brought in any new players over the summer. There had been rumours that if Huddersfield decided to change the manager, I might be in with a chance.

Halifax played Kettering Town the following day and after the match, I said to Mulhall and Kieran O'Regan, his number two, "I might not be around for much longer. I'm going for a chat with Huddersfield tomorrow about becoming their next manager. I wanted you to hear it from me first." They wished me all the best.

I was interviewed by Malcolm, the other three board members and Trevor Cherry, the ex-Town player and my former manager at Bradford City, at Malcolm's home. Trevor, an associate director who advised the board on football matters, had worked with Terry Yorath and me at Valley Parade and I suspect he recommended us as the new managerial team. As a raw, untried manager, I would need someone as my assistant who had a lot of experience and as well as being a top coach, Terry had been manager of Wales and Lebanon and also Swansea, Bradford City and Cardiff. I couldn't have had a better man alongside me, either then or when I rejoined the club in 2003. We had some tremendous times as a partnership.

I'd never been to an interview in my life. I'd no idea what to wear even and in the end opted for a suit and tie. I wasn't nervous really because after spending four years at Huddersfield as a player, I knew everybody in the room and they knew all about me and my personality…which is why they had invited me for an interview. It wasn't as if I was going in there cold and trying to impress a group of strangers. I don't think there were any other candidates but I suppose they must have had one or two people in mind in case I interviewed badly.

I was asked what I thought about the team and how I would set about turning things round if I got the job, the sort of players I would be looking to sign, how I would work within a fairly limited budget and so on. As I left, Malcolm said he'd give me a call later. The phone rang soon after I arrived home. He said they were impressed with what I had to offer and were prepared to give Terry and me a chance.

It had all happened so quickly, just three days in which I went from part-time footballer at non-league Halifax Town to manager of a famous First Division club. My life was about to change for ever.

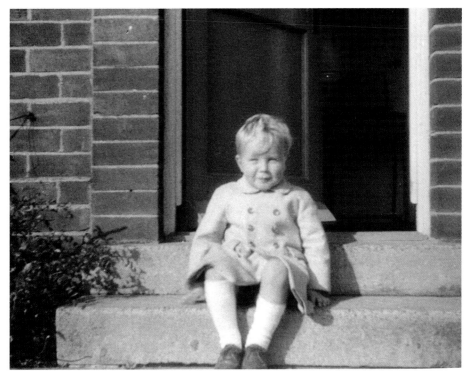

Watch the birdie! Peter, aged two, already has an eye for the camera.

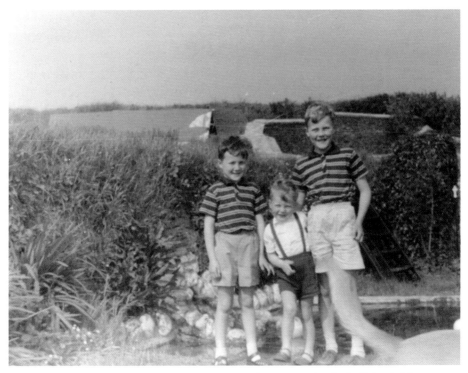

Sunshine boys. Peter with Gerard (left) and Anthony on a family holiday in Newquay.

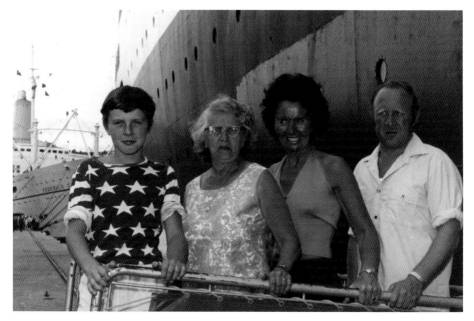

All aboard! Peter ready to set sail on a QE2 cruise to Madeira in 1973 with (from left) Auntie Cathy and his Mum and Dad.

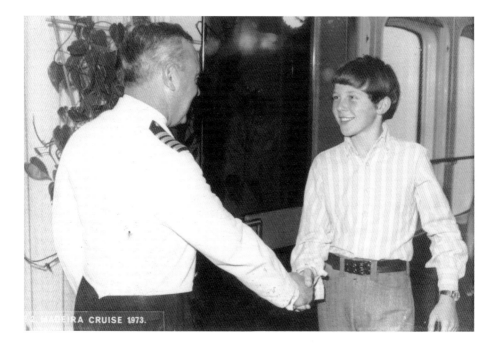

MADEIRA CRUISE 1973.

Cruise control: Peter meeting his namesake captain Peter Jackson on board the QE2.

Joker in the pack: The late Norman Collier, a keen Bradford City fan, hams it up with (from left) Mark Ellis, Peter and Barry Gallagher.

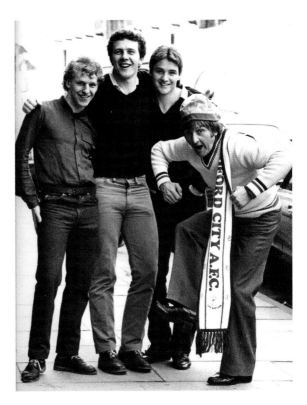

Words of wisdom: On the training ground with Terry Yorath, a major influence on Peter's early career at City and later his assistant manager at Huddersfield Town. (Picture House Ltd)

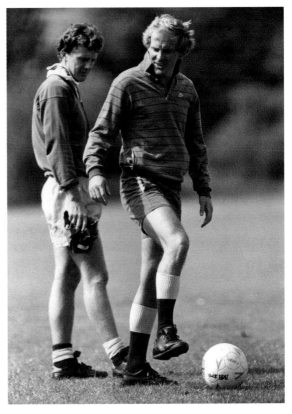

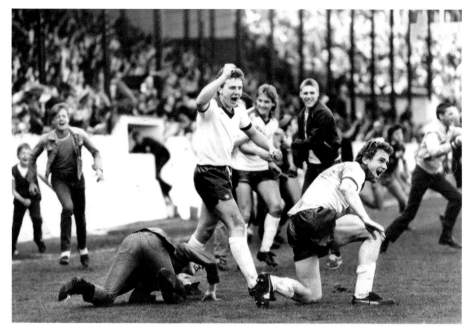

We've done it! Celebrating City's promotion to Division Three in 1981 with Bobby Campbell and the City fans.

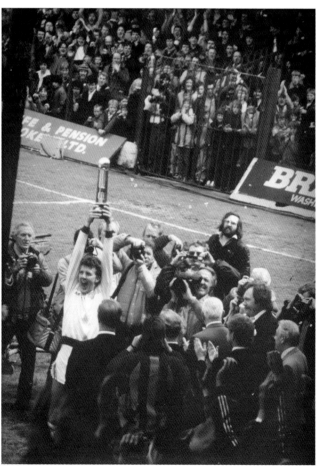

Triumph. Peter raises the Division Three Championship trophy before the game against Lincoln at Valley Parade on May 11, 1985.

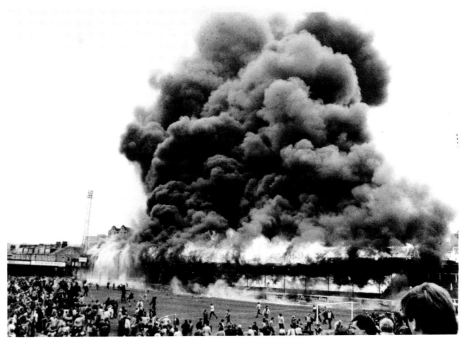

Tragedy. The scene around an hour later as flames engulf the main stand. Peter rescued Alison and Charlotte from the players' lounge immediately below the floodlight pylon on the left. (Yorkshire Post)

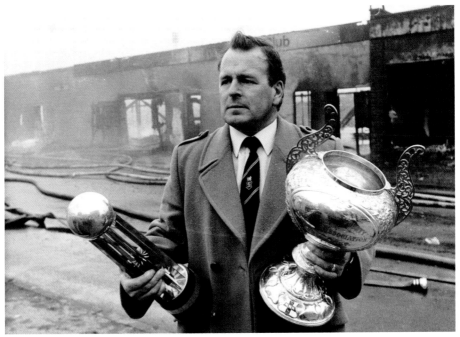

Aftermath: Mike Smith, a member of the Valley Parade commercial team who later worked with Alison at Appleyard Jaguar, with the Division Three Championship trophy and the West Riding Cup, both of which survived the blaze (Yorkshire Post)

Meet the boss: Peter with Willie McFaul soon after joining Newcastle in 1987 (Ian Dobson)

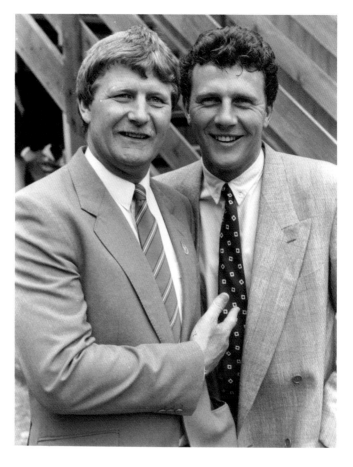

Samba time: With Mirandinha, the first Brazilian to play in the top flight when he joined Newcastle in 1987.

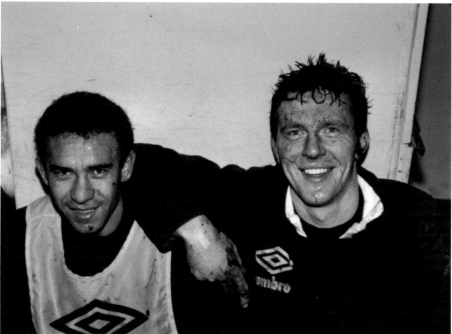

Heads I win: An aerial tussle with Wimbledon's John Fashanu in the 1988 FA Cup quarter-final at St James' Park, watched by Paul Gascoigne and Dennis Wise. (Julian Brannigan)

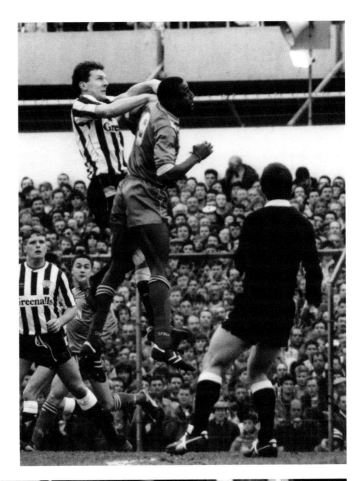

Talk of the Town. With Huddersfield manager Eion Hand after signing for Town in 1990. (Huddersfield Examiner)

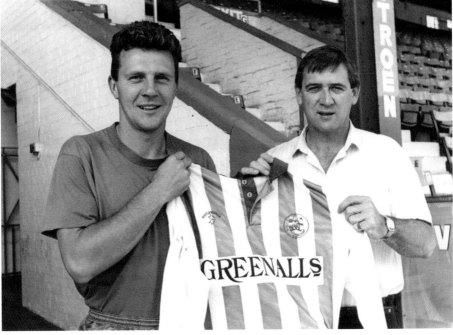

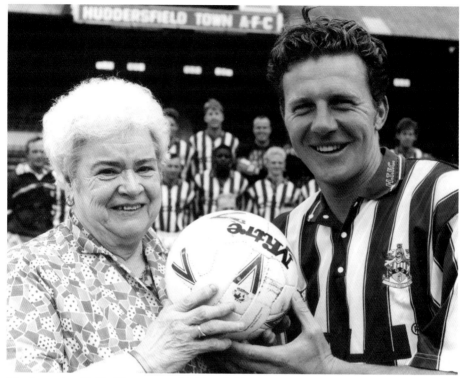

My favourite: Nellie Thompson, Huddersfield's laundry lady, steals the show at a pre-season photocall. (Huddersfield Examiner)

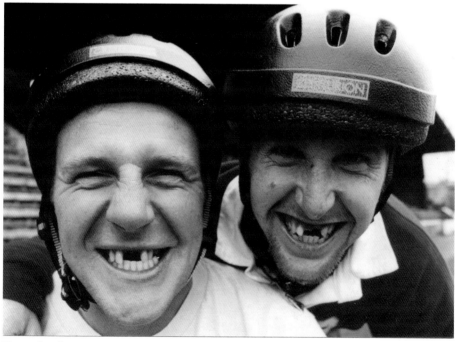

Fangs for the memory: Peter and Town and Wales striker Iwan Roberts don the helmets for a cycle safety awareness day.

On the dotted line: Signing a contract extension, watched by Town manager Neil Warnock and chairman Terry Fisher, in July, 1993. Peter joined Chester the following summer. (Huddersfield Examiner)

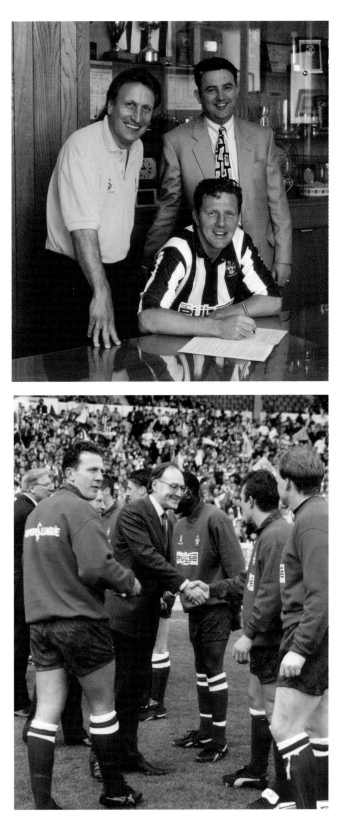

Shake on it: Introducing the Town players to Home Secretary Michael Howard, guest of honour at the 1994 Autoglass Trophy final at Wembley. Then Peter spent the entire match on the subs' bench (Huddersfield Examiner)

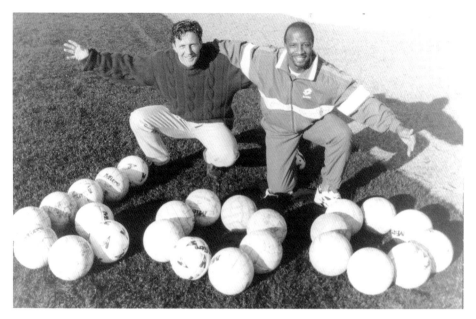

Milestones: With Cyrille Regis at Chester, where they both reached the 600 league appearance landmark.

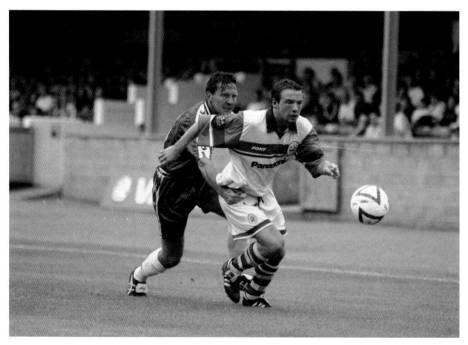

Final fling: A tussle with Huddersfield striker Marcus Stewart in a pre-season friendly at Halifax, one of Peter's last senior appearances. Two months later he was Stewart's manager! (Huddersfield Examiner)

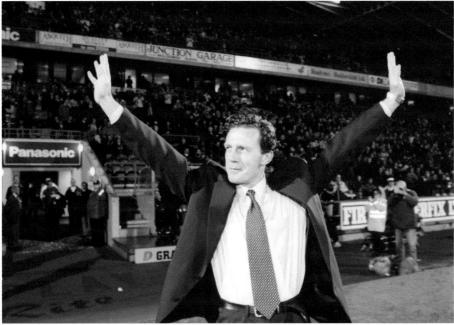

Management man: My first game in charge at Huddersfield, against Charlton on October 14, 1997. We lost 3-0. (Huddersfield Examiner)

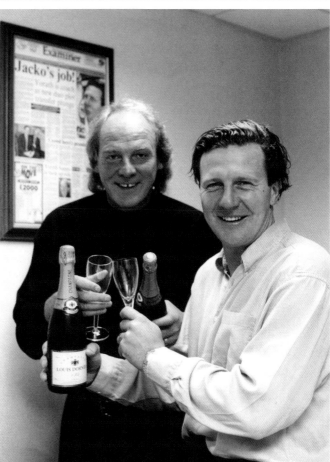

Bubbling over: Sharing a Manager of the Month award with Terry Yorath. (Huddersfield Examiner)

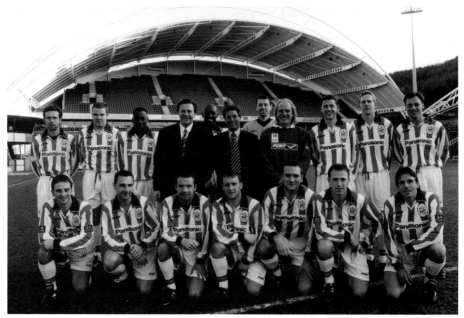

New man in charge: The Town squad with new owner Barry Rubery, pictured between Peter and Terry Yorath, after his takeover in January, 1999. (Huddersfield Examiner)

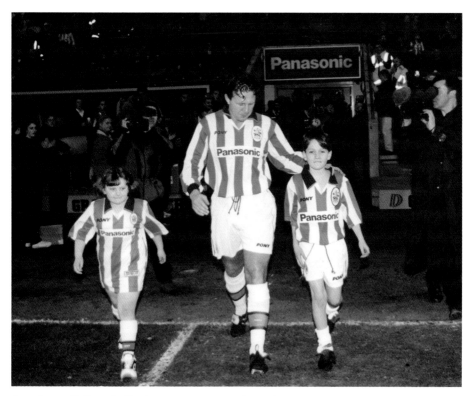

Last farewell: Peter's final appearance as a player, in a reserve match against West Brom at the end of the 1997-98 season. Oliver was one of the mascots.

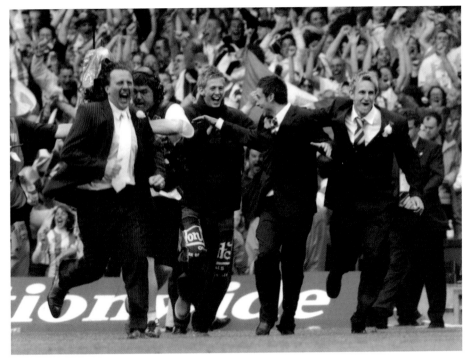

Finest hour: Huddersfield win the League Two play-off final at the Millennium Stadium – and the celebrations start in earnest. (Huddersfield Examiner)

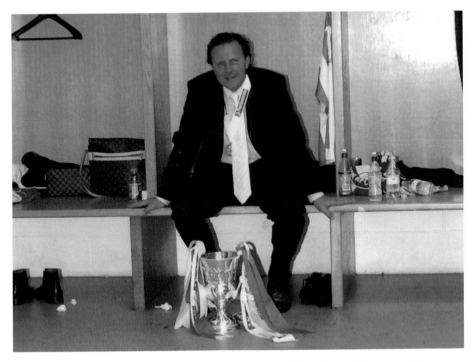

Pause for thought: Taking a breather with the League Two play-off trophy as the players celebrate on the pitch. (David Wright)

Young Guns: Huddersfield's pre-season corporate hospitality brochure. Brokeback Mountain, the film about two gay cowboys, was released soon afterwards… (Huddersfield Town)

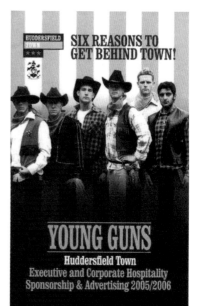

SIX REASONS TO
GET BEHIND TOWN!

YOUNG GUNS
Huddersfield Town
Executive and Corporate Hospitality
Sponsorship & Advertising 2005/2006

Old pals act: Re-united with Paul Gascoigne when Rangers met a Bradford City line-up in Stuart McCall's testimonial match at Valley Parade, April 2002. (Telegraph & Argus)

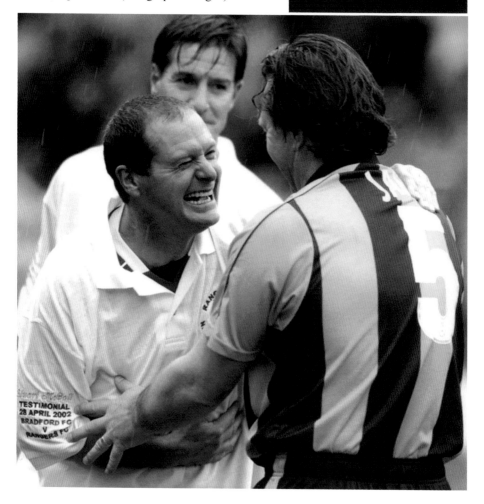

All the best, Jose: Meeting Mourinho before Huddersfield's FA Cup fourth round tie at Chelsea in January, 2006. (Huddersfield Examiner)

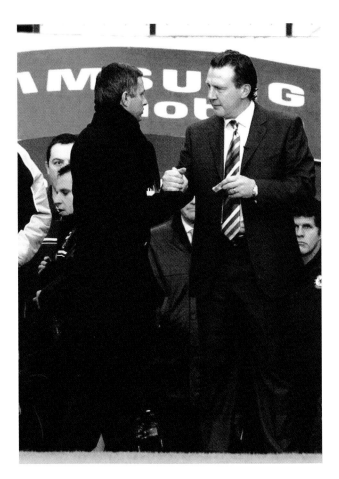

Au Revoir: With the Manager of the Month award before Lincoln's match against Wycombe on March 1, 2008. Peter's radiotherapy treatment began twelve days later. (Lincolnshire Echo)

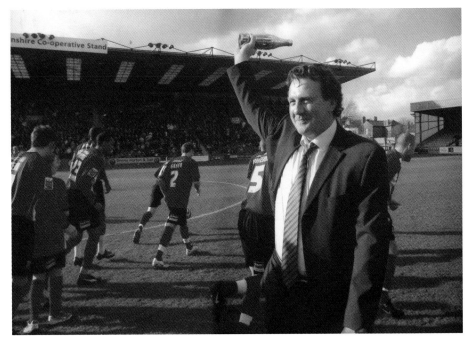

Back in the old routine: Peter with number two Iffy Onuora after returning to Lincoln (Lincolnshire Echo)

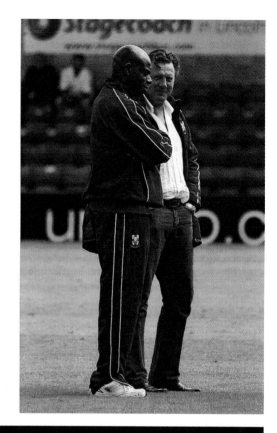

Lifesaver. Peter salutes Bradford City striker Jake Speight after his goal secured a crucial point against Burton Albion during the club's fight for league survival in April, 2011. (Telegraph & Argus)

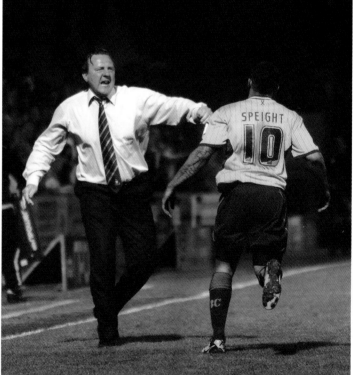

7. Managing nicely, thanks

In October, 1997, Peter was appointed manager of Huddersfield Town, a job he was to keep for 18 months. Alison, still running her Rosemary Conley franchises, was determined that whatever happened on the field, they should savour every minute of his time in charge. "I knew we had to make the most of it because the only certainty for football managers is that one day, sooner or later, they will be sacked."

Alison's Story

I call them my Harvey Nichols days, Peter's first spell as manager of Huddersfield Town. Days when I'd think nothing of going out in Leeds and spending a thousand pounds on designer handbags and shoes, Chloe, Chanel, Gucci, Prada. I look at those bags now and think, "God, how much did I pay for that?" It was a ridiculous amount of money and I have to say that those Harvey Nichols days are well and truly a thing of the past!

I wasn't showing off. It was something I felt I was somehow expected to do, a bit like our time in Newcastle when I felt I had to live up to the popular image of a footballer's wife. I thought I had a role to play as a manager's wife and had to look the part. I wasn't a Victoria Beckham by any means but I always had fantastic clothes with designer labels and spent a fortune on beauty treatments and on my hair.

It was my money, not Peter's. For the best part of twenty years I earned good money in various jobs and I spent it on my kids, myself and our family holidays. I never touched Peter's money except for paying bills, work on the house and entertaining.

But those 18 months when Peter was in charge at Huddersfield for the first time enabled us to enjoy a complete change of lifestyle before, inevitably, he was sacked. That's football, I'm afraid. Even if a manager is doing fantastically well, he can still find himself out of a job when a new owner comes along. And that's exactly what happened to Peter when Barry Rubery, a multi-millionaire businessman, bought Huddersfield Town in 1999.

A manager simply doesn't know what's just around the corner and that uncertainty was at the back of my mind from the start. I urged Peter to go out there and try to enjoy every single minute, although in the early euphoria, I don't think either of us realised how much our lives were going to change. We'd been through something similar at Newcastle, when almost overnight, Peter went from being a little-known lower division player to a high-profile performer in a soccer-mad city.

And now all of a sudden we started receiving invitations to all kinds of functions. Peter's gut reaction would be to turn them down. He'd say, "We're not going there. They're only asking us because I'm a football manager." And I'd reply, "Does it matter why we're being invited? You might not be a manager for much longer so let's make the most of it."

I was with my Rosemary Conley ladies on our annual trip to Springs Health Farm in Leicester when Peter went for his interview with the Town directors. It was all very cloak and dagger because we didn't want anyone to smell a rat. We weren't supposed to use mobile phones in the health farm so I had to keep mine on silent in my pocket. Every now and then I'd sneak off into a corner and ask what was happening but it wasn't until we were on the way home in the coach that the call finally came through to say he'd got the job. Even then, I couldn't tell anyone because it was top secret until the official announcement a couple of days later.

I was absolutely delighted, of course. And I never had any doubt at all that he'd be able to do it, particularly as Terry Yorath, his coach and mentor at Bradford City before he moved to Newcastle, would be working alongside him. I knew Peter's attitude would be absolutely spot-on, even though he'd go at it like a bull in a china shop.

That's his approach to any job he does and I believed the inevitable streak of naivety would work in his favour. He could just go in and be as loud and brash as he wanted because he would not be pre-conditioned about how a manager should operate. I could imagine Peter coming up with an idea, Terry telling him to be a bit cautious and think again and Peter going ahead anyway. But importantly, I also knew that Peter would accept Terry's advice on the really important issues and would also learn quickly from his mistakes.

As a family, we all accepted that we'd see less of Peter. He was being paid well as manager of Huddersfield Town and working long hours was part and parcel of the job. We had to adapt to that and I had never relied on Peter being around all the time anyway. I had learned to live with his mood swings when he was a player and it was no different now he was a manager, perhaps a bit more intense. Sometimes he'd be very quiet, sometimes giddy with excitement and we went along with that.

His appointment did not alter my own career with Rosemary Conley in any way. Peter would probably disagree but I would say that until I set up my care company, Caremark Calderdale, in 2010, he was never as supportive of me in my career as I was of him in his. That isn't being critical or unkind. It's just that I haven't needed the same kind of support. I always felt I had to be strong for him because of the extreme ups and downs he lived through in football. Before Caremark, I hadn't experienced the same kind of professional highs and lows in any of my jobs. At Caremark, however, I have endured similar levels of stress and he has always been there to support me. In fact, sometimes he worries himself to death about things that I feel I have under control.

I realised that in management, as in playing, there would be clearly defined areas where a wife would simply not be involved because the door carried a sign saying Men Only. So I saw my role as being there for Peter and supporting him in any way I could. As a player's wife, I'd been ready to move wherever and whenever the job dictated, although as it happened, Peter only moved away from Yorkshire once. But if he'd been offered a contract by Portsmouth, Plymouth, Port Vale or Peterborough, I would have gone along with it. Management would be the same.

For me, the big difference between Peter's two careers was that once he became a manager, I felt it was my duty to be present at the club on match days. When he was a player, I'd been very hit and miss, not least because I'd never particularly enjoyed football and, especially when the kids were young, I had other things to do on a Saturday afternoon or Tuesday night.

But I knew that as a manager's wife, the ground rules would have to change because I believed the manager's wife had a status within the club and therefore had a role to play, too. During Peter's playing career I would never have dared to speak to the manager or his wife unless they spoke to me first. They were important people in the club hierarchy who should be treated with respect. I hoped that I would receive the same kind of respect from the Huddersfield players and I did. If I passed any of them in the corridor, they would always call me Mrs Jackson. Which I have to say felt a bit odd at first.

Huddersfield always had a reputation for looking after their staff and their families and they treated me very well. On match days, I would arrive at the ground at about 12.30pm or one o'clock and go straight into the boardroom, where I would have a chat with the chairman and the other directors and then sit down for a meal. I was encouraged to take Charlotte and Oliver along and I could also invite a couple of guests if I wanted. Then we would watch the game from the directors' box. Of course, I knew that I would have to be very careful what I said because they were also Peter's employers and it was important that I didn't make any chance remarks that would compromise his position. So I had to be on my guard.

Before the match, everyone in the boardroom would be very positive and enthusiastic and so would the visiting directors when they arrived. There was usually a fairly friendly atmosphere between the two sets of directors and plenty of good luck messages before the kick-off. Perhaps that was the politically correct thing to do but even so, I don't recall occasions when there was any hostility before the game even started.

The atmosphere tended to change at half-time. If one of the teams was in front, their directors would be upbeat while the opposing directors would be showing signs of tension. Sometimes I would pick up comments about the manager, why did he do this or why didn't he try that? That was the signal to keep the smile in place, look positive and keep the mouth firmly shut, apart from perhaps reminding people that there was still 45 minutes to play.

Win or lose, I never went near the boardroom after the match. I believed it was important for the directors to be able to say exactly what they wanted without having to look over their shoulders to see if the manager's wife was listening in. And anyway, I had decided that there was another role that I should be playing on a match day: hostess in the manager's office.

As soon as the match ended, I'd go down to Peter's office, taking along Charlotte and Oliver and anyone I'd invited to the match. So sometimes there would be five or six of us waiting either to celebrate with Peter...or commiserate when he walked in with his face down to the floor after a defeat. He would have invited the opposition manager and his sidekick for a drink so when they walked in, sometimes when Peter was still doing his Press conferences, I'd do the honours while they checked the results on the telly before Peter arrived.

I never tried to discuss the finer points of the match, although Peter always tells me that after one match that Town won easily, I smiled at the opposing manager and said, "Wasn't that a great game?" He wasn't impressed. But talking football wasn't what they wanted anyway; professionals hate amateurs, particularly women, trying to pretend they know anything about the game. So instead I'd ask them about their families, if their wife or kids had come to the match, how long the journey home would be. Small talk.

I honestly thought that was the normal thing to do, that other managers' wives up and down the country were playing hostess at the same time. And it wasn't until a while later that I discovered it didn't happen very often elsewhere. I tried to create an open, relaxed atmosphere in which the managers and their assistants could wind down a bit for 15 or 20 minutes after all the tension of the match. And it seemed to work. I did the same thing during Peter's second spell at Huddersfield and again during his time at Lincoln.

However, it was completely different during his time in charge at Bradford City in 2011. I was never made welcome or encouraged to feel part of the club. There were no seats in the directors' box for me and the kids so instead we had to sit in the stand. The fans knew who we were but that didn't stop them having a go at Peter and giving us some stick as well. I don't think any family should have to be surrounded by people hurling abuse at their husband and father so after a couple of matches we just stopped going. Yes, we wanted to be there to support Peter but not in those circumstances.

Back at Huddersfield, everything was fine until Barry Rubery, a millionaire businessman, bought the club at the start of 1999. I think Barry must have woken up one morning and thought, "Today, I'm going to buy a football club." So he bought Huddersfield Town, more or less, it seemed, on a whim. He installed a right-hand man, Ian Ayre, who as far as I was concerned gave him some bad advice... but then I suppose I would be harsh about someone who played a part in the decision to sack my husband. It seemed to me that Barry knew little about the club's great traditions or if he did, he wasn't interested in them and wanted to change the traditional club badge on the players' blazers and the club shirt. He seemed to see the beautifully polished trophies and most of the memorabilia in the boardroom as relics from the past and not part of the club's future. And before long, Peter Jackson was history as well. "Peter Jackson, who's he? Never heard of him. Let's get rid of him and bring in a big name manager. Someone like Steve Bruce."

Peter suspected something was on the cards from the day Bruce was invited into the boardroom before a match – I was in there, too – and then spotted taking a seat in the directors' box. That was something Peter would never, ever have done to another manager. But even so, Peter had kept the club in the division in his first season and then challenged for a play-off place in his second. So he still thought he might be given an opportunity to build on the progress he'd made. Instead, one day, right after the end of his second season, Peter rang and said, "I've been sacked."

I couldn't believe it. I said, "What? After all the hard work, after the way you've lifted this club from the bottom of the table? Sacked?" Yes, I knew it was going to happen one day but surely that would be when results were bad and Huddersfield were struggling at the bottom of the division. In that situation, somebody has to be blamed and that person is the manager. But this was totally out of the blue.

The next three or four days were horrendous with Peter constantly asking what he could have done differently. I kept telling him that he couldn't have done any better and that nobody, apart from Rubery and Ayre, believed he should have been sacked. That was certainly the way it seemed from all the media coverage and the tremendous support Peter received from the Town supporters. In contrast, Rubery came in for an enormous amount of stick from the fans and a while later, he called Peter and said he felt dreadful about the way things had been handled.

On a personal level, though, I couldn't help but like Barry. What he did to Peter was totally wrong but he was likeable enough as a person, a bit of a cheeky chappie. One of the first things he did after he took over was promise us an end-of-season family holiday at his home in Barbados, using his private jet. And despite Peter's sacking and all the trouble it caused, he kept his promise, although in the end we stayed in a hotel instead of his house.

And at the beginning of April, he gave Peter a birthday treat, a couple of nights on his luxury yacht in the south of France. He said we could use the private jet to fly down to Nice, where his chauffeur would meet us and take us to a five-star hotel in Juan les Pins. Next morning, the chauffer would drive us to the yacht, which was moored nearby.

We flew out straight after the home match against Swindon on Easter

Monday. The hotel was fantastic and on the Tuesday morning, the chauffeur, I think he was called Jean Pierre and he also doubled up as captain of the yacht, came to collect us. As we approached the harbour, we saw that the smaller boats were moored at the jetties nearest the shore, where the sea was shallower, and the further out to sea we went, the boats got bigger. We had nearly reached the final jetty when the car stopped and we climbed out. The yacht was enormous and as we walked towards it, a remote-controlled gangway came down on to the jetty and we climbed aboard.

We asked Jean Pierre if he would be staying on board as well but no, we were to have the yacht to ourselves. He showed us where everything was and said the yacht was totally at our disposal. He'd come back in the morning when we'd decided where we'd like to go. Before leaving he showed us the massive control panel, it must have been about five feet by three feet, which operated everything on board. He said the only thing we might need overnight was the central heating as it could be a bit chilly in the evenings at that time of year. He showed Peter which switch operated the heating and added severely, "Do not, under any circumstances, touch any other switches." OK, we said.

When he'd gone, we made ourselves at home, relaxed on deck and late in the afternoon, decided to go for a stroll and buy something from a local deli for dinner on board. We stopped on the way back for a couple of drinks and by the time we returned to the harbour, it was about nine o'clock and quite dark. So much so that we couldn't work out which was our boat. We knew roughly where it should be but in the dark, they all looked more or less the same. So the only thing we could do was click the remote control for the gangway at every yacht we came to and eventually we found the right one.

We climbed on board and switched on the lights. "Jean Pierre was right," I said. "It's a bit chilly, isn't it?"

"Right, I'll switch the heating on," replied Peter, opening the control panel. "Which switch was it again?"

"I've no idea."

"Neither have I. I think it was this one." No luck. And no luck with the next switch. Or the next. Or the next. Then, to our horror, Peter tried one more switch and this deep rumbling noise started down below and the water at the back of the yacht began churning around. I said, "Peter, what have you done? You've switched the engine on. This yacht is worth millions of pounds and if we can't turn it off, the whole thing might blow up. Where's Jean Pierre's number?" But there was no number for Jean Pierre and the rumbling and churning continued all night.

He arrived as arranged at nine o'clock the next morning and, as we feared, he was not a happy man. In a mixture of French and English he had a real go at Peter, accusing him of not doing as he was told and saying he could easily have caused thousands of pounds worth of damage. Fortunately, when he checked, everything was OK and I think it was just the pumps that had been rumbling away and not the engine. Eventually he calmed down enough to ask us where we fancied going. "Oh, up the coast to Monaco or somewhere like that," I replied casually.

So off we went, opening a bottle of bubbly after a while. I was still in my designer fashion phase and kitted out in an Escada blouse, pants and plimsolls and felt pretty confident I looked the part as we cruised towards our destination. Even so, it started to get a bit cold after a while so I went downstairs and found a white polo neck M&S jumper to put over the top. That did the trick and I was still wearing it as we pulled into the harbour at Monte Carlo. On the jetty, there were all sorts of people taking pictures and I asked Jean Pierre who they were interested in. "You," he replied. "They see a yacht like this and think that everyone on board must be famous." Not in an M & S jumper I wasn't! So I ripped it off straight away to make sure we lived up to the right image.

That night we decided to go out but realised that the gangway was up and we didn't know how to lower it from on board the ship. Peter thought we should try and find the switch on the control panel but after the previous night's disaster, that was clearly a non-starter. So I said, "Peter, you're just going to have to take the remote control and jump on to the deck of the boat next door." He didn't seem totally thrilled about it but fair play, he clambered to the edge of our yacht and then launched himself on to the boat alongside us, which I ought to say, was unoccupied. No alarms went off, Peter pressed the remote control, down came the gangway and once Peter had made the return journey on to our yacht, we strolled on to the jetty and into town. This time making sure to remember where we were moored. How could we know as we boarded the private jet next morning that in a month's time, Peter would be out of a job?

The next time I crossed paths with Rubery was in a football club boardroom; I've no idea exactly where or when. I was with Peter and spotted Barry standing in the opposite corner from us. I hadn't actually spoken to him face to face since the sacking so I said to Peter, "I'm going over to tell him what I think."

"No, you can't…be careful what you say."

"Never mind that, I'll give him a piece of my mind." I walked across and said, "Hi Barry."

"Hello Alison, how are you doing?"

"Fine. What are you doing now?"

"I've just bought a diamond mine."

"Well, can I just say that I hope you know more about diamonds than you do about football clubs!"

He just laughed. So did I. "I'll tell you what, Alison," he said. "I haven't actually mined my first diamond yet. But when I do, I'll give it to you!"

I'm still waiting.

Peter's Story

The first thing I did as manager of Huddersfield Town was collect a Town shirt from the club shop and have it mounted and framed. It bore the inscription: Be Proud And Honoured To Wear The Shirt. The finished product was huge, around 3ft square, and within a few days of my arrival, it was fixed to the wall behind my desk in the manager's office. It dominated the room and every time a player, or anyone else for that matter, came to see me it was the first thing he saw. I wanted every single player to know how I felt about that shirt and, more important, to feel the same way, too.

I'd spent the four happiest years of my playing career at Huddersfield Town, wearing the famous blue and white stripes. Town, the first team to win three successive league titles in the Twenties, were steeped in tradition and I was immensely proud to wear that shirt; to be club captain was a huge honour. The framed shirt said it all.

The official Press conference to announce my appointment was held on Tuesday, October 7, the day after Brian Horton's departure, and when Terry Yorath and I walked into the room, I couldn't believe how many newspaper, television and radio journalists were there. At that moment, I realised what a big job it was going to be and how much media attention surrounded a club like Huddersfield Town, who were currently bottom of what is now the Championship.

Instead of answering after-match questions from one or two reporters in the corridor outside the dressing room, I was on a stage in front of the cameras and microphones, being grilled about my plans for the team. Who was I going to sign? Why had things gone wrong? How would I get Town out of the mess they were in? How did I feel about coming into such a big job without any managerial experience? These days, would-be managers receive media training as part of their courses but I was straight in at the deep end.

I was the youngest manager in the division and there were some big names around, people like Graham Taylor, Peter Reid, Alan Curbishley, Bruce Rioch, Joe Royle and George Burley. But I didn't feel fazed by the challenge, just excited. And I was determined to get across the message of how enthusiastic Terry and I were, that we couldn't wait to get started and failure was simply not an option. I never felt overawed or frightened.

One of my first one-to-one interviews was with Terry's daughter Gabby, now Gabby Logan. She had just started at Sky and I joked that as well as being the youngest manager in the division, I was better looking than Sunderland's Peter Reid and John Rudge at Port Vale. It was just a bit of fun and I had a laugh about it with both of them afterwards.

But before long, people in the media started referring to me as the best-looking manager in football so, working on the basis that any publicity is good publicity, I played along with it. It quickly snowballed to the point where match programmes for Town's away games would often carry a pen picture that would include a phrase like, "widely regarded as the game's best-looking manager." Ridiculous! It also became a bit of a joke with some of the other managers, who would say, "The best-looking manager's in town!" when I saw them before or after a match. Basically it was all tongue in cheek stuff but importantly, people started talking about Town with a smile on their face, which was what I'd intended all along…and I'm still better looking than Reid and Rudge today!

My first priority was to speak to all the players individually. Four, the goalkeeper Steve Francis and three defenders, Tom Cowan, Kevin Gray and Jon Dyson, had been in the dressing room when I was a player. To them I was Jacko, team-mate and captain, and I had to stamp my authority straight away. I told them that from now on I would be Gaffer.

I wanted to sit each player down across the desk, with the framed shirt behind me, talk about my approach to the job, what I expected from him and to hear his thoughts on why we were in such a mess. I needed to know how committed each of those players was to the shirt. It seemed straightforward enough but soon, I was learning about a very different side of football management: that as well as being my players' manager, I was also seen by some as a guardian or counsellor, someone who could help with any problems they might have away from the club.

As a player, I wouldn't have thought about talking to the manager about anything other than football, certainly not my personal troubles. But I learned very quickly that while a would-be manager can go on all the FA, PFA and UEFA courses, no training programme exists that can teach him how to deal with situations where he is helping players keep their lives together. There were drink problems, anger management problems, betting problems, wife problems, girlfriend problems, money problems, you name it. Two players just broke down in front of me in the office and sobbed uncontrollably. It was something I had simply never expected.

I didn't mind doing it. I reckoned that if I could help with their problems off the field, it might bring another five or ten per cent out of them on the field, which was something I would need. So I always spent time with any player who knocked on my door and wanted to talk, although I was quickly finding out that the pressures on a manager are ten times bigger than anything any player has to worry about. The chasm is massive. A player saunters into training for a couple of hours, plays 90 minutes then goes home and forgets about the game, win, lose or draw. If he has a problem, he can go and talk to his manager.

But who does the manager turn to when he has a problem? He soon finds out who are his true friends and who are the plastic hangers-on. He can never switch off, he can never relax, he's involved 24/7. The phone never stops ringing, there are training schedules, board meetings, press conferences. He always has to be planning ahead. It can be the best job in the world. Or the loneliest. There's no in-between. The stress levels are intense, Saturday's result dictates everything and any manager who claims he can switch off and forget about the football club when he goes home isn't telling the truth.

My first game was against Charlton at home. Alan Curbishley, their manager, made a point of talking to me beforehand, saying that if ever I needed any help or advice, all I had to do was give him a call. They were going well, we were low on confidence and were well-beaten 3-0. But in less than 12 hours I was given a reminder of life's real priorities when I received the call to tell me that my uncle Ronnie, my mother's brother, had died the previous night when he arrived home in Bradford after watching the match. It may be a cliché but a family tragedy like this really does put losing a football match into perspective.

Terry and I never had any doubt that we would keep Huddersfield in that division but four defeats in my first five games didn't exactly help our cause, even though they exposed the team's shortcomings and showed us exactly the size of the task we faced. But I vowed that I would never let anyone see me deflated. In only my third game in charge, we were turned over 4-1 at Port Vale. It was a depressing performance but afterwards on the coach home, Terry said, "Never let your head drop. Never let anyone see how you're really feeling." And from then on, I always wore the mask and did my best to look upbeat and positive. Only Terry knew how I was feeling deep down. But believe me, the dugout and the touchline can be lonely places when things are going badly.

Every day was a learning curve for a young manager who had only been in the job for seven days, then seven weeks then seven months. I was learning how to handle the players, how to approach board meetings, how to deal with agents when I wanted to sign a player, how to work with the media. I had to learn how to pace myself on days when I might be up at seven and not home again until midnight or later because I'd been watching a game. When you've been in management for a few years, all these things become second nature, you adapt and find a way to keep things on an even keel. But as a new manager, the highs and lows were enormous and every day presented a different challenge that I felt had to be tackled immediately.

Like signing new players. Obviously we had to bring in one or two people and there was a bit of money available. Above all, we needed experience, leadership on the pitch and in the dressing room and the first player we signed fulfilled all those requirements. Barry Horne was 35, he'd played over 50 times for Wales and most of his 600-plus league appearances had been in the top flight. On top of that Barry, a chemistry graduate who moved into teaching when he retired, was chairman of the Professional Footballers Association. Terry knew all about him from their time together with Wales and I made him captain straight away. He became a key figure in our fight for survival and a big influence throughout the club. The other players looked up to him and when Barry spoke, people listened.

My next signing was Lee Richardson from Oldham, another experienced midfield player who later moved into management, and he was followed by Wayne 'The Chief' Allison, the big striker who provided the power and strength we needed up front. I paid a club record £700,000 for The Chief and it wasn't easy persuading the board to part with that kind of money. But we probably wouldn't have stayed up without him.

The Chief played alongside Marcus Stewart who, in February, 2000, moved on to Ipswich for £2.5m and the following year was the leading scorer in the Premier League. Marcus played over 650 league games in a 20-year career and still says that The Chief was the best front line partner he had. When they were on song, they were unstoppable, with Stewart's movement allied to Allison's strength and aerial power.

He was followed by David Phillips, another experienced Welsh international who could fill several roles, Grant Johnson, a young Scottish midfield player, and goalkeeper Stephen Harper, who came in on loan from Newcastle until the end of the season. Stephen was outstanding for us and I was desperate to sign him on a permanent basis the following summer. Instead he went back to Newcastle and was second string there for the next ten years. I've always told him that he has wasted his career. OK, he played for a Premier League club and was earning top money but a goalkeeper with his ability should have been playing first team football, not languishing in the reserves or keeping the subs' bench warm. He was a fantastic kid and a fantastic keeper and he should have played five or six hundred games not around 200.

All the signings did well for the club and played a part in making sure we stayed in the division. But the real revelation for supporters was a man who had been signed by Brian Horton from Plymouth Argyle in the summer of 1995. Horton had paid £125,000 for Paul Dalton but he'd never really made much of an impact and when Terry and I arrived, he was little more than a fringe player.

Dalton was a confidence player, the sort who went into his shell as soon as the manager started to get on his back. But I realised after watching him in a practice match that he could make things happen for us. I told him, "You've got a special talent and I want you to use it. Don't be chasing back to make sliding tackles, there are people behind you who are paid to do that. You can win us matches. You might lose us some as well but we'll pick up a lot more points if we have you playing to the best of your ability."

He'd played out wide for most of his career but I gave him a free role just behind the front two and it was from there that he clinched that crucial first win in my sixth game in charge, 3-1 against Stoke at the McAlpine Stadium. It was an emotional day for everyone and years later, a guy came up to me and told me that he'd only cried twice in his life, once at a funeral and once when the referee blew the final whistle after that game against Stoke!

I can still see the dying seconds as if it was yesterday. We were winning 2-1 and hanging on when, deep into injury time, Stoke won a corner. They sent up the keeper, Carl Muggleton, so there were 22 bodies in our box and I just knew they were going to score. It seemed inevitable. The corner came over and somehow we managed to knock the ball away...as far as Dalton, just outside our penalty box. He set off, with every other player apart from our keeper, Vince Bartram, in pursuit. And, of course, the hounds on the trail of the fox included Muggleton, once a team-mate of Dalton at Hartlepool.

Dalton wasn't the quickest player in the world but he had a head start and just kept going. A while back, the goal featured on the What Happened Next? feature on the BBC quiz show A Question Of Sport and there on the touchline, running along with Dalton, were me and Wayne Burnett, one of our subs. As soon as Dalton crossed the halfway line, he took aim and fired...and for a few seconds, the world seemed to stand still. But he was bang on target and we'd won 3-1.

The place erupted and I knew from that moment, with absolute certainty, that we would stay up. Yes, there would be hiccoughs along the way and it wouldn't happen overnight. But the team and the club were on the rise, moving in the right direction. The Great Escape had begun and the theme tune from the film became an anthem for the fans.

Dalton went on to produce some of the best individual displays I have seen at that level. In the space of a few weeks he went from Huddersfield reserves to being rated as just about the top player in the division, perhaps second only to Paul Merson, the former England and Arsenal man, who was with Middlesbrough. Dalton's contract was due to expire at the end of the season and maybe that played its part, too. In fact, once I had given him a new contract his form dipped a bit. That can happen...but by the time he signed the new deal he'd done enough to keep us in the division.

Our first away win was at Manchester City, the following Friday night, in my first live Sky match as a manager. Exactly ten years earlier, Town had been beaten 10-1 at Maine Road, not surprisingly the biggest defeat in the club's history, so there was a bit of stick flying around about that before the game. We played really well, won 1-0 and Robbie Edwards, ironically a City fan, scored the goal of the season when he hit a 25-yarder into the top corner at the end of a move featuring 29 passes. It said everything about the spirit that was growing up that we went to a ground where we'd once been humiliated and gave such a good performance.

It was a night to remember. I travelled back from Manchester with Alison and her brother Jonathan and his wife Joanne and we stopped off and had a sandwich and a couple of drinks. Well perhaps more than a couple...even though I'd agreed to do an interview with Yorkshire Television at nine o'clock the following morning. I had one of the biggest hangovers ever and I still can't believe how rough I looked on the telly next day. But after a win like that, it was worth it.

Survival was guaranteed with a 1-0 win over West Brom two weeks before the end of the season and as it happened, a couple of weeks earlier, West Brom had been the opponents for my final professional appearance, a 75-minute 'cameo' (or that's how I remember it anyway) in a reserve match. I'd been saying for a while that I fancied playing one last game around my birthday at the beginning of April and, as luck would have it, my old Chester team-mate Cyrille Regis was West Brom's reserve coach at the time.

We had a shirt printed with Jackson and number six on the back and there was a bit of publicity in the local press. On the day of the match, I said to Ann Hough, the assistant secretary, "How many do you think will turn up?" She said she reckoned around a thousand, 1,500 maximum. I thought she must be joking. But in fact there were nearly 6,000 there. It was unbelievable, such an emotional night.

All my family and neighbours came and I also invited a lot of the people who'd helped me into the professional game. Schoolteachers like Mr Jackson from Greenhead School and some of the other coaches in junior football who'd pushed me. With 15 minutes to go, Terry held aloft a huge board that told number six to come in, his time was up, and as I trudged off the pitch, I kissed the shirt and threw it into the crowd. My competitive career was over.

For our final league match, at home to Port Vale, loads of fans turned up in army uniform to celebrate the Great Escape. It was a game that meant nothing to us but to Port Vale it meant everything. They were two places above the relegation zone, on the same points as Stoke and one ahead of Manchester City. City were away to Stoke so if they won and we beat Port Vale, City would be safe.

Instead we got beat 4-1 and even though City won 5-2, they were relegated along with Stoke. I was bombarded with hate mail from City fans all summer but we didn't send them down. They had 46 games to stay up and couldn't do it. The afternoon was a bit of an anti-climax for everyone at Huddersfield, too. We desperately wanted to end the season with a win but even so, we could all look back on an incredible seven months.

I made two signings in the summer: keeper Nico Vaesen, who played for the Belgian club Eendracht Aalst, and Manchester United winger Ben Thornley. And Chris Beech, a goalscoring midfield player, arrived from Hartlepool in November. Nico had been spotted playing in Belgium by Jeff Lee, our chief scout. He watched him from the stand a couple of times and then paid at the turnstile to have a look at him from behind the goal. The next morning, Jeff said, "I think I've found you a keeper."

We brought Nico over for a trial and signed him straight away. A keeper is judged by his mistakes and Nico couldn't have made a worse start. In his first game, at Bury, he was sent off for handling the ball outside the area. Inevitably, he struggled for a while and Oliver, who had a nickname for all the players, christened him Nico Vaseline. But I believed in Nico and before long, that changed to Nico Velcro…and three years later, he moved to Birmingham for £750,000, ten times what we'd paid for him.

We made a good start and on September 11, eleven months after I took over with Huddersfield rock bottom of Division One, we beat Tranmere 3-2 at Prenton Park to go top of the table. The match was played on a Friday night and was televised live on Sky. What an incredible turnaround! From a nowhere team heading for relegation to leading the race for a place in the Premiership. It was down to a lot of hard work by a lot of people: the board, the players, Terry, reserve coach Terry Dolan and Jeff Lee. And the fans, of course. It's something I have always been immensely proud of. To take over a club at rock bottom and give people the belief to go to the top of the league in such a short time was an immense achievement by us all.

As we drove away from Tranmere, Terry and I were laughing that we'd better enjoy it while it lasted because other clubs were bound to overtake us the following day. But incredibly, all the results went in our favour and, apart from one week when Sunderland knocked us into second place, we stayed on top for six weeks. We stopped the coach on the way home from Tranmere and bought champagne for all the players.

We were due to play Everton in the League Cup the following week so next day I decided to go and watch them play Leeds at Goodison Park. I took Oliver along in my new club Mercedes, parked in the official car park and then we took our seats in the directors' box. Living the dream. A year ago, I'd been playing for Halifax Town and now here I was, manager of the leading side outside the Premier League, sitting in the directors' box at Goodison Park!

A few weeks later, I wanted to watch a player in an Arsenal reserve match at Highbury so I took Alison with me to London. We travelled down on the train, took a taxi to the ground and strolled through the famous marble halls towards the directors' box. It was a sunny afternoon and as I settled down to watch the match, Alison put on her sunglasses…and started to read the book she'd brought along specially for the occasion. Women!

Being a successful manager meant that all of a sudden I was a wanted commodity. People I hardly knew, and sometimes complete strangers, would recognise me and want to talk. If Alison and I were out shopping, people would make a fuss of us. If we went out for a meal, we would be given the best table. For years, once a month on a Saturday night, we'd been going to Bibi's restaurant in Leeds for a meal with friends. You couldn't reserve a table on a Saturday and even though we sometimes turned up at around seven o'clock, they'd be queuing out the doors and it could be half ten before we got sat down.

We'd stand in line, watching the privileged few ease their way to the front of the queue and be shown to a table straight away. Maybe a past or present Leeds United player, maybe a showbiz personality or a prominent local businessman. Of course, Terry was an ex-Leeds player, too, and soon after we took over, I asked him, "Terry, we're going to Bibi's on Saturday night, you don't know anyone there, do you?"

"Sure," he replied, picked up the phone, dialled a Leeds number and asked for Angelo. "OK, you'll be all right on Saturday," he said as he put the phone down again. Sure enough, as soon as the head waiter spotted us as we by-passed the queue, he came over and said, "Good evening, Mr Jackson. Your table is over here!" I thought, "Yeees, made it!" I realised things like this were the trappings of success and that one day, the escalator would stop going upwards. But I was young and happy to enjoy it while it lasted.

Town had reached the top by playing with an energy and passion that reflected the atmosphere right through the club. There were some big sides around us like Sunderland, Wolves, Bolton, Birmingham, West Brom, Norwich and Sheffield United. But we were more than just competing with them, we were top of the league.

However, unlike some of our rivals, Town were never going to have the kind of money to buy players in the £1m bracket; in fact, we were still looking to pick up free transfers in the bargain basement. The only big money I'd been able to spend was the £700,000 on Allison and that had been a one-off that swallowed up virtually all the budget. And without major investment, we would struggle to hold on to our place in the top three or four. We were punching well above our weight.

And then the rumours started…there was a businessman called Barry Rubery, who had built Pace, a micro technology company based in Saltaire on the outskirts of Bradford, into a multi-million pound global giant. There was speculation that Rubery was keen to get his hands on a Football League club and that Huddersfield were ripe for a takeover. And, the whispers added, if Rubery moved in, Peter Jackson would move out and be replaced by a 'big name' manager. Just rumours, just speculation, just whispers but they refused to go away.

I tried not to let them affect me and in mid-November, we beat Bradford City, who had spent a lot of money and were promoted at the end of the season, at the McAlpine. It was a good performance and kept us right up there in the mix. As I was leaving the ground afterwards, a young chap came up to me and said, "When this Rubery chap takes over, he's going to sack you and bring in Steve Bruce. I know because I service his cars." I tried to laugh it off. After all, wasn't I living the dream? In charge of the club I loved and challenging for a place in the Premiership? Why would anyone want to get rid of me? But the rumours, the whispers continued, the speculation grew and our form started to dip. We were still in the top seven or eight but now looking more at a play-off place than automatic promotion. Then finally, on January 2, 1999, Barry Rubery was unveiled as the new owner of Huddersfield Town.

His arrival, 15 months into my time in charge, marked the beginning of the end for me…but also the start of my only experience of what life might be like as a Premiership manager. OK, Town were a Division One club but thanks to Rubery, I started to live the privileged lifestyle of a top-flight manager. On a personal level, it was the use of his private eight-seater Lear Jet for a few days' ski-ing for the family in Courchevel and my birthday treat on his yacht in the South of France.

On a professional level, the plane was available for me and Jeff Lee if we wanted to look at players anywhere in Europe. We'd set off from Leeds Bradford airport at teatime, watch a match in Holland, Norway, Sweden, Denmark or wherever, hop back on board afterwards and be tucked up in bed by midnight…earlier than if we'd driven up the A1 to Sunderland. Barry and I would sometimes meet in top-class restaurants and discuss Town's affairs over a slap-up meal and he would usually order the most expensive bottle of wine on the list, something I'd never aspired to in my life.

At the start of the Rubery era, everything was geared to Town becoming a Premiership club sooner rather than later and he told the media that money would be available for new players. At one of our first meetings, he said I must never go to the papers and tell them we couldn't afford a player we fancied. He said, "If we want a player then he's in our price range."

I tested the water by trying to sign Neil Redfearn from Charlton. In 1997, Redfearn had led Barnsley into the Premier League and done well in the top flight the following year, even though Barnsley were relegated. He'd moved on to Charlton, also a Premier League club, for £1m but hadn't settled in London and was looking to return north. But when the crunch came, the deal never materialised. Then I lined up Ade Akinbiyi, the Bristol City striker, for £1.3m. But Barry said he wasn't worth it, although six months later, Akinbiyi went to Wolves for £3.5m. I started to wonder who was advising Rubery about his transfer policy.

One or two things didn't add up. Before we played Bradford City at Valley Parade in April, we'd drawn three and lost three of our previous six matches. But Rubery was saying that if we won at Bradford he'd pay for the players to go to Turin for the Champions League semi-final second leg between Juventus and Manchester United. We won 3-2, played really well and afterwards all the lads were going mental about the trip to Turin. Then Barry's line changed: only the man of the match could make the trip and in the end, I don't think anyone bothered.

When I arrived at the club the following Monday morning, one of the secretaries came into the office and handed me a fax that Barry had sent to the general office. Anyone in there could have read it, even though I believed the contents were confidential. He said my performance over the previous few weeks had been shocking, asking how I could inspire a team to win at Bradford City, who were heading for promotion, but lose at home to Swindon, who were struggling near the bottom. I realised I was in trouble.

Town finished in tenth position, a disappointment after the way we'd started the season but a big improvement on the year before. We hadn't been able to maintain our flying start but I knew we'd made real progress and I was convinced that with the kind of investment Barry had at his disposal, we had a genuine platform for a serious challenge the following season. That was my feeling when, on May 10, the day after the end of the league season, Terry and I met Town's chief executive Ian Ayre, who became the managing director of Liverpool in 2011. On the agenda were the plans for the 1999-2000 season, investment in new training facilities and generally putting in place the long-term groundwork for a really strong football club. It was a productive meeting.

However, because there was still speculation about my position, there was one thing I needed to know. So as we left the meeting, I turned to Ayre and said, "Can I have a quick word, please? There's still speculation about my future..." I didn't get any further. "We're sacking you in the morning," he said. Just like that. Just as if I'd been an office junior or temporary bar staff. Then he added, "Barry will see you in Leeds tomorrow." I was utterly devastated. I rang Alison straight away and then drove home in a daze. Terry, Terry Dolan and Jeff Lee arrived soon afterwards with a few cans of Stella. I just felt numb. I thought I'd been building myself up for the moment, at the same time hoping it wouldn't happen. But then the job was just swept away from me in one sentence. Everyone, Alison, the kids, the coaching staff, the players, the office staff, knew how much I'd given to that job and how much I cared about them. But because the season was over, a lot of people, particularly the players, weren't even around to say goodbye. Next day I met Rubery and Ayre at the Hilton Hotel in Leeds to sort out a settlement.

The 'big name' manager Rubery had been seeking arrived on May 24. Steve Bruce left Sheffield United on May 17 and was appointed Town manager a week later. He'd been to a couple of our games towards the end of the season, sitting in the directors' box, and I couldn't help but spot him from the touchline. I wasn't happy about that. Over the next few months, he spent an estimated £3m on new players but Town finished eighth at the end of his first season. He left the club in October, 2000, with Town back where they'd been when I'd taken over three years earlier: bottom of the table.

I was bitterly, bitterly disappointed at the way it ended. I never had a problem with Barry as a person. I had my ups and downs with him, of course, but I liked him as a man. I was less happy with some of the people around him and the advice he received. And if I had been given the kind of money Bruce received, would I have done any better? Who can tell?

What I do know is that I didn't let myself or the club down in that first spell as manager. It was a wonderful experience and no one can ever take away so many happy memories. And little did I know that for Peter Jackson and Huddersfield Town, the best was still to come.

8. Highs and lows

For Alison, a new decade also meant a new career, moving from slimline to airline as she exchanged her Rosemary Conley franchises for life as an air stewardess. For Peter, out of work after losing his job at Huddersfield, the wilderness years had begun. "Now I was Peter Jackson, ex-football manager. And to some, the 'ex factor' meant I was no longer flavour of the month."

Alison's Story

"Is there a doctor on board?" I was on a flight from Manchester to Tenerife, a member of the cabin crew working for the JMC airline, part of the Thomas Cook group. A passenger had been taken seriously ill during the flight.

No, there wasn't a doctor on board. But there was a nurse. Me. At first, the passenger said he was feeling breathless so I gave him oxygen and tried to keep him relaxed. But soon he was also complaining of increasingly severe chest pains and I was pretty sure he was having a heart attack. I told the purser, the head of the cabin crew, what was happening and that I didn't think he would survive unless he received hospital treatment as soon as possible. In other words, we would have to divert to the nearest airport.

Diverting and landing an aircraft in an emergency is a massively expensive business for an airline and something a captain will try to avoid if possible. But obviously if it is a matter of life or death, it has to be done. "I'll tell the captain," she said.

The captain came out of the cockpit and walked down the cabin to where I was treating our sick passenger. He took me to one side and said quietly, "You say he's having a heart attack?" he asked.

"Yes."

"Are you sure?"

"Yes."

"If so, I will have to divert the plane, land and have the emergency paramedics waiting on the tarmac. Are you absolutely certain? It's your call, Alison."

No pressure then.

"Yes. We have no other choice. If we go all the way to Tenerife we'll land with a dead body on board."

So the captain radioed ahead and was given a destination. The passenger was strapped upright into his seat to be secure for landing and I went back to my own position in the cabin. That is flight procedure. No one can be allowed to lie in the aisle or across a seat, however ill he may be; a crew member cannot leave his or her landing position, even to look after a sick passenger. That may sound harsh but in the event of a major emergency during landing, the safety of 300 fit passengers has to be more important than one sick passenger and the priorities cannot be changed.

We made our unscheduled landing at the nearest available airport in France, don't ask me where, and the paramedics were waiting. The sick passenger and his wife left the plane. He had indeed suffered a heart attack and was treated on the spot before being taken to hospital. He survived.

I'd joined JMC two years after Peter had been sacked by Huddersfield in 1999, also the year my father died. For a while, Peter and I were both pretty low and our reaction was to go on loads of holidays. If the kids were off school, we'd all go along; if not, our next door neighbour Rachel, who lived on the other side from Pam and Fergie, moved in and stayed with them.

But you can have too much of anything, I suppose, and one day, soon after returning from one of our trips, I was sitting on the step at the back of the house, having yet another look at Peter's pride and joy of a garden. He was driving me mad at home. When he's not working, he's an absolute pain to live with, horrendous! He was totally bored and moaning all the time. "All I've ever known is football so I can't do anything else." And I suddenly thought, "God, this is boring! Too many holidays, too much time doing nothing. Time for a new job."

I started scouring the jobs pages in the local papers and soon spotted an advert for the manager of the Clarins fragrance counter in Harvey's department store in Halifax. I had no experience as a beautician or of working in a shop but thought, "Yes, I can do that, no problem." So I applied, went for an interview and told my interviewer everything she wanted to hear. I'd been to enough interviews before to know what to expect and I sold myself as a manager, assuring her that once I'd received the training, I wouldn't have a problem working as a beautician or in selling the products. A week later I was away on another course, this time at Clarins House in London, just behind Oxford Street.

It was a one-week residential course in which I learned all about the products, specific sales techniques and, of course, how to do facials, make-up and body treatments. By the time the course ended, I knew all about persuading clients that buying just one product was no good, they should also have another two products to complement it and then, in the long-term, perhaps three more to complete the treatment. In fairness, they were beautiful and I still use Clarins to this day.

There were two of us in the department, myself as manager and Sharon, a twin, who was my assistant. She would be around 20. I'd never worked the nine to five routine before and after operating for so long on my own initiative, it was a massive culture shock. Harvey's was, and still is, a family-run department store with traditional values and the owners were very hands-on. All the staff knew one another and it seemed most of them had worked in the store for years and years. It felt a bit like working for Grace Brothers in the old television series, Are You Being Served?

I was the new kid on the block but it didn't take long for me to get to know the other members of staff, first on the beauty floor and then throughout the store. We all had to get changed in a little locker room on the top floor and there was a staff room alongside where people ate their lunch. I never ate there. Instead, I either met Peter or my friend Christine for lunch in town or just wandered about for an hour. Members of staff weren't allowed to use the store restaurant even if they were with friends or family.

I soon noticed that while everybody seemed to enjoy their job once they got started, most of them would arrive for work moaning or complaining about some aspect of the job or the prospects for the day ahead. At first, I used to think, "Well, if it's that bad, find something else that you enjoy." That had always been my philosophy. But I soon realised that the complaints were more of a ritual than anything else, the automatic response if anything went slightly wrong. And the most minor incident, like a till roll breaking or a couple of pence missing when we cashed up, would become a major trauma. After once working in the life or death atmosphere of a cancer ward, I just could not believe how people could become so heated about nothing.

I went straight in at the deep end, doing facials on my first morning, and I quickly found a sales routine that seemed to work pretty well. Sales figures were certainly good. But without wishing to sound unkind, because of the day-to-day routine, it was probably the most boring job I have ever done and inevitably it was pretty short-lived, less than a year.

My escape route came early in 2002 while I was having a chat with Sharon during a quiet spell in the department. She was telling me that her twin sister was working as an air stewardess and straight away, I thought, "That's it! That's the next job for me." I began writing letters to all sorts of airlines and before long, had an interview with JMC in Manchester. I was offered a job…provided I came through their six-week training programme.

It was a tough six weeks, based at Manchester Airport. We stayed in a hotel overnight although we had weekends off so I was able get home for a couple of days' rest. People seem to think that airline cabin crew have a doddle of a job, that they are just there to serve the drinks and pander to the whims of the passengers. But that is the smallest, least significant part of the job. OK, we have to know how to organise the cabin service on each flight but the bottom line is that the crew are there purely and simply to ensure the safety of the passengers. That was what the training was about; not how to serve a glass of wine with a smile and without spilling it in the passenger's lap. After six weeks, it was pass or fail and anyone who did not come up to scratch was not given a second chance.

I was going to fly on two different aircraft, the Airbus 320 and Boeing 757, and I had to prove that I was absolutely up to speed with all the emergency procedures and safety drills and to know where every single piece of essential equipment was situated on both aircraft. In an emergency everything has to happen quickly and efficiently with not a split second wasted and the last thing you need is a member of the cabin crew who doesn't know automatically where a vital piece of equipment is stored.

To learn about emergency landings on water, we would spend whole days in a swimming pool, learning how to inflate a life raft or dinghy, how to drag all the occupants on board and how to keep them calm until rescue arrived. Or we'd be in a mock-up cockpit going through the fire emergency procedures, wearing a smoke mask with visibility down to nil; it was claustrophobic and not easy to stay calm even though we knew it was only a trial. Some of the trainees would panic and the rest of us had to calm them down, just as we would calm down passengers in a real emergency. We were taught how to use escape chutes and to help other people, pushing them through the door and down the chute as fast as possible. I've never had a head for heights so standing at the top of the chute and throwing myself down was a tough one. And, of course, we had to learn how to give the safety demonstration before take-off.

I've flown a lot since leaving JMC in 2004 and I always, always watch the safety demo intently…and not just out of respect to the crew. The people who can't be bothered to listen are the ones who panic most if there happens to be an emergency. I never presume that I will know what to do just because I once worked as cabin crew. It is vital that passengers take time to watch and listen to pre-condition their brain to know what they will have to do in an emergency.

I make sure that I know exactly where the fire doors are and which one is most appropriate for me, exactly where my life jacket is, exactly how my oxygen mask will work and remind myself what to do it if it doesn't drop automatically. I never store baggage underneath the seat in front because it can hinder my escape from my seat. I always use the overhead locker. My seatbelt is always fastened tightly across my hips, I remember the brace position properly and I'm always conscious on take-off and landing that both feet are together and firmly on the floor. Simple precautions but they could save my life.

I only flew to European destinations but I don't think I ever worked with exactly the same people two days running. That was so refreshing after life in a department store, when I worked alongside the same people, moaning and groaning about the job, day in and day out. We were a team of nine: captain, co-pilot, purser and six crew. And even though the potential risks were high, it was probably the least stressful job I have ever done in my life because it was so enjoyable.

We all got on so well together and had such a laugh, both with the passengers and among ourselves. Sometimes, it was like working on a light entertainment programme. The one physically hard thing about the job was the sheer wear and tear on my feet because I would be standing on them for most of a 15-hour day. At the time, I was driving a BMW convertible automatic so on the drive back from Manchester to Brighouse I just used to switch on cruise control and let the car do the rest. I could hardly bear to put my feet on the pedals because they ached so much.

We did three flights a week although we were also on 90-minute standby if a problem arose. We had to report 90 minutes before the departure time and there would be a half-hour briefing in which we'd be reminded of the secret emergency codes. On every flight the captain has pre-arranged sentences to alert the crew to a potential emergency without alarming the passengers. When the crew hear those words, they go to their stations and await instructions. There are different codes for each emergency: a possible landing on water, the landing gear not coming down, missing the runway and even a disruptive passenger in the cabin. I can't honestly recall what the codes were…and even if I could I wouldn't repeat them now. Imagine the panic on a flight if the passengers knew in advance what the emergency codes might be!

At the briefing, the purser would also ask if any of us had any particular skills and I would always say I was a qualified nurse. So if any other crew members had to deal with a medical problem they would call me. We had oxygen on board and all aircraft were equipped with a defibrillator because at 36,000 feet, any crisis would be a life or death situation and we would need the best equipment.

Thankfully, I was never involved in a major emergency but I did have a couple of really rough landings and once, when we hit a patch of turbulence, one of the crew broke her leg when she couldn't lock the wheels of her trolley in time and it rolled forward out of control. I was working at the other end of the cabin at the time but there was a doctor on board and I helped him put her leg in a splint. She then lay on the back seat until it was time to prepare for landing.

The flights were not always straightforward. Sometimes, if there had been delays or technical hitches elsewhere, we would have to fly an empty aircraft to another airport to start a journey. Once we flew over to Cork to collect the Munsters, a travelling army of Irish Rugby Union supporters who had chartered a flight to go and watch Munster play in France. Once they were all in their seats, they started to unfurl a massive Munster flag from the front of the cabin. The idea was to roll the flag right out to the back of the cabin before take-off but that had to be kicked into touch straight away. We flew them to France, off they went to watch the match, no doubt unfurling the flag at the stadium, and then we flew them back to Cork that night. I've no idea whether they won or lost.

I was almost always the oldest member of crew so on Friday night flights to Majorca, Ibiza or Tenerife, I would be stationed at the back of the cabin, where the rowdiest passengers were likely to be. People with mobility problems would be seated at the front, then families, then older people and so on until the lads or lasses heading off for a stag or hen weekend would be right at the back. Even before our cabin stations were announced during the briefing, I knew with absolute certainty that on those flights, I would be stationed at the back. "Alison can sort them out," was the thinking.

The kids would usually have been drinking in the departure lounge and they'd be shouting, swearing and generally making a nuisance of themselves. Sometimes there would be youngsters who'd never been on a flight before and when we took the food round, they'd press their buzzer and shout, "I haven't got an effing table."

"Yes you have," I'd reply, and patiently show them how to pull the table down from the back of the seat in front.

Sometimes, one or two of the lads would start making offensive remarks to the younger girls in the crew and that was the signal for Alison to go on to the attack. On one occasion, one of the girls ended up in tears and asked me to help. I marched down the cabin and stood in front of the lads, hands on hips like a headmistress. "Right," I said, "I want each of you to hand me your passports this minute. Unless you apologise to the stewardess you have insulted, they will be confiscated by the captain.

"If you don't behave yourselves on the rest of the flight, he will keep them, you will not be allowed into the country and this airline will refuse to fly you home or ever again in the future." That would usually nip any trouble in the bud and before long, one of the ringleaders would come down the cabin and, ever so meekly, apologise and plead for their passports back. I would hand them over with a severe expression and a dire warning about their behaviour on the rest of the flight. We rarely had any trouble on the return journey, mainly because they would stagger on board looking as white as a sheet, ask for bottles of water, fall asleep and be dead to the world until we landed.

At the end of every flight, when all the passengers had left the aircraft, we had to carry out a security check for anything that may have been left behind. First and foremost we were looking for bombs but also for personal belongings like wallets, glasses, passports, tickets. You would be amazed at the things people forget. We had to lift everything off the seats, blankets, pillows and so on, and also check under the seats and in the overhead lockers. It was a routine business that became second nature before we headed off to the crew room to complete all the in-flight admin.

One night we landed in Manchester after a very late flight from Spain. It was absolutely pouring down and for some reason, the air bridge into the terminal wasn't working so the passengers had to disembark down a gangway on to the tarmac. As luck would have it, we'd had on board what must have been the original family from hell; well Liverpool, actually. The party should have been a couple, the wife's father and about six children of all ages but the husband had been barred from boarding the plane because he was too drunk. They were brash, rowdy, argumentative and to make matters worse, the grandfather also suffered from incontinence problems.

So we all breathed a sigh of relief as they headed down the gangway and we began the security check. When we reached their seats, I lifted up a blanket and there, underneath, was a little toddler, fast asleep. He must have been over two because he was wearing his own seat belt…but only just. I thought, "This can't be possible," picked up the toddler, who was starting to wake up, and promised I'd find his mum. I was just asking another crew member how anyone could leave a baby on board when she picked up a blanket from the row in front to reveal a little five-year-old, also fast asleep. We assumed he would be frightened at being woken by a stranger in a funny uniform but he just gave us a knowing look as if to say, "Don't worry, it's happened before and it will happen again."

Mother and children were soon reunited in passport control although I don't recall her being shocked, ashamed or embarrassed. Or, for that matter, eternally grateful. We were just glad we'd carried out a thorough security check or the kids would have been locked on board all night.

The other crew members were great. The purser would usually be around my age but all the rest were much younger. Even so, they never seemed to regard me as a mother figure or agony aunt. I was just accepted as one of the team and I'd always be invited when they had a party. They worked hard and partied hard and needless to say most of them had a few tales to tell about their love lives; some of the lads were gay and they seemed to live a very colourful existence. But I took most of it with a pinch of salt. After all, we've all been young, haven't we?

I stayed with JMC for two years and would probably have worked there for longer if they hadn't ask me to switch to long haul. That would have been a completely different kettle of fish and simply would not have worked. Having to spend four or five nights a week jetting off to some exotic corner of the world might sound like the perfect job…but not for a wife with two kids and a husband at home. And from a professional point of view, while spending a ten-hour day with a young crew was a lot of fun, five days on end would have been a different story. Would I have wanted to spend a whole week with a group of people half my age? No. It was time for a change.

Peter's Story

Gradually the phone stopped ringing. At first, it seemed everyone wanted to commiserate or sympathise about being sacked by Huddersfield but after a while, my calls weren't returned any more and so-called mates didn't want to know me. They wanted to be associated with people who were doing well, people whose names were in the papers or on the television, people who were popular.

I was still the same man, being out of the public eye didn't all of a sudden make me a worse person…but that's football. It's a world full of hangers-on who pretend to be friends. Alison had always been grounded about it, warning me that the good life would eventually come to an end and then my 'friends' wouldn't be there for me any more. I knew it was true. But that didn't make it any easier to handle when it happened.

The first few days are still a bit of a blur. Alison, Charlotte and Oliver were going on a family holiday to Majorca with her brother Paul and their kids. Her mum was supposed to be going as well but she was taken ill at the last minute so I went instead. One or two holidaymakers recognised me and wanted to talk but it was all pretty low-key and I was thankful for that. Funnily enough, I've always found that football rears its head in the most unlikely places when we're on holiday. Hardly anybody seems to notice us in Majorca or on the Algarve but once, Alison and I went to a barbecue in Fiji and all sorts of people wanted an autograph and tried to talk football all night!

There was a bit of money from Huddersfield although, as my contract didn't have long to run, it wasn't a fortune. But that wasn't really a worry because I was confident I would get back in pretty quickly. And sure enough, almost straight away, I had a call from Halifax Town chairman Doug Tate. Halifax had parted company with George Mulhall after finishing tenth in Division Three and wanted me to take over. If I'd let my heart rule my head, I would have jumped at the chance because I'd been so happy there as a player two years earlier.

But I saw myself as a First Division manager, a man who'd taken over a struggling club and done really well. I was sure something bigger than Halifax would be just around the corner. If I'd known then what would happen in the next four years, I would have probably said yes and hopefully lifted Halifax out of the bottom flight. But instead, I chose to wait.

Over the next few months I was linked in the media with one or two clubs, including, ironically, Sheffield United, the club Steve Bruce left before succeeding me at Huddersfield. And I applied for the jobs at Blackpool, when Nigel Worthington left at the end of 1999, and Bristol City, when Tony Fawthrop departed at the end of the 1999-2000 season, soon after succeeding Tony Pulis. I had interviews at both clubs, meeting Blackpool chairman Karl Oyston at the Tickled Trout hotel near Preston, and the Bristol directors in a hotel room in the city.

My interview at Huddersfield had been a pretty informal affair as we all knew one another but these two were quite daunting because, apart from my record as a manager, they didn't know much about me or my personality. I would have an hour or so to convince them I was the man for the job, which was a lot to do in a short time. I'd no idea who else was in the running for either job, although as I was walking in for my interview with Oyston, Steve Thompson, the former Lincoln, Southend and Sheffield United manager, was walking out. It was a bit embarrassing for us both. In the end, Blackpool opted for Steve McMahon and Bristol chose Danny Wilson. I've no idea how close I was but before long my name stopped being mentioned when a managerial vacancy arose and the self-doubts began.

In a year, I'd gone from figurehead to also ran, from being in the public eye and working virtually all day, every day to being out of work. It was just so frustrating because I knew I could do the job that had been taken away from me. I'd done it once and I could do it again, if only someone would give me a chance. And in those circumstances, it was easy to lose self-respect and allow the despair to kick in.

There were times when I was very low. I've always tended to keep things to myself and it takes a lot for me to open up to anybody. So I never really told even Alison how lonely I was feeling, particularly after she started working as an air stewardess. She was away a lot of the time, the kids were at school and I was at home, on my own with nowhere to go, nothing to do. Sometimes I used to sit on the steps leading on to the patio at the back of the house and just cry. Of course, there were people a lot worse off than me – and I would be in a far darker place in 2008 when I was diagnosed with cancer – but they were bad days.

I don't really know how I would have coped if Hayden Evans, owner of the HN Sports Agency, had not come along. I'd first had contact with Hayden early in my time at Huddersfield because he was Wayne Allison's agent and acted for The Chief when he moved to Huddersfield in 1997. The agency was based in state-of-the-art offices in the grounds of Harewood House, the stately home halfway between Leeds and Harrogate. Hayden was a good boss and it was a good business. We had over 100 clients and it was one of the top agencies in the country at the time. Joining HN Sports gave me something to get up for in a morning and helped me back into football.

The job was only part-time at first and Hayden was happy for me to work from home. But it gave me an opportunity to start going to matches again and talking with players and managers. It opened my eyes to a different side of the game. For the best part of two years, I'd been a manager, now I was one of the dreaded football agents! It was a complete about-turn. Whereas before I'd been negotiating with agents to sign players within my club's wage structure, now I was the agent trying to get the best deal for my players.

Back then a lot of players still used to negotiate their own transfers whereas these days, just about every transfer involves an agent. He's part of a negotiating group that also includes the selling club, the buying club, the buying manager and the player. Nowadays a transfer at the top end of the market operates on an even higher level because the bigger clubs all have a chief executive in overall control and sometimes a director of football as well. A manager will tell his chief exec which player he wants and then it's down to the chief exec to sort out the fee, the terms and the contract and tie up a deal. But at the start of the new millennium, not every player had a representative and competition between agencies to sign up good young players was pretty intense. Hayden probably saw my experience as a manager as a useful bargaining tool with potential clients.

David Batty, Gary Speed and Simon Grayson, who were or had been Leeds United players, were the three biggest names on our books alongside another half dozen or so top-flight players. And I soon found out that dealing with top players like that was rarely a problem. They were playing regularly at first team level, weren't looking to get away and it was just a case of keeping the relationship ticking over, making sure they had everything they needed.

It was the lesser players and the ones who weren't involved every week who provided all the hard work. They seemed to assume that an agent was also a miracle worker, that he could just click his fingers and organise a move that would guarantee first team football, usually at a higher level. The phone would ring and the player would say, "I've been dropped, I want a move." Or "I'm fed up of playing in the reserves, can you find me another club?" Or maybe, "Can you have a word with the manager and find out what's going on?"

I'd reply, "How can I get you a move when you're not even playing in the first team? Why have you been dropped? Take a long, hard look at yourself. You earn yourself a move by playing first team football and when that happens I'll see what I can do." It wasn't what they wanted to hear, of course, because you won't find too many footballers who admit they deserve to be dropped. But it was a forthright, up front answer. Players at all levels were, and still are, pampered too much. Instead of getting on and doing things for themselves, they expect agents to be all things to all players. "Can you bring me a new pair of boots over?" was a regular request.

One player in the reserves at Newcastle rang me straight after the end of one season. He was one for the future so we needed to keep him on board but even so this was one request too far. "Peter," he said. "I'm supposed to be going away to America with the girlfriend on Friday but we've just split up. Can you get me a doctor's note to say I've got a bad back and can't fly?"

I went to a lot of games and my prime responsibility was to identify young players with potential, talk to them and try to persuade them to join our agency. A young player can make an agency a lot of money if he makes the grade and gets a big money move. But the jewels were few and far between and for every ten players we signed up, one, perhaps two, would make money for the agency through a transfer. Others might make a bit with a boot deal or some other kind of sponsorship. The secret was spotting the young ones who might go on and make it big.

As time went by and I hadn't got back into management, I took more of a hands-on role, working more or less full-time alongside other agents in Hayden's team like Ian Baird, Imre Varadi and John Pearson, who had all played a lot of league football. It was hard work but when I finally went back into management I knew from first-hand experience where the agents were coming from.

I spoke to managers on a regular basis, asking if they might be interested in signing one of our players or taking him on loan. Or sometimes a manager would call me and say he wanted to get a player off his wage bill and could I find him a club.

Managers are renowned for not calling agents back but they were more inclined to accept a call from me because I'd been a manager myself. And similarly, when I became a manager again, I always tried to answer an agent's call because I'd worked on their side of the fence, too. I knew from personal experience that it was a difficult job and a hard way to make a living.

Working for Hayden was an important part of the learning curve for me and I also picked up a new skill in the media as a radio summariser, travelling up and down the country to grounds where once I had played or managed. Instead of giving Press conferences, I was working alongside the media, seeing how the job looked from their side of the fence. I'd always been pretty comfortable with the Press as a player and manager but I had a few misgivings at first about the reception I would receive. I needn't have worried, everybody was fine.

Mostly I worked for The Pulse, a local radio station covering West Yorkshire. At the start of the 1999-2000 season, they asked if I fancied covering Bradford City's matches, home and away. City had just been promoted to the Premiership, I was a Bradford lad and an ex-City player so I jumped at the chance to be involved in what was an exciting time for the club. The money wasn't brilliant but it was good to get out and watch Premier League football and instead of shouting and bawling on the touchline, trying to give a more considered view from the commentary box.

Home or away, commentator Chris Cooper and I would be at the ground at around half past twelve on a Saturday to set up all the equipment. We'd go on air at two o'clock for the pre-match discussion, cover the match and do an hour's phone-in afterwards. I also went to the managers' press conferences with Chris and then afterwards we'd discuss their verdicts.

It's easy for an ex-manager to feel a bit of an outcast in that kind of situation but most of the managers would give me a nod or come over and say hello afterwards. Some went further. Once, standing outside Leicester City's old Filbert Street stadium, I was spotted by Martin O'Neill, Leicester's manager at the time. He came straight over, asked how I was doing and invited me into his office for a coffee. That was a nice touch. He also said I could go down to his office for a drink when I'd finished but I didn't want to keep Chris waiting.

I tried to be as objective as I could in my comments and give listeners a professional insight about what was going on tactically and how the managers might be thinking. A lot of pundits and summarisers are frustrated football managers themselves, ex-players who have wanted to go into management at some stage but never made it. Similarly a lot of the high profile television pundits have never been a manager. So while they know about football, they don't know about management from the inside, how the job works and the pressures involved.

However, I knew what the men on the touchline were experiencing and how, for better or worse, one decision could alter the course of a match. And I tried to get across how managers might have reached those decisions. If I'm totally honest, there were times when I tempered my criticism because I knew what the managers were going through. And, of course, I also wanted to get back into management myself and I knew that it wouldn't do me any good if I became known as someone who ranted and raved about the men in a job. I didn't want to burn any bridges. So, rightly or wrongly, it was always a bit of a balancing act.

Then on Christmas Eve, 2001, the chance to return to management finally came along. With Bradford City, my hometown club. They had been relegated from the Premiership at the end of the previous season and had just parted company with Jim Jefferies after 13 months in charge. Out of the blue, I received a call from Geoffrey Richmond, the Bradford chairman. Richmond had been the driving force in taking City into the Premier League from the old Second Division and transforming Valley Parade into a top-class stadium. He'd hired and fired six managers in seven years and there were people in the game who didn't have a good word to say about him. But I'd never had a problem.

He called me at HN Sports and invited me round to his home in Shadwell, on the outskirts of Leeds. We had a long chat and on the face of it, I was being offered the perfect opportunity, the job I'd been waiting for. I agreed to call Richmond with my decision on Christmas Day but even as I drove away from his house, I had reservations. For some reason, it just didn't feel the right move at the right time.

I'd left Huddersfield nearly two years earlier but during my time as manager, relations between the two clubs and their supporters had not been good. In February, 1997, before I took over, City striker Gordon Watson suffered a broken leg in a challenge from Town defender Kevin Gray and sued Gray for negligence. Watson was eventually awarded substantial damages and there had been bad feeling between the two sets of supporters ever since. And as Huddersfield manager, I was always seen as the villain by Bradford fans when we played at Valley Parade. I was the man who'd left City to play for and then manage their closest rivals. Would the hostility from my time as a Huddersfield player and manager still be a bit raw? Would everybody at the club, especially the fans, be behind me, particularly if things didn't work out at first?

On a more personal level, Charlotte and Oliver went to schools more or less halfway between Huddersfield and Bradford. Most of their schoolmates supported Huddersfield but a lot of the others followed Bradford and both the kids were on the receiving end because I was the Town manager. Around six weeks before Huddersfield were due to play Bradford, they would start to come home and say, "Dad, you can't lose this one, you really can't." And as the match got nearer, it would become more intense. "Dad, they're going to do this or that to me if Town don't win."

Not losing to Bradford became a huge issue for them and within the family. The way that tension can build up in the household of a football manager is obviously a side of the job people don't see. But I used to feel physically sick as I walked to the dugout knowing the kind of pressure the kids would be under if we lost. Thankfully we won two of my three games against City in my first spell as Town manager…and drew the other.

All these things were nagging away as I drove away from Richmond's house that Christmas Eve. I talked it over with Alison who said that it had to be my decision. And my first thought when I woke up on Christmas morning was that it still didn't feel right. It was a gut feeling. So I called Richmond before we even opened the presents and told him I was turning down his offer. He wasn't happy. Nicky Law was given the job instead and I carried on working for HN Sports, convinced I had made the right decision, even though it would be another 18 months before I finally returned to management.

Meanwhile Huddersfield were sinking fast. Everything happened so quickly: in September, 1998 they were top of the old First Division; in May, 2003, I was in the commentary box when a draw against Charlton condemned them to relegation into the bottom tier. It was desperately sad to see the club decline, decline and keep declining.

The following week, I had a call from Terry Fisher, the former chairman who had presided over Neil Warnock's successful promotion campaign in 1995. He told me the club was in grave danger of going under and he was involved in takeover talks. Would I be interested in going back as manager? He didn't have to ask twice. I packed up my job at HN Sports and worked unofficially without pay or any kind of security, talking to a few players totally off the record, telling them I was going back to Huddersfield. Would they be interested in playing for me?

Then right at the last minute, there was a hitch, Terry pulled out of the deal and Huddersfield Town were 24 hours away from going out of business. Enter Ken Davy, owner of Huddersfield Giants Rugby League club, who shared the stadium with Town. He was taking charge of both clubs and yes, he wanted me to go back as manager. At the Press Conference to announce the appointment, one of the journalists told me straight that I must be mad. I thought, "You know what, you're probably right." But so what? I never questioned my decision for a second, never doubted my ability to turn the club round. This was my dream job and I just couldn't wait to get started.

9. Fast cars and the fast lane

After living the high life for two years, it's back down to earth and a switch to four wheels for Alison. For Peter, on his return to Huddersfield Town in June, 2003, it's time to shoot for the stars, even though the portents are not good. "We had eight registered professionals, no coaches, no physio, no pre-season programme, no sponsorship, no season ticket sales...and as far as outsiders were concerned, no future."

Alison's Story

From my first day training as a nurse back in 1974, I was convinced that I would never spend my working life sitting at a telephone switchboard. Simply not my scene, I'm afraid. But it just shows how wrong you can be. And how was I to know when I started my stint as a part-time receptionist at the Appleyard Jaguar dealership in Bradford that I was on my way to yet another career swerve? This time into the world of corporate car sales.

It all began at the end of 2004. Peter was back in charge at Huddersfield by this time, I'd given up the high life with JMC and our daughter Charlotte was studying for a degree in television production and media studies at Huddersfield University. She was also earning some money as a weekend receptionist at Appleyard and one day came home and said, "Mum, the weekday receptionist is going on maternity leave and they're absolutely desperate..." She didn't get any further.

"No chance, Charlotte! I could never learn how to operate some great big switchboard."

"But mum, can't you just come and help out until they find someone else?"

"No."

As it happened, I hadn't worked for a couple of weeks and was starting to wonder what I might do next. Should I go back on the airlines after all? Should I find something completely different? If so, what? I needed a bit of time to think it all over, so I relented. "OK, but only on a temporary basis until everything is sorted out. Maybe a couple of weeks. No more."

"Thanks Mum. You'll be all right, it's really easy."

It was not easy. The switchboard looked more like the pilot's controls in the cockpit of a Boeing 757 than a (part-time) office receptionist's work station. There were dials, knobs, switches, buttons, electric leads, all the paraphernalia that meant I could, theoretically, connect callers to every office or workshop extension in the building. Easy? For an 18-year-old student, maybe. For me, it was totally daunting and within half an hour of clocking in, I was thinking, "Right, it's back to the airlines for you, Alison!" But I don't give up that easily.

The motor trade is a close-knit community and as my brothers Mark and Jonathan and my sister Lizzy worked in car sales, people knew who I was and I fitted in quite easily on a personal level. That helped me get away with putting calls through to the managing director's office instead of the service department or vice versa. And in fairness to Charlotte, operating the switchboard turned out to be pretty straightforward after all; just a question of getting used to it. Before long, it became second nature.

As well as handling all the telephone calls, I was also dealing face-to-face with our walk-in customers…and talking to a person rather than a voice on the other end of a phone was much more my line. I enjoyed being in the environment of car sales, so much so that before long, I decided that while life as a receptionist was never going to be for me, actually selling cars just might be.

So if a customer came in and there wasn't a salesman immediately available, I'd step in, show him the cars, hand out the brochures and take all his details. Or if someone was hanging about in the waiting room while his car was in the workshop, I'd make time to have a chat. He'd usually be thumbing through a brochure anyway so I'd wander over and ask when his car was due for renewal, had he looked at the new models and did he know he could finance a brand new car for the same kind of money as he was paying now?

The sales manager, Phil Norfolk, was not impressed by what I saw as using my initiative. "Alison," he'd say. "Selling cars is not your job. Stick to being a receptionist and leave it to the professionals." I didn't take the slightest notice and carried on as before. I knew there would be more to being a full-time salesperson than just chatting up customers, not least acquiring expert technical knowledge about the cars, but it wasn't long before I was thinking very seriously about moving in that direction. But how to make the switch? I knew Phil would be hostile to the idea of me invading his territory. He was more of an old-fashioned type of car salesman, a real man's man who didn't seem to think women had a place in car sales. And I suspect he also thought that because of Peter's football, I wouldn't want to work weekends. So he was never going to agree to me moving into his team.

However the dealer principal, a guy called John Fickling, was more sympathetic and I sensed that he might be prepared to give me a chance. John, who had worked with my brother Mark before joining Jaguar, had also spotted the potential in my brother Jonathan and later our son Oliver went to work for him in an apprenticeship. He has since worked for Volkswagen in Leeds and Mini and BMW in Bradford, where he is now business sales manager. All the sales people John has nurtured have gone on to do well. As it happened, the corporate sales manager, a lovely man called Mike Smith, was not far away from retirement and John asked if I fancied moving into corporate sales and learning the ropes from Mike. He said it would be a

Monday to Friday job so it would fit in well with Peter's football and the family. Would I like to give it a go? Too right I would!

Until I walked into that job, I knew nothing about cars and even less about computers. I didn't even know how to switch a computer on. So I had to learn fast on both fronts. I went on a corporate management training course in Reading, which gave me a basic grounding, and I picked up a lot of knowledge as I went along. I was working in an environment where my colleagues were talking about Jaguars for most of the working day and while I might not have known how a particular engine actually worked, I knew what it was capable of and what its advantages would be. And I was, after all, working only with Jaguars. I could imagine how difficult it must be for a general used car salesman who had to learn about all the various makes and models of cars he might be dealing with.

It was the first time I had worked in an almost entirely male environment so I also had to learn to handle the jokes and the innuendo. It was pretty sexist stuff sometimes but basically innocent, friendly banter and water off a duck's back. No one could work in the motor industry if they took offence to that kind of thing and I soon had a stock of one-liners to give back. I never saw it as a problem.

Everybody knew Mike Smith as Mr Jaguar. He'd been with the company for over twenty years and seemed to have contacts with every business, large or small, in the city. What he didn't know about Jaguar cars wasn't worth knowing either and he was more than happy to pass on the technical information. It seemed as if I was being groomed to step into his shoes and my time as a corporate sales consultant would be used to prepare me for the step up. So I shadowed Mike, going to events like corporate golf days or black tie sportsmen's dinners where I would often be the only woman present. But both were the perfect opportunity to talk to businessmen about Jaguar cars.

My job also involved cold calling local businesses, large and small, and explaining the advantages of buying their company car fleet from Jaguar. "How many company cars do you have? What range of cars is involved? How are they funded? Do you know you could have so many cars for so much funding?" I approached people who had perhaps always seen Jaguar as a very elite marque and not suitable for company cars. So it was down to me to convince them otherwise. I had to put myself out there, get my name known, stay in touch regularly with potential customers and then, hopefully, when the time came for a change of company cars, they would come to Jaguar.

And when it came to agreeing a deal, there was absolutely no room for error. For example, a business might order six company cars, each one a different model with a particular specification…and there could be anything up to sixty different specs. If a car with the wrong spec arrived on the forecourt, the company had the right to cancel the order and Appleyard would be thousands of pounds out of pocket.

I took over from Mike when he was appointed brand manager in June, 2004. In around six months, I'd moved from part-time receptionist to corporate sales manager and I ran the operation for the next eight months. I had to sell my BMW convertible, which was a blow, and instead started driving a top-of-the-range Jaguar, cleaned and valeted every day, which wasn't a blow! And there were more training courses down in Reading. Whenever I set off on another course, I'd ask myself, "Why are you doing this? Why are you punishing yourself?" But I'd just get on and do it anyway because I enjoyed the work so much.

Peter was driving a Range Rover at the time and I did my best to persuade him to have a Jaguar instead. The Range Rover wasn't a company car as such but he had an allowance from Huddersfield Town to buy the car of his choice. He loved his Range Rovers and although I tried very hard to convince him a Jag would be a better bet, he wasn't having it.

I didn't have any success either when I tried to convince Huddersfield's former owner Barry Rubery that the thing he most wanted in the world was the brand new XJR, Jaguar's first aluminium model. Jaguar had an incentive scheme for sales personnel and there was a bonus for anyone who could arrange a genuine test drive with a client who was seriously considering the car. I hadn't spoken to Barry since he'd jokingly promised me his first diamond but he came along, had a test drive and said he liked the car. But in the end, decided against it. No diamond, no Jaguar. Can't win 'em all, I suppose.

But I had better luck with one of Richard Branson's right hand men at Virgin Atlantic. He wanted a brand new XJR in black and we were one of the few dealerships who had the car in stock. He insisted that there must be no miles on the clock so instead of driving it down to the nearest showroom to his office near Gatwick Airport, I arranged for it to be delivered on a transporter and flew down to Gatwick to complete the deal. The dealership was on his doorstep so I checked that the car had been valeted and was absolutely immaculate and then presented myself at the Virgin HQ.

He came into reception straight away. He was about 6ft 7in tall and was clearly in no mood for small talk. "Morning, Alison," he said. "Where's the car then?" I explained that it was waiting for him at the showroom down the road. "Right, let's go," and he bounded out of the door, taking giant strides towards his new car with me teetering along behind in my little suit and high heels. We dealt with the paperwork and then I told him we had to complete the handover with a full check of all the controls and their functions. That's a legal requirement so that if someone drives a new car away and ploughs into a brick wall, he can't complain he hasn't been told how to drive the car.

He wasn't having any of that. "What do you mean?" he asked. "Look, I've got a Ferrari, a Porsche and a Bentley at home in Brighton and this is just going to be a comfy car for the journey to work and back. So forget all these knobs and dials. I'll take you out for lunch instead and find out about the controls on the way. What time's your flight back?" So off we went. He was a really nice gentleman in his fifties, he wasn't trying to chat me up, we had lunch at a pub nearby, talked about our families and then he dropped me off at departures for the flight back. "That can be classed as your test drive," I said, as I closed the passenger door.

That first year at Jaguar was a really rewarding time and I felt sure that I was in there for the long haul. Then on Valentine's Day, 2005, I received the call at ten to eleven in the morning from Halifax General Hospital. Mum, who had been admitted three days earlier, was not looking too good and could I get there as soon as possible. I dropped everything, ran out of the showroom and rushed to the hospital. I was a couple of minutes late. All five kids arrived within twenty minutes of one another.

She had been a diabetic since the age of 45. She lived on her own in a five-bedroomed house and would never have considered leaving. We'd moved everything downstairs so that she could live on one floor because she was very breathless, had heart problems and her legs were badly ulcerated. Until a short time before, she'd lived an active life with her own group of friends with whom she went on holiday. She was out and about just about every day and always looked immaculate. She was a really bubbly person and was so proud that we had all done so well. Everybody loved her.

But over the past few months, her health had deteriorated, her eyesight was failing because of the diabetes and she couldn't enjoy the kind of lifestyle she'd always led. As well as her medication for diabetes and heart problems, she had a weekly supply of oxygen to help her breathing. Then one day she had a fall as she was looking for an oxygen cylinder and cut her shin. The leg became infected and soon the infection spread to the other leg. She wasn't silly and I'm sure she realised that before long the only option would be an amputation, something she would not be prepared to go through because of the problems it would cause her family.

She had always said that if she ever became very ill, people would have to spend their time looking after her and she wouldn't want that. So after her fall, she simply stopped taking her medication. Her legs and her general condition deteriorated rapidly and within a few days she was taken into hospital. She never told any of us what she was doing and we didn't find out until it was too late. But she knew exactly what would happen.

For some reason best known to myself, I actually went back to work the following day, thinking that was what mum would have wanted and that I couldn't let people down by staying off. But it was all too much. I was grieving and there was a funeral to arrange so I took a week off. But I decided to go to work the day after the funeral to tackle the pile of work on my desk that would have built up.

Soon after I arrived, the new dealer principal, Chris Gardner, called me in. He told me that the general sales staff were struggling for business and suggested that I might transfer some of my potential corporate deals to them, deals that could have been regarded as general sales rather than corporate. But these were deals that I'd worked so hard to set up, customers I'd spent hours developing. I wasn't going to have them snatched away from me. I just blew my top. I said, "If that's what you think of all the business I've built up, general sales can have the lot." And I walked out. I never went back.

Peter's Story

Before the first home match of the 2003-04 season against Cambridge United, we played a video on the big screen at the McAlpine Stadium, filmed the previous day, with me as master of ceremonies. On the film, I called over each of the players who would be facing Cambridge and asked him to introduce himself to the supporters who, a few weeks before, had barely heard of him. And they all concluded their speech by saying what a great club Huddersfield was and how fantastic it was to be there. As they walked away, I called after them, "Keep the faith and believe!" It became a catch phrase throughout the club.

OK, it was a PR exercise to launch the season but there was a serious message, too. A few weeks earlier, Huddersfield Town had been within 24 hours of going out of business. Instead, the Supporters Trust raised £150,000 and the club was able to go into administration instead of being wound up. Chairman Ken Davy had secured the club's future and on my first day, I called the handful of professionals together along with the academy players. I said, "Just being where we are now has been a big challenge for everyone. But that's in the past. The important thing is, where will we be at the end of the season? I believe we will win promotion." Did they believe me? Who knows? But that first team meeting was the start of an incredible journey for Huddersfield Town, for those players and for me.

When I was appointed in June, 2003, the club was on the brink of extinction. In May 2006, we were within a whisker of a place in what is now the Championship. In March, 2007, I was back on the outside looking in. Sacked, given 45 minutes to clear my desk and escorted out of the ground. Talk about the highs and lows of football management!

There was a fantastic atmosphere from the start. The administrative staff behind the scenes probably knew better than anyone how close we had been to going under and that seemed to inspire them to work doubly hard to make sure we would never be in that situation again. The manager and the players are the ones who receive the plaudits when things go well but believe me, every single person at that club deserved enormous credit for the way we clawed ourselves back from the precipice.

As the new manager, there was a plus side: I didn't have to go in and clear out a lot of senior players to bring in new faces…because virtually all the senior players had been released. But I had some promising young pros and some good kids coming through from the academy. I knew that if I got hold of the right kind of players to operate alongside them, I could build up a spirit in the squad and we'd have a chance.

I'd already tipped off Terry Yorath that I might be going back and he'd agreed to return as my number two. Then I brought in Lee Martin, a former Town keeper, as physio…and I had a backroom staff. I made Rob Edwards club captain. He'd played for me at Huddersfield before, he loved the club and I knew exactly what to expect from him: the 100 per cent commitment that I would need from every player. We're still in touch today.

All sorts of people came for trials and eventually I signed 14 players, people who'd been released in the summer and who nobody else wanted. They were desperate to find a club and I was desperate to find players. Apart from Efe Sodje, the Nigerian international defender who had been released by Crewe, none of them were well-known. That didn't worry me. It was their personality I was looking at, not their reputation.

Sodje was a colourful character renowned for always wearing a bandana during matches bearing the slogan, Against All Odds. He was 30 but he'd started his league career late, making his name with Stevenage in the Conference before joining Macclesfield in 1997. He had a reputation as a maverick but he'd made over 100 appearances for Crewe, most of them in what is now the Championship. I made a few calls about him and the feedback was that he was a bit of a one-off, an individual who had his own warm-up and cool-down routines, didn't take part in shoot-ins and wasn't always seen as a team player. But he was a good defender who'd proved himself at a much higher level and been a member of the Nigerian squad in the African Cup of Nations in 2000 and the 2002 World Cup. When we met, I took to him straight away. I felt he could be a key man provided I let him know right from the start who was the boss.

I didn't have to wait long. He was late for training on his first morning and while I pretended to make a bit of a joke about the transpennine train service, I left him in no doubt that I'd come down on him like a ton of bricks if it happened again. And after that, he was never a minute's bother. In fact, every morning, without fail, he used to knock on my office door, pop his head round and say, "Morning, Gaffer!" just to let me know he was on time. I made him my team captain. He was unavailable for our first league game but his performance in the Carling Cup-tie against Derby three days later was one of the finest debuts I've ever seen. At Boston on the Saturday he had just about the worst league debut imaginable! But that was Sodje and the vital thing was that straight away, he'd taken on board what we were trying to achieve.

I drilled it into all the lads that they were playing for the best club they would ever play for. It was something I believed passionately after my years there as a player and manager and I reckoned that if I told them often enough, they would start believing it, too. "Keep the faith and believe!" It was a joy to manage that group of players.

In an attempt to give the club a bit of a profile, I told the media before the start of the season that while I had to admit I was no longer the best-looking manager around, as I'd boasted in 1997, I would be the best-dressed and always wear a suit and collar and tie on the touchline. Again there was a serious message because I have always felt that a manager should set an example by looking professional and I wanted supporters to think that if I went about my job in a professional manner, so would my team. Sod's Law, our first game was played in heatwave conditions and I had to abandon the shirt and tie at half-time in favour of a tee shirt.

We made a reasonable start in the league but victories in the Carling Cup over First Division sides Derby and Sunderland, who had just been relegated from the Premiership, gave us the early momentum we were looking for. The 4-1 victory over Sunderland at the Stadium of Light was the breakthrough game for Jon Stead, who was 20 at the time. Until then, he'd been a promising young striker who had attracted a bit of attention. But that night he really tortured the Sunderland defence and people began to sit up and take notice. All of a sudden, Huddersfield had a player who was being watched by Premiership clubs and that cranked up our profile a bit more.

We came down to earth with a bang at Macclesfield in December, losing 4-0, and for the first time our fans gave us a bit of stick. I tore into the players afterwards. "That was an embarrassment. If that's what you think of me and this football club, I'll go." It needed saying, they responded and our season took off at Christmas when we won 1-0 at Darlington, sparking a run of six straight wins that lifted us from tenth to fifth. By which time we'd lost Stead.

I didn't want him to go. I wanted promotion and thought his departure would be a body blow. Seven years earlier, in Steve Bruce's first season, Huddersfield had sold Marcus Stewart, their leading scorer, when they were in with a realistic chance of promotion into the top flight. It sounded all the wrong notes about the club's ambitions and they dropped out of contention. I was afraid the same thing might happen if Stead was sold. On the other hand, we were a Division Two club and if the right offer came along from a Premiership side, Jon deserved the chance to better himself. Who were we to stand in his way?

The offers started before Christmas with Sunderland first in at £800,000. Ken Davy was ready to accept there and then but I knew clubs would be prepared to go a lot higher. "They'll come back," I insisted as the bids increased and we kept saying no. Eventually, Blackburn came up with £1.3m, a record for a player at our level. Our first home game after he left was against Darlington, who were struggling against relegation. We played badly and the score was 0-0 just before half-time when a message flashed up on the big screen: Stead scores for Blackburn! We lost 2-0 and if I'd had anything to do with it, the scoreboard operator would have been sacked there and then!

In fairness, the Stead money was a windfall and we spent some of it on Pawel Abbott, a striker who was born in York but had a Polish mother, from Preston. Initially, we brought in Pawel on loan but after he'd scored four goals in six appearances, I called Craig Brown, the former Scotland manager who was in charge at Preston, to ask about a permanent move.

"How much do you want for him?"

"I'll put you on to Clive Middlemass, he deals with that sort of thing." Middlemass was the chief scout and how he came to be handling transfers was beyond me. He quoted a fee of £200,000, way over the top, and eventually we agreed on £125,000.

With two matches to go, it was in our hands. We were third, three points ahead of Torquay, who had a better goal difference. All we had to do to be promoted automatically was match their results. We lost our last home game against Mansfield, who were also challenging for the play-offs, while Torquay drew to reduce the gap to two points. But we would still go up if, once again, we matched Torquay's result on the last day. I was invited to appear on Soccer AM on the morning of our match at Cheltenham, interviewed live by presenter Helen Chamberlain…a fanatical Torquay supporter.

Over 2,000 Town fans came to Cheltenham and another 6,000 watched the match live on the big screen back at the stadium. With 15 minutes to go, we were winning 1-0 and Torquay were 2-1 up at Southend. All we had to do was hold our nerve. Then Abbott chose to attempt a 35-yard backpass to Paul Rachubka, our keeper, Kayode Odejayi intercepted, laid it into the path of Shane Duff and Cheltenham were level. Utter disbelief. We couldn't force a winner, Torquay held on at Southend and we were condemned to the play-offs.

When the final whistle went we were in a state of shock. How could we have missed out? For most of the match we were heading for promotion. The players were in tears, the fans were stunned, I was in bits. With the players sitting crestfallen in the centre circle, I went back into the dressing room. I lit a fag. Yes, that's right. I'd started smoking two years earlier and couldn't kick the habit. How mad was that?

I could have cried, too, but I knew that I had to put on a positive front. I waited as the players trudged in, one by one, and when every single member of the squad was in the room, I said, "Listen, you might feel as if you've blown it but we're still in there fighting. Think how far we've come since last summer: from eight players to the play-offs. Did any of you think that was possible? Enjoy your weekend and we'll re-group on Monday. It will be hard but we can do it. Never lose your self-belief." I left them and walked on to the boardroom to see the directors and my family. No one uttered a word. Charlotte was crying, Oliver was crying and didn't speak for two days.

It was Andy Booth who broke the ice when the players reported back on Monday. "Don't worry about the backpass, Pav," he said to Abbott. "It's only cost me a £3,000 holiday!" Abbott laughed, everyone else laughed and we were back in business with a play-off semi-final at Lincoln on the horizon five days later. Lincoln were a good side and it was going to be tough. We won 2-1 at their place then in front of a full house at the Galpharm, we were two down at half-time, I tried to stay calm. "One goal is all we need," I said. "One goal. If we get that goal we'll piss this."

Fifteen minutes into the second-half we were awarded a penalty. Danny Schofield scored. The stadium erupted. With seven minutes left, Edwards equalised and we were leading 3-2 on aggregate. No mistakes this time and we were on our way to the Millennium Stadium for the final against Mansfield. It was a night I'll never forget and I always say that lifting those players from the despair of Cheltenham to the delight of reaching the Millennium Stadium was my biggest achievement as a manager.

The three play-off finals were to be staged over the Spring Bank Holiday weekend, with our match scheduled for the Monday. We travelled down on the Friday and stayed in a hotel in the centre of Cardiff. It was full of West Ham fans who were there for the Division One final against Crystal Palace and on our way back from training on the Saturday morning, a couple of bottles were flung at our coach. We were due to watch the match that afternoon but the driver said he wasn't prepared to risk driving through the West Ham fans without a proper escort. So only one option: walk. I told all the players to wear their club blazers and hold their heads up. I said, "We're Huddersfield Town. We'll go to this match as a team and we'll come back as a team."

Let's just say that the walk to the stadium was character building. We came in for a load of abuse and all sorts of stuff was thrown in our direction but we finally arrived in one piece. Our seats were directly behind the dugouts so the players got a real sense of what it was going to be like on the Monday.

I'd decided that on the big day, all the players would wear their blue club suits and ties and have the White Rose of Yorkshire in their buttonholes and they all reported for our pre-match meal looking fantastic. There was only one exception, Sodje, my captain, who never, ever wore a tie. And he wasn't going to make an exception, even for a play-off final. I spotted him as he walked into the dinning room. "Where's your tie, Sodj?"

"Gaff, I don't wear a tie."

"Don't wear a tie?"

"No, Gaff."

"Right, well if you don't wear a tie, you're not fucking playing." He went and put his tie on.

As we stood in the tunnel before the match, I just felt so proud of those players and what we'd all achieved together. We'd been a tight group from day one and to prove it, Jon Stead, who'd played in 26 league matches before his move to Blackburn, was back with us for the day, sitting on the bench. His presence summed up the togetherness that was such a vital part of our success. Our wives, girlfriends and families were in the stand and as we all sang the National Anthem together, I just knew we were not going to lose, never more so than when Mansfield had a goal disallowed in the 93rd minute.

It ended goalless after extra-time and it was all down to penalties. Before the match Keith Curle, the Mansfield manager, was quoted as saying that his side would not be practising penalties, that professional footballers shouldn't need to practise. Try telling that to our players, who had practised, practised and practised for hours.

And it pays off. Edwards scores Town's first, Paul Rachukba saves from Wayne Cordon, 1-0. Schofield nets Town's second, Liam Lawrence hits the bar, 2-0. Tony Carss scores, so does Neil MacKenzie, 3-1. If Lee Fowler scores, Town are promoted. Paul Ogden, commentating on Radio Leeds, tells his listeners, "West Yorkshire is holding its breath." Not for much longer…Fowler hits the jackpot. Town are up!

It's hard to put into words how I felt afterwards and I think everybody else would say the same thing. It was magical, it really was. We'd come from nowhere to win promotion, 25,000 fans had followed us down to Cardiff and even before the final, season tickets were flying out of the club. We'd sent out a message that Huddersfield Town were on the way back.

There was champagne in the dressing room and we had a whip round on the coach as we were leaving Cardiff. I think it was probably a tenner a head. We stopped at an off licence on the outskirts of the city and me and three or four players bought as much as beer and wine as we could. The shop owner spotted the badges on our suits and said, "Celebrating promotion then? Well done, lads!" He must have thought it was his birthday because we just about cleaned him out.

Only the players were on board and it was just like a school trip. I wasn't the manager any more, I was just one of the lads and there to enjoy myself. We sang all the way back to Huddersfield and when we landed, I grabbed the trophy and took it home with me as the lads set off for a night on the town. It had pride of place in the bedroom that night, accompanied me to the office the next day and then took centre stage again when we had a celebration down the pub with family and friends. Eventually, someone at the club happened to ask where it was and it was put into the trophy cabinet.

It had been a wonderful few days yet throughout the play-off campaign, I had been nursing a secret: an approach from Leeds United. They had parted company with Peter Reid the previous November and Eddie Gray, the caretaker manager, left at the end of the season after Leeds had been relegated from the top flight. I had two calls from their chairman David Richmond between our final league match at Cheltenham and the first leg of the play-off semi-final at Lincoln. I'd supported Leeds as a kid, followed them as far as the European Cup final in Paris in 1975 and here was an opportunity to become their manager.

But I couldn't do it. Everybody at Huddersfield had stuck by me during the season so I felt it would be a betrayal. How could I have tried to motivate the Town players when all the time I was talking to another club? I would have forever been labelled a fake and a Judas by the Town fans. So I said no. Inevitably the news leaked out and even though I had turned down that initial approach, a lot of Town supporters were furious. In fact one fan in Brighouse said, "I love you for what you've done for this club, Peter. But I know where you live and if you go to Leeds now, I'll burn your house down." He wasn't smiling either.

But Leeds persisted. They rang again before and after the second leg of the play-off semi-final. They would meet me wherever I wanted, somewhere totally discreet. I said no. And they even called me on the team coach when we were on our way to Cardiff for the final. Once again, I said I couldn't even consider talking to them until after the final. I never heard from them again and soon afterwards they appointed Kevin Blackwell, who had been Reid and Gray's number two. With hindsight, did I do the right thing? Let's say I never look back and think, "What if…?" I just know that nothing could ever take away the feeling of leading Huddersfield Town to victory in that play-off final.

I still don't think that we received the full credit we deserved. When I go down to the stadium now, there's not much in the way of memorabilia about the 2003-04 season. The club even sent the trophy back to the Football League rather than pay £6,000 to keep it for ever. OK, we hadn't won three Championships or the FA Cup like the team of the twenties or, for that matter, won promotion to the top flight like they did in 1953 and 1970. But everybody at the club had been through hell and high water for that trophy and all we ended up with was a little replica instead of the real thing.

By the summer of 2005, Huddersfield Town were really on the move. We'd ended our first season back in what is now League One by winning eight of our last nine matches, missing out on the play-offs by a single point. Now it was time for a new way of promoting and marketing the club and boosting the corporate hospitality business. We were looking for something really high profile, something that would make us the talk of the Town and beyond.

As most of the players who'd done so well over the last couple of seasons were still just kids, we looked first at Jacko's Young Guns. Then we decided to leave Jacko out of it and just promote The Young Guns, take their pictures wearing cowboy outfits and put it all together as a corporate hospitality brochure and then a 2006 calendar. It was a great idea and as a bit of a laugh, Terry and I said we'd feature as a couple of ageing gunslingers.

The photographers arrived first thing one morning during pre-season, armed with what looked like hundreds of cowboy outfits, gun belts, the lot. The only things we didn't have were horses and Red Indians. The dressing room looked like a scene from a Western movie set as the lads tried on all the outfits and the shoot took a whole day. We all had a load of fun, corporate hospitality sales jumped and when the calendars reached the club shop for Christmas, they flew off the shelves. Then early in the New Year, Brokeback Mountain, the film about two gay cowboys, was released in the UK! There was a fair bit of stick flying around after that.

Initially our target after winning promotion twelve months earlier had been consolidation but in the end, I was disappointed not to go up. On March 19, we were in fifteenth place, not a million miles away from the relegation zone, but then we went on that run of eight wins in our last nine matches. If we'd won the other one, instead of drawing 1-1 at home against Colchester, we would have made the play-offs as the form team.

Finishing that first season so strongly gave everyone at the club a huge lift and the Young Guns started the 2005-06 campaign as one of the favourites for promotion. For the first time since I'd returned to the club, expectations were high. That didn't worry me but I was very conscious that while some of our potential rivals had been able to invest, we hadn't really spent much at all by the time the new season got under way. Some clubs had been spending up to £500,000 and more on players while we were still looking at the bargain basement and free transfers. I'd signed a couple of defenders, Danny Adams and Martin McIntosh, midfielder Mark Hudson and also Gary Taylor-Fletcher, who could play up front or in midfield. But most of the £1.3m we'd received for Jon Stead 18 months earlier had not been spent on new players.

We flew out of the blocks, winning nine of our first 14 matches, with only two defeats, and topped the table in mid-October. The club's Patrons Association used to hold a monthly meeting and the manager would be invited before, during and after the season. I strolled into the mid-season meeting expecting to see a bumper attendance. Instead there were only twenty or thirty. I said to Darren Herbert, one of the association's officials, "What's going on? Where is everybody? We're flying, we've been in the top three all season, I've just won the Manager of the Month award and there's nobody here to talk to about it." He replied, "That's the problem, Peter, you're doing too well. There'd be far more if they had anything to grumble about!"

And it wasn't just in the league that people were sitting up and starting to take notice of Huddersfield Town. An FA Cup run was in our sights, too, with the dream of drawing a Big One if we could make it through to the third round. After seeing off Welling at home 4-1 all we had to do was beat Conference North side Worcester City away and we'd be in the hat for the third round draw. The conditions at Worcester were atrocious. Walking to the dugout, I trudged through about six inches of mud, wrecked my shoes and didn't do my suit any favours either. Best-dressed manager? Not that day. The match was televised live and it was a poor game but we won 1-0.

The draw was due to be televised soon after the final whistle so the interviewer asked me to go on camera live from Worcester for my comments. The draw started and before long one of the giants came out of the bag. "Chelsea…" the champions, Jose Mourinho's megastars. I held my breath. "Will play…Huddersfield Town." I couldn't believe it. Chelsea away? Talk about wanting a Big One! Not only were Chelsea the reigning champions, they were top of the Premiership and had lost only once in the league. Everybody was talking about Chelsea, everybody was talking about Mourinho. And now everybody would be talking about Huddersfield Town as well. Fantastic!

As soon as the draw had finished and I'd given my verdict on camera, I rushed back to the dressing room to tell the players, who didn't have a TV or radio. "Who've we got, gaffer?"

"Cheltenham away."

Silence.

"Sorry, I got that wrong. Not Cheltenham…Chelsea!"

Pandemonium.

When I spoke to the Press boys afterwards, I joked, "If I'm going to be standing alongside Mourinho on the touchline, I'll have to buy myself a new suit!" They milked that one for all it was worth and yes, I headed off to Jimmy the Suit's in Huddersfield town centre. He stocked all the top brands and I went for a Pal Zileri in grey and completed the outfit with a new shirt, tie and shoes. All through the build-up to the match there were stories about Mourinho, the self-styled Special One, and this Yorkshireman who claimed to be the best-dressed manager. Mourinho reckoned to be a pretty sharp dresser himself and at one stage, it looked as if the match would be more of a fashion contest than a third round FA Cup-tie.

I loved every minute and made sure the players enjoyed it, too. It was the first time most of them had been in the spotlight and I wanted them to take it all on board. And the fans. They'd been through some dark times but now we'd turned the corner, we'd won promotion from the bottom tier, we were gunning for a place in what is now the Championship and we'd been drawn at Chelsea, arguably the most glamorous side in the land, in the FA Cup. We sold our allocation of 6,000 tickets straight away and at our next home game, against Southend, a new chant started: "Who needs Mourinho when we've got Jacko!" The whole club was buzzing.

And there was a football match to be played. On paper, we had no chance. By the time we arrived at Stamford Bridge on January 7, Chelsea had won nine Premiership matches on the bounce, were 14 points ahead of Manchester United and looked certainties for a second title in a row. But I kept hammering away at the players. "This is the FA Cup. There will be a shock in the third round. Why can't it be us?"

Before the kick-off, I wanted to do something a bit different and maybe take some of the attention away from Mourinho on his home territory. I needed to make sure that Mourinho emerged from the tunnel first. All the cameras would be on him and if I was first, they'd switch away from me as soon as he appeared. So I lurked around as he climbed up the steps. Then when he paused at the top, I started to climb the steps behind him. For a few moments we were standing together on the touchline with the cameras on both of us and the Town fans chanting, "Who needs Mourinho when we've got Jacko?"

I hadn't spoken to him before the match and as we shook hands, I couldn't really think of anything to say, other than, "Would you like a piece of chewing gum?" I've no idea why…and I can't remember whether he took a piece or not. But full credit to Mourinho. He walked straight over to our bench and shook hands with Terry and the staff, the substitutes and my lad Oliver, who was on the bench with us. I couldn't let him miss that one, could I?

We went in at half-time 1-0 down after an early goal from Carlton Cole. It could have been more but we'd started to get it together and surprise Chelsea towards the end of the half. I told the players that they could go on and win and to keep believing. I said, "Some of you might play in the Premiership one day, others might never have another chance to play against a top side at a top stadium with over 40,000 fans in the ground. So for the next forty-five minutes, make the most of it, enjoy it and whatever you do, don't come away thinking you could have done better."

They gave everything in that second-half and when Gary Taylor-Fletcher equalised after 75 minutes, I was convinced we'd hold on for a replay. But with eight minutes left, Arjan Robben broke clear on the left and crossed for Eidur Gudjohnsen to hit the winner. We'd lost but I was so, so proud of my players and I knew I had to be the first to tell them. Mourinho obviously had the same idea. He was walking towards the Huddersfield players as they left the pitch after applauding our travelling fans but I pushed in front of him and shook each player by the hand. Back in the dressing room, I sat them all down, told them how well they'd played, how they could be proud of their performance and how they should enjoy the moment and the weekend. Then I added, "But we'll come in on Monday and be ready to push on in the league again, starting at…"

At that point, the Chelsea kit man came into the dressing room and shouted, "Well played, lads, Jose says you can come into the dressing room for some players' shirts…"

My words "Scunthorpe on Saturday" fell on deaf ears as they all rushed across the corridor to the home dressing room. I whispered to the kit man, "Make sure you get me one, too," sat down and waited for them all to come back. They returned with stories of a chef cooking pasta for the Chelsea players, of Mourinho wrapped in a towel and how the players had handed over shirts, boots, anything to satisfy the northern invaders.

I headed off to the Press conference. My average meeting with the media lads involved a bit of a natter in the corridor or a small Press room with a maximum of ten or a dozen journalists. At Stamford Bridge that day, there must have been 80 or 90 writers, radio reporters and television interviewers from all over the world and the verdict from the journalists was that we'd given a good account of ourselves. I can't recall anyone asking about my new suit, though!

As he headed for his own media conference, Mourinho invited me into his office for a glass of wine. The office was pretty minimalist with a small desk, a picture of Mourinho and his wife and not much else apart from a television and a fridge. I was asked what I'd like to drink. "A glass of white wine, thanks," I replied, thinking, "Yes, I'm really looking forward to this, nothing but the best Chablis for Mourinho." Disappointment. The label just read Chelsea Chardonnay. Mourinho arrived a few minutes later. He'd been wearing a collar and tie during the match but now he was sporting his casual look, a brown leather jacket, jeans and a scarf. Maybe I shaded it in the fashion stakes, maybe not.

Before we left I asked if he'd mind sending me the in-depth scouting report on my players that Chelsea had used in their match preparations. I thought it would be useful to learn what a top club thought about the way we went about things. It arrived a few days later together with a letter saying how nice it had been to meet me and that the team were a credit to me. You deserved a replay, he added. That was a nice touch…and I still have the letter.

My only regret was that we didn't get the replay we deserved. The match would have been live on Sky, we would have pocketed over a million pounds and I would have had some cash to spend on the thing that really mattered: winning promotion. And we should have gone up. Instead, after winning only one of our last six matches, we ended up fourth, six points away from an automatic slot.

So it was the play-offs again, with the semi-final against our Yorkshire rivals Barnsley. We did really well at their place, won 1-0 with a Taylor-Fletcher goal in the 85th minute and hit the woodwork a couple of times. We looked comfortable and should have wrapped it up in that first leg. Instead we were beaten 3-1 at the Galpharm Stadium, which had been re-named at the start of the season, four days later, a crushing blow. Were we complacent? No. Were Barnsley better on the night? Yes…and they also had that little bit of luck that we didn't have in the first leg. The first goal was always going to be crucial. If we'd scored it, we would have been two up with an away goal. Game over. But we didn't. They went in front with a penalty after 58 minutes and although Jon Worthington equalised in the 65th minute, the momentum was with Barnsley and we under-performed all night.

Defeat hit me like a bullet. Ten months' hard work thrown away with the finishing line in sight. I didn't sleep for three nights. I discovered that if losing in the play-offs is a huge blow for a player, it's ten times worse for a manager. He's spent a whole season picking the sides and choosing the tactics and to get so near but so far is a numbing experience. The players can shrug their shoulders and go off on holiday; the manager spends the next fortnight wondering, "Where did I go wrong? Could I have done this or that better?" And then, instead of thinking about the players he might bring in to consolidate in a higher division, it's back to the drawing board to find players who could help him go one better next time.

I have to admit that I was in two minds about whether to carry on. In three years, I'd won promotion, just missed out on the play-offs and then lost a play-off semi-final. With the financial backing available, had I taken the club as far as I could? The board obviously didn't think so because I was offered a new contract straight after our defeat by Barnsley. And despite my misgivings, I signed it because, in the end, I could never have just walked away from Huddersfield Town with unfinished business to attend to.

We started the 2006-07 campaign as promotion favourites, even though once again there hadn't been any real investment. I'd brought in Luke Beckett, a striker, and Matt Glennon, a keeper, without spending much money and one or two more kids had come through from the academy. But we'd fallen short the previous season and we needed better players to reinforce what we already had. We'd all like a Ferrari but if you haven't got any money, you have to settle for a second hand Ford Fiesta. And that was our situation.

In our first home match of the season, against Rotherham on August 8, we secured a place in the record books when Taylor-Fletcher scored the 500,000th goal in English league football. I don't think any of the 10,161 fans, and certainly none of the players, knew about it. I found out when I went into my office afterwards, switched on the television and heard the presenter talking about a historic moment. Then they showed the re-run of Gary's goal, our third in a 3-1 win. The referee's changing room was just down the corridor so I dashed in and asked the ref, Paul Robinson, for the match ball. Brooky, the kit man, inscribed it with a felt tip pen, Gary signed it and for the next six months it took pride of place in my office. To this day, Fletch insists it should be his but try getting me to part with it now!

I'd known about Gary from my time as an agent when we picked him up at Northwich Victoria, who were in the Conference. He went out on loan to Hull in 2001 and soon afterwards joined Leyton Orient, where apparently he was voted the worst player ever to appear for the club. I bet they aren't saying that now! He had loan spells with Grays in the Isthmian league and Dagenham and Redbridge in the Conference before joining Lincoln in 2003. He played in the Division Three play-off final against Bournemouth at Cardiff at the end of that season and I was working as a summariser that day. I was also keeping an eye on Gary. So, I suspected, was Bristol City manager

Gary Johnson. "Are you watching Taylor-Fletcher, then?" I asked him.

"No, I don't think he'd hack it any higher up the league." Six years later, Taylor-Fletcher notched the first goal ever scored in the Premier League by Blackpool, the club he joined for a snip from Town in 2007. That made him the first player to score a goal in the six top divisions of the English football pyramid, a fantastic achievement. Gary invited Alison and I to Blackpool's final Premier League home match of the 2010-11 season, against Bolton at Bloomfield Road. It was a tremendous match and Blackpool won 4-3. We joined his family and friends for a meal before the game and then five minutes after the final whistle, Gary appeared in the hospitality lounge, still wearing his tangerine shirt. He came over to our table, stripped off his shirt and presented it to me, his first agent. It was a fantastic gesture and I was so proud to see a player I'd picked up in non-league football performing at the highest level. People are quick to give professional footballers a bad name but I like to think there are still a few around like Gary, a credit to his profession.

High expectations mean the pressure on the manager is cranked up a notch or two and even though we were as high as fifth in the table in mid-October, there were whispers that if we didn't make it this time I'd be on thin ice. And in truth, we never really got going. Perhaps the decisive moment came in early December when Terry had to quit as my number two because of ill-health. There was no way he would be working again in the foreseeable future and he was a serious loss. Terry had been with me throughout my managerial career but his health was more important than Huddersfield Town. I should have brought in someone from outside the club, something I'd planned to do in the summer when I approached Neil McDonald, my former Newcastle team-mate, to become first team coach, working alongside me and Terry.

Instead, he was appointed manager of Carlisle and I decided to continue with just Terry and myself. When he was taken ill, Andrew Watson, our chief executive, urged me to bring in a replacement from outside but I decided to stay in-house and promoted John Dungworth, our academy coach. With hindsight, it was a mistake…but hindsight is a wonderful thing. John was a decent enough coach and we had one or two good results to start with. But I should have moved outside the club and appointed a right hand man I knew really well.

For the first time as a manager, I felt I was starting to lose my way a bit. A couple of players, McIntosh and Adams, wanted contract extensions but McIntosh was 36 and Adams 31 and I thought it would be better to move them on. Hudson was out of the side and unhappy and I was aware of a disruptive element in the dressing room. Cracks were appearing and without Terry, I started to feel lonely and isolated. I didn't have a number two I could turn to and took it all on my own shoulders. But even though results were not what we'd expected, there had been a lot of highs over the previous three seasons and I thought I'd pull through.

The axe fell on March 5, two days after we'd lost 5-1 at Nottingham Forest. We'd been beaten in our previous two home matches but the day before the Forest match, I'd received a text from Ken Davy. He wished me good luck and said that victory at the City Ground could give us an outside chance of the play-offs. Instead, defeat left us 14 points adrift with ten games to play.

Andrew Watson always used to call me on the Saturday night or Sunday morning after a match but that weekend the phone stayed ominously silent. I was in my office at eight am on Monday as usual and ten minutes later, I was just having a cigarette when there was a knock on the door. Ralph Rimmer, one of the directors. "Can you come up to the boardroom, Peter?" I didn't need anyone to tell me it was rocky news; let's put it this way, I wasn't expecting a new three-year contract. I walked up the stairs, into the boardroom, closed the door and sat down. There was me, Ann Hough, the secretary, who is now a director and a good friend, Davy, Rimmer and Roger Armitage, another director. Davy spoke. "Your contract has been terminated, Peter. Sign this termination agreement." And that was it. One blip in four seasons and I was out.

At the very least, I deserved to leave with my self-respect and dignity intact. But instead of being told to take my time and say my farewells to all the staff, I was given 45 minutes to pack my bags and go. I was treated like a criminal. Ann was asked to escort me back to my office and oversee me clearing my desk. She was in tears, the office staff were in tears and I wasn't a million miles away from crying, either. Before doing anything, I rang Alison and the kids because Huddersfield Town was part of their life too. I wanted to make sure they heard the news from me first.

Then I got to work. All I had in my drawers and on the walls was some personal memorabilia, a few of my favourite things: pictures, shirts, the Taylor-Fletcher ball, programmes, that sort of thing. And a few packets of fags no doubt. But anyone watching would have thought I'd been working for the Ministry of Defence and was under suspicion of selling top secret information. Soul destroying. When everything was packed up in boxes, Brooky helped me pile it all into the Range Rover...and I drove away.

I organised a Press conference for the local media in a hotel nearby at 11 o'clock the following morning. The club had issued the usual, "We'd like to thank Peter for his efforts" rubbish but I wanted to get across how special my time at Town had been. The club could take away my job but no one could take away the memories. It went well and it wasn't until midday that the last reporter left and I found myself alone in an empty meeting room. Just 48 hours earlier, I'd been preparing my players for an important match in front of 19,070 fans. Now I was out in the cold once more.

10. Into the storm

Peter did not stay out of work for long, returning to management with Lincoln City seven months after leaving Huddersfield. New surroundings for Alison, too, this time as a corporate headhunter. Life was good. How was either to know that their new world was about to fall apart? "In February, 2008, we were told that Peter had throat cancer," says Alison. "Our life changed overnight."

Alison's Story

Looking back, I should really have had more time off after mum's funeral and maybe I wouldn't have behaved as I did and walked out of Appleyard Jaguar. It might also have been different if my mentor Mike Smith had still been around; he might have been able to calm down the situation. But I'd worked so hard, along with Tracey Asquith who had done all the admin for me, to build up a business portfolio and now a chunk of it was going to be taken away. I couldn't sit back and let that happen. Soon after I left, the corporate sales department closed down, Tracey was made redundant and all the business was transferred to the general sales staff.

I wasn't out of work for long; a few days, no more. And it was another change of direction, this time into the world of corporate headhunting. A couple of weeks before mum died, a man called Mike Sheard had come into the showroom. He asked at reception if Mike Smith was around, because they'd had dealings before, so he was pointed in my direction.

His previous car, an Aston Martin, had been stolen to order from his home and was eventually traced to China. After the theft, he'd installed extra security but his wife June was frightened that the same thing might happen again if he invested in another brand new luxury car. So he was understandably unsure about what to do next. He'd already done the rounds of the dealers in leading marques: Ferrari, Mercedes, Porsche, Audi, Aston Martin, BMW. Now he wanted to find out what Jaguar might have to offer… but I could tell that he wouldn't be making up his mind in a hurry. Money was no object and he needed a car. But he just didn't know what to do next.

He'd already traipsed June round the other dealerships and by the time they arrived at Jaguar, she'd had enough and stayed in her car, a silver VW Beetle Convertible automatic, a really unusual car. He explained the situation and I said, "Look, you've no idea what kind of car you really want so why spend fifty, sixty, seventy thousand pounds on a car that might not be right for you? There's a fantastic used XJ6 on our forecourt, £25,000, two years old, low mileage, drives like a dream. Take it for six months until you've got over the shock of what's happened and you're ready to start again. You'll easily get your money back if you want to change it. Let's take it out for a spin."

He was probably in his early sixties and when he told me he travelled down to his head office in London once a week, I said, "Well, the last thing you want at your great age is a hard, sporty drive on a round trip of nearly 400 miles. You need a bit of comfort!" He laughed and bought the XJ6 on the spot. He said, "In every other dealership, someone has tried to sell me the most expensive car in the place, even though I told them I didn't really know what I wanted. You're the first person who's come up with a really practical solution." We did all the paperwork, shook hands and as he walked away, he said, "And now you've got to come and work for me." So I did.

His firm was MGMS International, a recruitment agency and part of the Norman Broadbent Group, a massive headhunting organisation based on Fleet Street in London. His office was just two left turns away from the bottom of our road in Brighouse. I'd passed the building many times and sometimes wondered what they did. I went for an interview and he offered me a job in recruitment, persuading companies to use MGMS if they were looking to appoint a new executive. The company car? June's Beetle Convertible…although I threw away the trademark purple vase and pink artificial flower fixed alongside the steering wheel!

Their recruitment work was done by cold calling over the phone and I was soon arguing against that. I claimed until the cows came home that in the first instance it was essential to make personal contact with potential customers, that no one could develop a relationship over the phone without first meeting the person at the other end of the line. I urged Mike to send his team out to meet potential customers face to face and eventually he agreed. The ones who had the confidence to do that ended up being very successful; the others went back to the telephone.

I was selling people to people and dealing in senior management-plus, on salaries of over £80,000. You can't just advertise on a recruitment site or in a newspaper for that kind of job, you also need someone who can make sure you have found exactly the right person. So let's say one of our clients was a haulage company and was looking for a finance director. We would phone every single comparable haulage company within a 50-mile radius and sometimes beyond to find out the name of their finance director. Of course, the companies were aware of the existence of headhunters and their reception staff would be on their guard. So like all headhunting companies, we would have to use all sorts of ploys to find the information we were looking for. For example, one of the younger members of the team might pretend to be a university student planning a career in finance. "Is it OK for me to write to the finance director for a bit of advice, please?"

"Yes, of course, that won't be a problem."

"Thanks, could you give me his name, please?" Trade unions and data protection companies were quite good camouflage, too.

With the info on board, we'd call all the finance directors direct, explain our position, assure them that we were working on behalf of a respectable headhunting company and ask if it was a good time to talk. The answer was usually no so we'd fix an appropriate time.

Very often, people would tell us they were perfectly happy in their job, earning a good salary with no plans to move on. But if a new job meant an extra £50,000 a year plus benefits, that tended to make a difference. Well it would, wouldn't it? We would eventually narrow down the potential candidates to ten or a dozen and arrange formal interviews, sometimes at our head office in Fleet Street. Then we'd select the crème de la crème candidates, usually the best three, and hand their names and details over to the commissioning company. After that it was down to them.

Life was good. Peter had been manager of Lincoln City for four months and was doing well, I loved working at MGMS. Then, in February 2008 and just a few months into my new job, the bombshell exploded. Peter was diagnosed with throat cancer. Nothing can prepare you for that. I vowed I'd be strong for Peter and the kids and at home, I was. But at work I just kept breaking up and bursting into tears. There was no way I could carry on long-term. In that job, I needed to be totally driven, bright, sparky, chatty, outgoing, pleasant and there was no room for an agent who wasn't totally focussed, whose mind was elsewhere. And for the foreseeable future there would be only one focus for me: Peter.

Peter's Story

Believe in me whoever you may be
Coz I'm the Lord of the Imps, said he
And you won't go wrong if you follow me
Coz I'm the Lord of the Imps, said he

Not exactly top of the charts material but it meant so much when the Lincoln fans christened me Lord of the Imps soon after I arrived in October, 2007. They had taken me to their hearts…and I felt exactly the same way about Lincoln City, or the Imps as they are known by their supporters. The nickname came via Hollywood and the film adaptation of The Lord of the Rings, directed by Peter Jackson. And the fans adapted the words to the tune of Lord of the Dance. Even my car parking space at the stadium was given a new id, changing from Manager to Lord of the Imps!

Joining Lincoln was the start of an incredible journey for me, on a personal and a professional level. A journey that would see me diagnosed with throat cancer just four months later and, after I returned following successful treatment, a journey that I believe finally banished my unwanted reputation, in some quarters at least, of being a one-club manager,

Huddersfield Town.

When I joined Lincoln, they were rock bottom of the Football League and on my first day, I joked to Steff Wright, the chairman, "The only way is up!" And it was. We finished my first season in 15th place and improved to 13th the following year. After I was sacked in October, 2009, the decline began that ended with relegation to the Blue Square Bet Premier League in 2011. That hit me hard because Lincoln City will always have a very special place in my heart. The sooner they are back where they belong in the Football League the better.

Unlike my first sacking by Huddersfield in 1999, when I was in the wilderness for four years, I was only out of work for five months after the axe fell for the second time. In the immediate aftermath there were the same phone calls and empty promises that I'd received eight years earlier but it wasn't long before I was back tending the garden with only family and close friends around. It hurt…but less than before. I was older, more mature and yes, a bit harder, I suppose. I knew that if and when I got back in, the same people who'd turned away now would be back with the same promises. But when and where would that next opportunity be?

In the end, two came along at the same time. In October, Millwall, who were bottom of League One, parted company with Willie Donachie. Around the same time, John Schofield and John Deehan, Lincoln's manager and director of football, left Sincil Bank. I sent Millwall my CV and even though there were some pretty high-profile candidates, my first interview went well and I was invited back to meet the chairman, John Berylson, when he flew in from the States a few days later. After that meeting, I was one of two candidates asked to return for a third time. On Friday, November 2.

I never actually sent Lincoln a CV. Instead, Steff Wright rang and asked why I hadn't applied for the job. I replied, "I'm talking to Millwall, I've had two interviews and they want me to go down next Friday for a third time."

"Well come and talk to us anyway, let's make it Monday."

Steff and the Lincoln directors outlined their plans for the future and I was impressed. It certainly didn't feel like a club in trouble. Then, after an hour or so, Steff asked if I wanted to see their new training ground, a few minutes' drive away, before having another chat. Obviously I was keen to have a quick look at what training facilities they had to offer but couldn't quite work out why Steff was dawdling around after leaving the stadium. And, when we reached the training ground, he seemed to want to show me every blade of grass and every piece of equipment. Eventually, I suggested that it might be time to go back to the ground and talk a bit more about the nuts and bolts of the job. He agreed but once again, we crawled along at a snail's pace all the way back.

I found out why a few weeks afterwards. I was Lincoln's first choice but they had also arranged to see Willie Donachie in case my interview went belly up. So while Steff was showing me the training facilities, the other board members were talking to Donachie at the stadium…and in fact, our paths crossed, literally: as Steff and I were driving back into the car park, Willie was driving away, although we didn't actually see one another.

Lincoln offered me the job there and then and I asked for 24 hours to think it over. But anyone who's ever had a job interview will know that sometimes you leave thinking, "This is the one for me." I felt like that about Lincoln. So it was a dilemma: Millwall, a bigger club and a division higher, might offer me a job and the money would be better. On the other hand, they might not…and Lincoln's offer was on the table. The nagging fear was, "What if I turn down Lincoln and miss out at Millwall?" I could have been out of work for another six months, twelve months, who knows how long?

Decision time: I rang Steff on the Tuesday and said, "I'll come to Lincoln." Then I spoke to Andy Ambler, the chief exec at Millwall, and explained the situation. He wished me luck and the following week, Kenny Jackett was appointed manager of Millwall. He stayed at the club until May, 2013, by which time he was one of the longest-serving managers outside the Premier League. Any regrets? No.

Lincoln may be out on a limb and a bit off most fans' radar but it was a well-run club with a nice little stadium, just outside the city centre, and the new training facilities were excellent. There was a hard core of three or four thousand fans who were proud of their club and even though they were bottom of the table, the potential was there to establish the club at a higher level. We even had our own world-class aerobatics squadron…the Red Arrows were based just down the road at Scampton and used to fly over the training pitch every day. It sounds odd but in the end we just took them for granted.

And the city of Lincoln itself is beautiful, dominated by the cathedral quarter, where the film, the Da Vinci Code, was set. Steff wanted me to move there and asked me again when I signed a new deal in January, 2009. It was certainly a city I could easily have lived in but as a football manager, you have to look at job security and whether it's worth uprooting your family when you might be out of work and looking for another job in twelve months' time.

Steff was around the same age as me and ran a successful construction business. He loved his football, he was fanatical about Lincoln City and was prepared to go the extra mile for his club. We got on straight away, we were honest with one another and he was never moody, like some chairmen. Win, lose or draw, he would either come into the office or call me and we would discuss the game in a sensible way. I really appreciated that. He didn't interfere, never questioned why I wanted to bring in a player and was happy to trust my judgement on football issues. He was probably the best chairman I worked with and we still speak regularly.

However we were after all 92nd in the league so there were clearly big problems to tackle, not least the club's profile. I said to Steff, "Right, there's

91 clubs above us and everybody out there sees Lincoln as a backwater. We need to raise our image in the media. Let's try and get a mention on the newsreel strip on Sky Sport at least once a week." It was never going to happen that often for a club in the bottom division but we managed a few newsworthy lines that put our name in lights once or twice.

Steff was also keen to take the club out of Lincoln and into the county, after Yorkshire the second largest in England. He asked if I'd be prepared to go with him to pubs and clubs all over Lincolnshire to promote the Imps. Of course! We went to loads of venues; sometimes twenty would turn up, sometimes a hundred and twenty but the response was always positive. And on the back of that campaign, we sold record season ticket sales the following summer.

I was a bit apprehensive about the reception I might receive from the fans. At Huddersfield, we'd had some raw rumbles with Lincoln during our Division Three promotion season, particularly the two play-off semi-finals in 2004. At the end of the second semi, one of their players, Kevin Ellison, was flat out on the turf when he was trampled on by an exuberant Town fan who had invaded the pitch, along with thousands more. Kevin picked himself up, chased after the fan and let's just say an altercation took place. In fact, seven years later I managed Kevin at Bradford and he remembered the incident vividly, admitting, "I gave him a bit of a slap!" But I needn't have worried about the fans. They took to me straight away and I felt from the start that everybody connected with the club really believed in me.

However the reality was that I'd taken over an unsuccessful team, low on confidence with just two wins out of 13. But part of a manager's job is to make average players good players and turn good players into very good players. To do that they have to believe in themselves and their manager and at a club like Lincoln, where a new man doesn't have the cash to chuck out half a dozen players and bring in his own men, belief is so important.

My first move was to recruit my former Newcastle team-mate Neil McDonald as number two. Neil had been working in Sweden after his spell as Carlisle manager and started on a week-to-week basis in case he was offered a bigger job. He said, "Look, Peter, I don't want a contract. I could be with you three days, three months or three years." But before long, he was enjoying it so much he was happy to sign a contract.

Whether he was quite so happy about our long-distance commute is another matter. Neil lived in Bolton and used to get up at around 4.30am to arrive at my house between half past five and six o'clock. They were long days and sometimes, if we went to a match at night, it would be after midnight before we got to bed. Then we'd have to be up and off again before dawn next morning. There are days, not many, when being a football manager isn't full-on and there's a chance to chill out. But for the most part, it's tough work, long hours and hard miles.

Neil and I took it in turns with the driving. We headed off from Brighouse via the M62, A1M, A1 and then the A57, a journey of around 90 miles. It was vital that we beat the morning rush hour traffic into Lincoln because that can be a nightmare. Nightmare or not, however, nothing would stop us from dropping in at Carol's Caff, a little portakabin in a lay-by about five miles outside the city. Without fail, when we arrived at around quarter past seven, Carol would have a mug of coffee and a bacon butty waiting for us, together with a selection of the morning papers. She was a City fan so we gave her a couple of tickets for home games and in return she wanted a signed picture to put on the wall of the cabin. The place would be full of truck drivers and farmers, who parked their tractors outside, and we had some real laughs with them. Breakfast with truckers wouldn't normally be on the menu for a football manager but for me, no day was complete without one of Carol's bacon butties.

Then one teatime, as we were setting off home, we spotted a sign in the lay-by saying, "Café closed due to fire." We screeched to a halt but there was no one around to tell us what had happened. We feared the worst. Was life as we knew it about to come to an end? As it happened, I was on my own next morning and sure enough, as I slowed down approaching the lay-by I could see that the tell-tale sign was still outside. Disaster! Then, just as I started to accelerate away, Carol appeared from nowhere and flagged me down. She said, "Peter, I've got your bacon sandwich and a flask of coffee." She must have got them ready at home but she'd no real idea what time I might be passing and might have been waiting for ages. The café re-opened soon afterwards and normal service resumed. No wonder I loved the people at Lincoln and desperately wanted to do well for them.

My first game in charge was against Chester, one of my old clubs. It wasn't the best of starts. The kick-off was delayed for nearly an hour because Chester were stuck in a traffic jam on the A1, we lost 1-0 to a controversial penalty and I ended up having an altercation with the referee, Trevor Kettle, after the final whistle. An FA tribunal, a two-match touchline ban and a £300 fine. But at least my row with Kettle demonstrated to the fans how much I cared about their club. And in December, while I was serving my ban, they even gave me a standing ovation after we'd lost 4-0 to Darlington!

We had to wait four games for our first win, against Notts County at home, but with that victory we climbed off the bottom and I knew for certain that we'd absolutely cruise up the table. We suffered a bit of a blip around Christmas, with three straight defeats, but after drawing with Bury on New Year's Day, we won two of our next four matches before embarking on a run of five straight wins that rocketed us up to 14th place, sixteen points off the bottom and ten points away from the play-offs. Maybe I was getting a bit carried away when I claimed we might even scrape into the top seven but what's wrong with a bit of optimism? And the fans loved it. Little did they know that for me, the good times had juddered to a halt.

11. The nightmare begins

"I started smoking at the age of 40," says Peter. "How crazy was that? We were on holiday in Majorca, Alison was just about to start work as cabin crew and was trying to lose a bit of weight. I suggested that instead of having a pudding after dinner, we'd have one of those menthol cigarettes. We'd stop the minute we got home. Alison stopped, I didn't. I went straight to the shop and bought a packet of fags and discovered that once the drug has hold of you, it never lets go. Non-smokers will say giving up is easy; just stop. But it isn't easy. In the end, I was on thirty and then forty a day, telling Alison I was on twenty maximum. People used to bring me two hundred back from holiday."

Alison's Story

In those days when you went on holiday in Europe, everybody seemed to sit outside after dinner and have a glass of wine and a cigarette, the done thing. So when Peter said, "Why don't we have a fag instead of a pudding?" I replied, "OK, let's have a minty one." I never inhaled, I just took a few puffs and then put it out so I couldn't see how anyone could possibly become addicted. The problem was that Peter had smoked a few furtive fags behind the bike sheds at school and maybe enjoyed it more than he cared to admit.

I was aware that he carried on smoking after we got home and I nagged him about it. The trouble is that nobody is going to stop smoking when you natter them. Everything you say about cost, health implications, what the children will think is like water off a duck's back. When somebody is hooked they can't give up unless they absolutely want to do so.

But I never really knew how many he was smoking, although I did realise that if he was saying 20 a day I could probably double it. Let's put it this way, he'd have a cigarette first thing in the morning and last thing at night so there must have been a few in between. I carried on nagging him but I was banging my head against a brick wall. How many times can you tell someone, "It's not my life, it's not my body but if it was me I'd be doing something about it. I've been a nurse, I can give you health advice so please take advantage of someone who's worked in a medical environment." But no.

I first noticed the split on his lower lip in 2002 when he returned from a European trip during his time as an agent. I asked if he'd been in a fight, although as far as I know he's never been in a fight in his life. I kept an eye on it and there was a recurring pattern: it would go away for a couple of weeks and then return. I knew he should go to the doctor but he refused. He was back in charge at Huddersfield by this time and said he was too busy, even though the doctor's surgery was only a few hundred yards away from our house and he could also have had a word with the club doctor.

But he wouldn't...and you can't drag a 40-year-old kicking and screaming to the doctors about a sore on his lip. You think to yourself, "What a bloody idiot you are, you're killing yourself," although you don't really believe he is.

Eventually, however, even Peter realised this one wasn't going to go away and it was time to see the doctor. He was referred to a consultant dermatologist and a biopsy revealed the presence of dysplasic cells, not cancerous but not good news. He had to start putting on a cream that was going to burn off the cells. It was massively painful and for a while all his lip was blistered. He used it for a month by which time the sore had disappeared.

Things improved for a couple of years and then the sore started to re-appear. In 2007, after he had been sacked by Huddersfield for the second time, I insisted that he went back to the doctor. He was referred to the consultant again and had another biopsy. Straight afterwards, we set off on a round-the-world trip for the whole of August. It was a bit of a spur-of-the-moment thing. We didn't know how long it would be before we received the results of the biopsy and said, "You know what, let's spend some of our savings." Maybe at the back of Peter's mind, where he hides everything, there was a bit of 'What if? What if?' but he never said so. I wasn't really worrying about it. I have always believed that the time to start worrying is when you have something to worry about, not before.

We went to a travel agent in Cleckheaton, someone involved with Huddersfield Town, who organised bespoke trips. We flew to Shanghai, where we went up the Jin Mao Tower, at the time the tallest skyscraper in China. Then on to Sydney, the Blue Mountains, where we stayed at the Lily Ann Fell Hotel, one of the best in the world. After that it was Cairns and the Barrier Reef, Ayers Rock, Fiji and finally California and the Regent Beverley Hills Hotel in Los Angeles.

There were loads of celebs coming in and out of the hotel and a strict rule that no one was allowed to take photos in the foyer. Anyone who tried was suspected of being one of the paparazzi, surrounded by heavies, hauled off and, for all we knew, never seen again. It didn't worry me because, quite honestly, I'm terrible at recognising people. I just don't have a clue...and I don't exactly look like one of the paparazzi anyway. The hotel had several limos available for guests, complete with liveried chauffeurs, and one of them took us on a tour of the movie stars' houses and Beverly Hills' version of Millionaires' Row before another trip off into the mountains.

It was in Beverly Hills that I finally fulfilled my dream of owning a Chanel handbag, a 2.55 Traditional Handbag in black leather to be exact and bought from the Chanel store in Rodeo Drive. At first, our chauffeur said he couldn't drop us off at the main entrance because it was on double yellow lines. But I pleaded that I'd spent the last few weeks dreaming of climbing out of a limo and walking through the front door of Chanel, so he agreed to take a chance...and got away with it.

After I'd chosen the handbag, the assistant insisted on showing us around the shoe and clothes departments - she must have thought we were loaded. While they were packing up the bag in a cardboard box and wrapping it in Chanel paper, Peter decided it was time for a cigarette. Yes, he was still smoking despite everything. I had a cup of coffee, soaked up the atmosphere for a while longer and then, after about an hour, the chauffeur strode into the store and called out in a loud voice, "Mrs Jackson, Regent Beverly Hills, please." I stood up. "May I carry your luggage, please Ma'am?" The assistant handed him the package and out we went to the car park at the back of the store. He put my shopping in the boot and off we went, with me full of myself and chatting ten to the dozen as we drove away. It wasn't until we were halfway back to the hotel that I remembered Peter, having a fag on the pavement...

When we returned home, the letter was waiting, asking us to make an appointment for the results of the biopsy. Thankfully we never open one another's mail so the children hadn't seen the NHS postmark and decided to take a look...just in case. Had we happened to ring home and ask if there was a letter from the NHS for Dad it might have been a different story. The letter was blunt and to the point, almost like, "Congratulations, you've got cancer. Please attend the hospital on such and such a date."

We were told this time that the cells were cancerous and needed to be removed immediately. The consultant said the cancer had been caused by two things: prolonged unprotected exposure to the sun – footballers didn't wear sun block when they trained and I don't suppose they do today – and, of course, by smoking. Peter stopped straight away and has never smoked another cigarette to this day. Instead, he started using Nicorette patches and chewing gum immediately.

Almost straight away, his voice became hoarse. He ignored it and said it was a side-effect of the Nicorette, insisting it would go away. It didn't. I made another appointment for him to see the GP, who arranged for his throat to be checked out at Halifax Infirmary. A scope was passed into his throat but Peter didn't tolerate it very well and he was told to make another appointment for a laryngoscopy under general anaesthetic. That was at the beginning of February, 2008.

I tried to be optimistic about the outcome. I've always believed that if you think negative thoughts, negative things are going to happen. But at the back of my mind, I was frightened. So was Peter. He said afterwards that lying in the hospital room waiting for the verdict was horrendous, one of the worst days in his life. Time seemed to stand still and he just felt helpless and alone. He knew deep down what the verdict was going to be but still prayed he might be wrong. He wasn't.

When I arrived to collect him, he'd been back from theatre for about twenty minutes. He had only been under the anaesthetic for a very short time but he was still really sleepy. He'd already seen the surgeon and told me he had some bad news. He shed one tear as he told me the news we were both dreading, the first time he'd cried in front of me. Then the consultant, Mr Martin-Hirsch, came in and showed us the x-ray pictures. He said he couldn't believe how Peter's condition had changed so quickly in a few weeks. For the first time the word oncologist was mentioned.

We left the hospital, walking slowly, hands held tightly. Then we had to tell the kids. Obviously they knew he was going for the check-up but they thought it would be good news. They were shattered but brave, asked a few questions and then left it at that. They were very quiet for a while. I printed lots of information from the Internet and told Peter, Charlotte and Oliver where it was if they wanted to read it. Both kids asked a lot more questions over the next couple of weeks although Peter dug his head into the sand. If either of the kids asked him if he was going to be all right, he just said, "Of course I will be, I'm Peter Jackson!"

He was doing his best to be positive in front of me and the kids but I could see that inside he was frightened to death. I wanted him to open up, to tell me what his real feelings were but that's never been his style. He sees it as his duty to remain strong in front of the family. My 50th birthday on February 10th was particularly difficult for him. We went out for a meal with all the family but he was far quieter than usual and when we got home, he disappeared upstairs. He later told me he'd been crying, sitting on the bed and telling himself he was too young to die.

Peter went back to Lincoln and I stayed on at work until we had a week in Tenerife just before he started his treatment on March 13. That was the worst time. The uncertainty. Once we had a full prognosis of what the treatment would be we could be ready to go. But the waiting seemed interminable. I would just burst into tears for no reason. I could see people were shocked. Alison burst into tears? No, she's the strong one, hard as a rock.

And once the treatment started, I was. It became a mission. I was going to put my own life on hold and look after him from start to finish. See it through. I convinced myself he would get better and then we'd go back to living a normal life. It was like a military operation. Plan it, work out how long it's going to take, know what's likely to be coming our way and what the outcome will be if all goes to plan. And then get on with it. I never had any doubts about whether I should be doing it. None at all.

Peter's Story

I was diagnosed with throat cancer on January 16. In early February, I was told I'd have to undergo twenty sessions of radiotherapy over a four-week period, starting in March. I was going to be away from Lincoln for the rest of the season and beyond so needed to find someone to take over while I was away. Someone I could trust with my life. Someone like Iffy Onuora, my former team-mate at Huddersfield Town, who was an experienced and highly-qualified coach and had also been caretaker-manager at Swindon and Gillingham. Iffy is not just one of my best mates, he's a beautiful person and I knew I could reply on him absolutely while I was away.

He was one of a small group of people who knew I had cancer. Alison and the kids knew, so did Steff Wright. So did Neil McDonald, my number two, who would have stepped in while I was away but instead opted to join Leeds United, where Gary McAllister had just been appointed manager, as first team coach. But otherwise it was a closely-guarded secret that very soon would have to go out into the public domain.

That time came before training on February 14, Valentine's Day of all things, when I introduced Iffy to the squad as Neil's successor. I called all 25 players into the dressing room and said, "This is Iffy Onuora, my new number two. In fact, he'll be more than a number two for the rest of the season. I've got throat cancer and in two weeks' time I'll be starting four weeks of radiotherapy treatment. The doctors say I've got a good chance of making a full recovery but I won't be around again until the summer at the earliest. Iffy will be in charge until I come back." The players were stunned. I broke down. It was awful.

By the time we returned from training, my cancer was public knowledge. The place was awash with television crews, radio men, newspaper reporters, all wanting an interview. I'd always enjoyed being the centre of attention as a manager. I'd usually gone along with any request for an interview and been ready to go the extra mile with the media because I believed virtually any publicity was good publicity for the club. But not this. I simply couldn't face touting around from one interview to the next so I asked everyone if they would agree to one interview on camera that they could all use. Even that was an ordeal.

I couldn't believe the reaction. Soon after I arrived home that night, there was a knock on the door. I vaguely recognised the chap standing there, a Huddersfield fan. He just stood there crying. He never said a word. One of Alison's workmates told her how, on the same night, she'd gone into a pub in a village just outside Huddersfield. She was sitting in the bar with a friend when the sports newsreader said on television that Lincoln manager Peter Jackson had been diagnosed with throat cancer. Apparently two women in the bar burst into tears. Two women I suppose I'd never met in my life and almost certainly will never meet in the future. No one can have any idea how humbling things like that can be.

Normally a person's serious illness is a private matter for himself, his family and friends but for a while, it seemed as if mine was everyone else's business, too. The cards and emails started arriving the next day. I thought there might be a few, mainly from Huddersfield. And perhaps some from Newcastle and Bradford, although I was still regarded as a villain there because of my Huddersfield connections. But there were hundreds of goodwill messages from all over the country, a lot from people I'd never met who'd been through a similar ordeal or nursed a loved one back to health. And more from Bradford than anywhere else.

One of my first callers was Jimmy Armfield, the former England captain and Leeds United manager and one of the best-known voices in football in his role as a BBC radio summariser. Jim was recovering from throat cancer himself and to know one of the game's most respected figures was rooting for me meant so much.

Lincoln's first game after the news broke was at Rotherham. I drove to the ground straight from home and arrived before the team coach. Then, after handing in the teamsheet to the referee, I went for a coffee in the boardroom with Steff. On my way back to the dressing room, I was stopped by loads of Rotherham fans, all wishing me well. One woman was in tears and gave me a big kiss. Another chap came over and said, "Peter, I've always admired you as a player and manager. Good luck, we're with you all the way." Then he shook my hand and a group of fans around him gave me a round of applause. It really was a moving moment.

I went into the dressing room, gave the players their team talk, watched as they went out for what would be my last away game for the foreseeable future and then followed them out of the tunnel. I was greeted by a barrage of, "Peter Jackson is a w****r, is a w****r!" And who was leading the chorus? The chap who'd just wished me all the best on behalf of the Rotherham fans! And would you believe, after the match, he made a point of coming over and shaking my hand again...but maybe that was because we'd lost 3-2, ending our run of five straight wins.

My last game was against Wycombe Wanderers at Sincil Bank a week later. They were going well under Peter Taylor and ended the season in the play-offs. After our winning run, we were flying, too, and before the match, Steff presented me with the Coca Cola League Two Manager of the Month award, with the players lined up behind us. The fans gave me a tremendous reception as I walked to the dug-out and I was presented with a good luck card from the supporters. It was the size of a settee, with what looked like thousands of signatures. Someone had written, "Jacko, I hope you don't die, you're too much of a legend!"

In my team talk, I said to the players, "Please, it's my last game. Go out and win it for me." And they did. Those lads gave me everything against a good side and we sneaked it with a late goal from Louis Dodds. I was in tears as I thanked them afterwards and then I invited them all into my office for a drink. I'd put a few cans of beer in the fridge. As I handed round the drinks, I noticed they were all shuffling around a bit and realised there was going to be a speech of some kind. I thought, "Oh no, more tears..." Eventually Scott Kerr, the captain, said, "Well, all the best gaffer. On behalf of the players, I'd like to thank you for this and that..."

"This and that, Scott," I chipped in. "What's this and that?" That broke the ice a bit and kept my tears away. And then Scott presented me with a pair of Gucci cufflinks and a Hugo Boss tie. It was a lovely gesture because those players weren't on thousands of pounds a week and had made a bit of a sacrifice for me. Eventually we all said our farewells and the players drifted off. But as Alison was driving me away from the ground, with my Manager of the Month award on my lap, I couldn't help thinking, "I may never be coming back." It was a long drive home.

I'll never forget the support I received from Steff, the players and everyone at Lincoln City. And from the wider football world as well. All those cards and messages told me how many people were behind me and I went into my treatment thinking it would be a breeze. I was very wrong there but I've no doubt that the support I received from Lincoln and everwhere else helped me pull through in the end.

12. Alison's diary

Alison kept a diary throughout Peter's treatment and recovery. "I wanted to write a true life, day-to-day account about the 20 days of radiotherapy and what we thought would be a 20-day recovery period. In fact, Peter was much worse than we had expected and was in recovery for 38 days. When his cancer was first diagnosed we had hundreds of letters and emails from people who had been through a similar experience. Their support helped us enormously and I wanted to do something that might help other people in the same way in the future. Something like writing a diary…"

Peter: *"I've never been able to bring myself to read it. I don't know if I ever will."*

Wednesday, March 12:

We arrived back from Tenerife at 1am. Five star hotel with spa, sauna, everything to help us wind down. With all the media attention and organising Peter's treatment, we were both drained and needed to recharge the batteries. On the first day, Peter just slept on a sunbed and soon had a suntan he swore made him look like George Clooney. I wasn't so sure! Instead I ensured he was well covered in a high sun factor and applied sun block every hour to his lip. It was coloured pink, but he didn't seem to mind. We had lots of walks, ate well, didn't drink too much alcohol and enjoyed a lot of early nights. But, just as we were trying to forget our problems, Peter's voice would prove a constant reminder of the cancer. It seems to be getting worse and I struggle to understand what he is saying sometimes, which can get a bit frustrating for both of us. When he has his back to me or is speaking through a wall or door, I really find it difficult. I try not to mention it too much, but I do just say 'yes' quite a lot of the time. And although his throat is sore most of the time, he does not like taking painkillers. I don't push him to take any now but I'm sure it will be a very different matter when the treatment starts.

Thursday, March 13: Day Zero

Day Zero at St James's. This is it, the treatment is about to get under way. We arrived early, read the papers and Peter took the opportunity to make a few football phone calls. Even when he is preparing for radiotherapy, Lincoln City still manages to dominate his thoughts.

We checked into reception and then went to sit in a quiet room, while Peter waited for his turn to undergo treatment in room number nine. We're going to see a lot more of the quiet room and room number nine over the next few weeks.

The duty radiographer introduced herself, telling us she would be part of

Smile, please! Alison (left), aged two, with her elder sister, Lizzy.

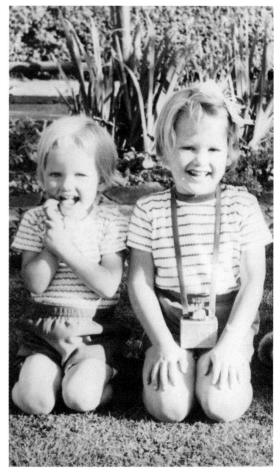

Beside the seaside. Alison (second right) with Lizzy, Mark, Paul and Jonathan on a family holiday in Filey.

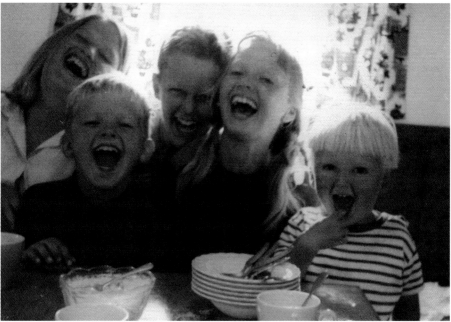

New girl. Alison's first day at Shelf County Primary School, aged nine.

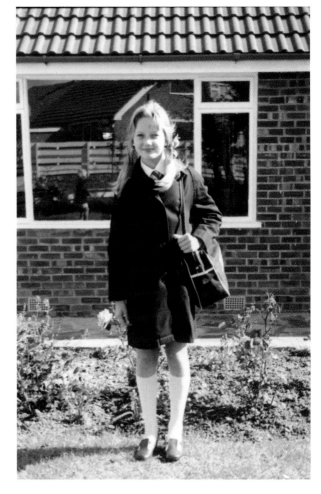

Flares and floaty hair. Alison (right) aged 14, with lifelong friend Christine Patterson.

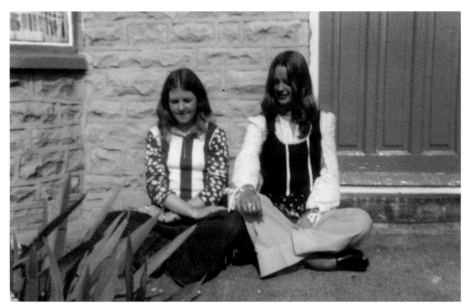

Carry on, nurse! Alison (right) embarks on her career as a student nurse at Bradford Royal Infirmary in 1976.

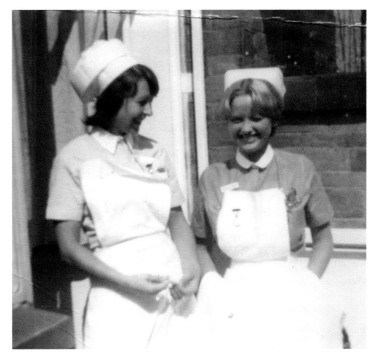

Happy couple. Peter and Alison celebrate their engagement at Silks wine bar in Bradford on December 13, 1980.

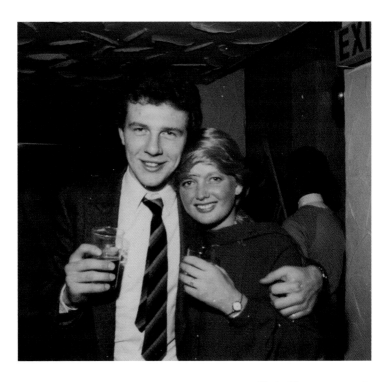

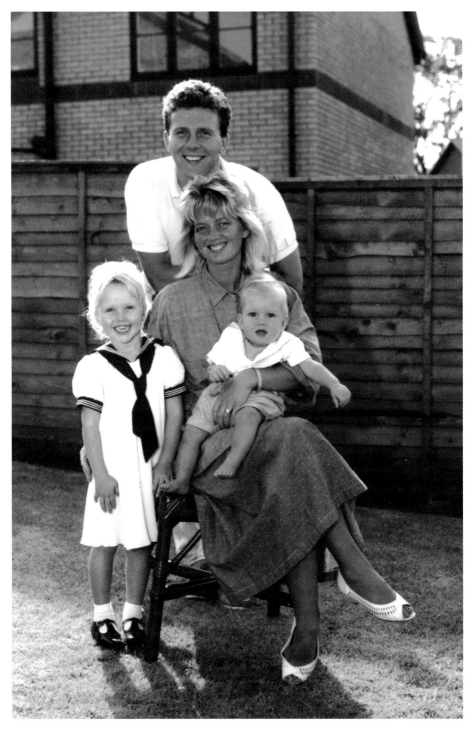

Footballer's wife. Alison with Peter, Charlotte and Oliver at home in Gosforth during their two-year stay on Tyneside.

Back home.
Oliver's first day
at St Michael's
Junior and Infants
School, Brighouse,
after the family
moved into their
new home.

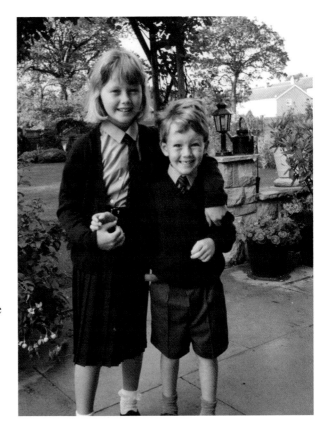

Model family: In 1994, the
Jacksons were named
Family of the Year in a
competition run by
Petroleum jeans – which
explains why they are all
wearing their gear!
(Halifax Courier)

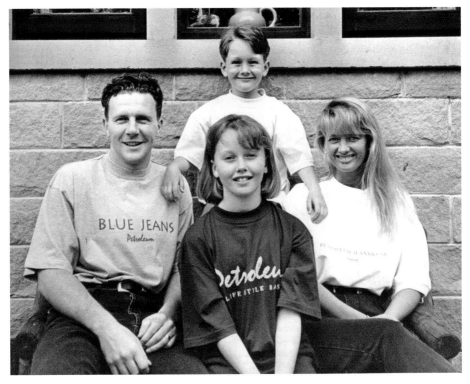

Samba time. Brazil star Emerson with Oliver, Chester's mascot in an FA Cup-tie at Middlesbrough in January, 1997.

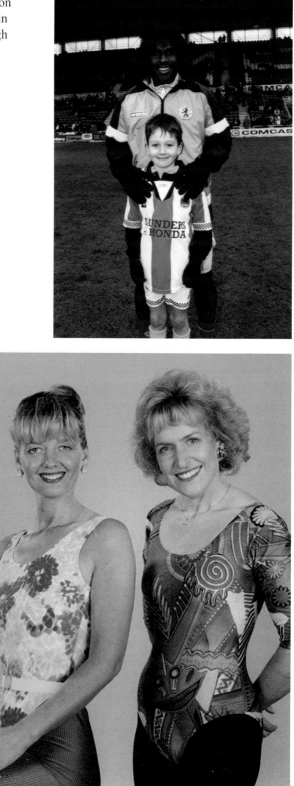

Ladies in Lycra. Alison and Rosemary Conley. (Rosemary Conley Diet & Fitness)

Getting to know you. Rosemary Conley with Charlotte and Oliver on a family day at Rosemary's HQ in Leicestershire.

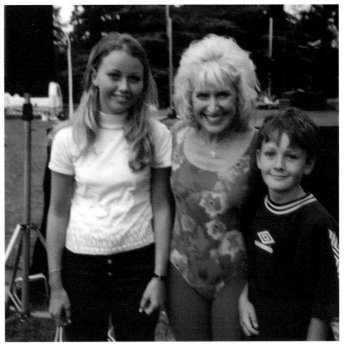

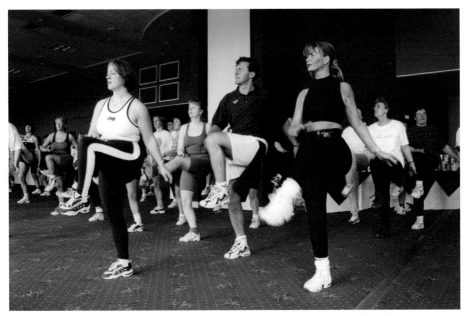

A rose among thorns. Best foot forward for Peter at a Rosemary Conley day at the McAlpine Stadium during Peter's first spell as Huddersfield manager. (Huddersfield Examiner)

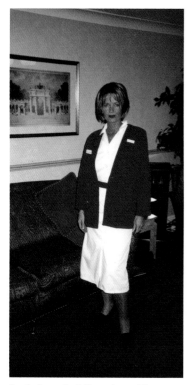

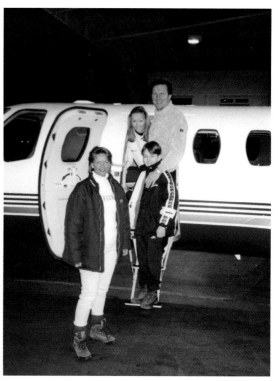

Lady in red. Alison in uniform during her spell as manageress of the Clarins counter at a Halifax department store.

Jet setters. Setting out on a ski-ing weekend in the private jet owned by Barry Rubery, who bought Huddersfield Town in 1999 during Peter's first stint as manager.

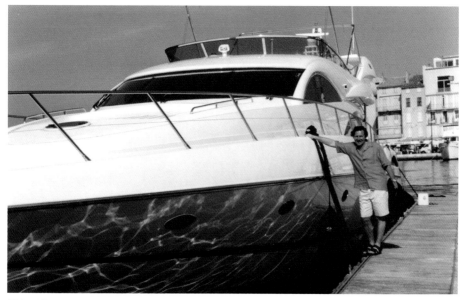

Ship Ahoy! Peter's 38th birthday present from Barry Rubery was a weekend aboard his luxury yacht in the south of France.

Words of wisdom. Peter and Charlotte, during her Television Production and Media Studies course at Huddersfield University, where she produced a programme about her father, the football manager.

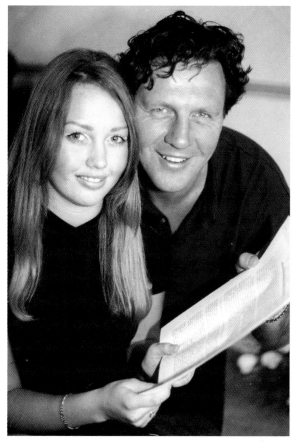

Over my shoulder. Alison learns all about the fireman's lift while training as aircrew for JMC Airline in 2002.

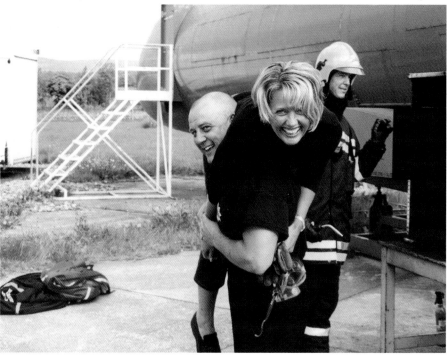

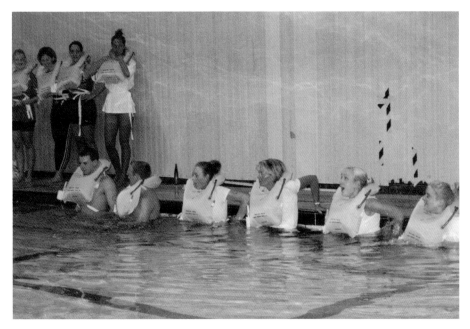

In the swim. More aircrew training for Alison (third from right), this time on water survival.

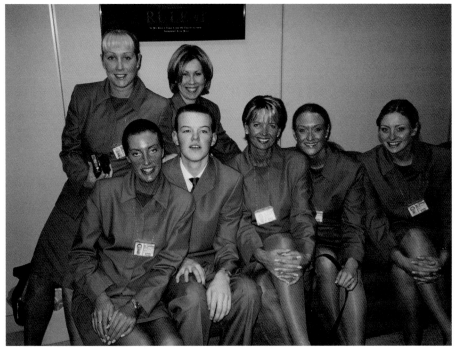

Meet the team. Alison with her JMC colleagues after gaining their 'wings' as qualified cabin crew.

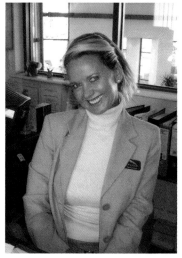

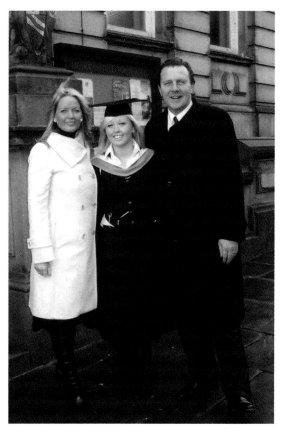

Corporate lady. Alison after her appointment as corporate sales manager for Appleyard Jaguar in Bradford in 2004 (Appleyard Jaguar).

The graduate. With Charlotte on her graduation day in 2004.

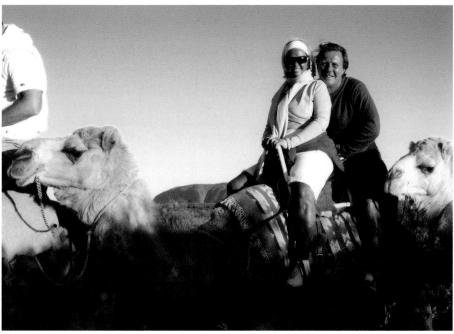

On top Down Under. Taking a camel ride at Ayers Rock in the Australian outback in 2007.

Dark Days. Peter had to be fed though a nasal tube during his recovery from throat cancer treatment, which started in March 2008.

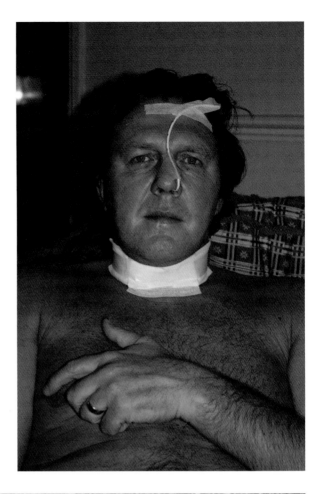

Struggling on. Peter with the 'Roy Cropper' backpack feeding device he renamed after the Coronation Street character.

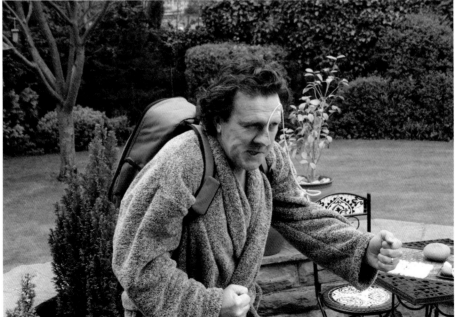

Leap of faith. Peter bouncing back during a break in Cornwall after his treatment, May 2008

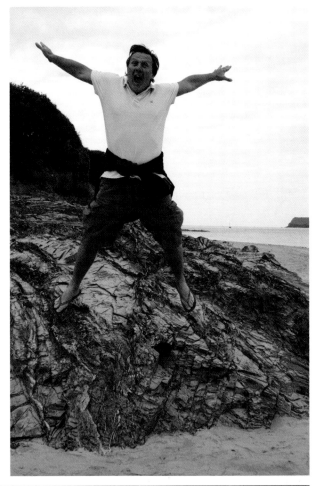

When you're smiling. A breather on a coastal walk at Rock in Cornwall as Peter and Alison near the end of the nightmare.

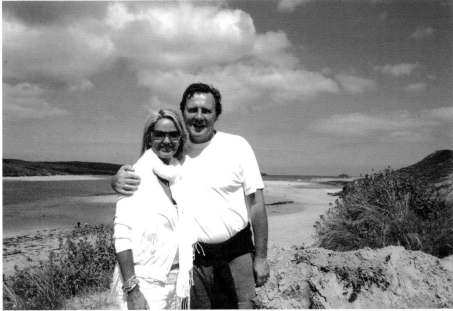

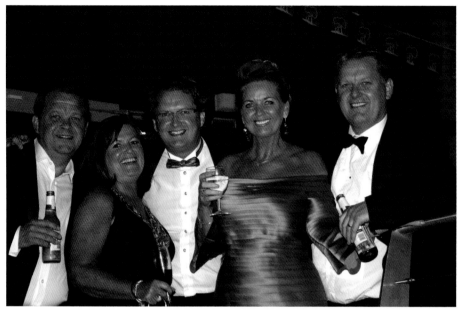

Happy families 1. Mark, Lizzy, Jonathan, Alison and Paul celebrate Oliver's engagement.

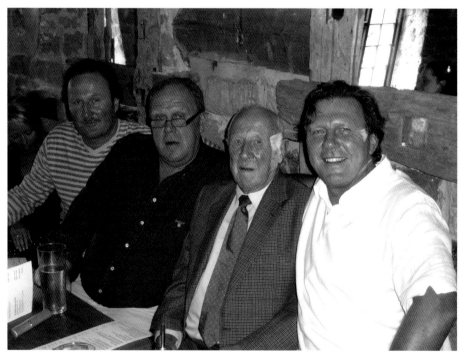

Happy families 2. Peter with his father and brothers Gerrard (left) and Anthony.

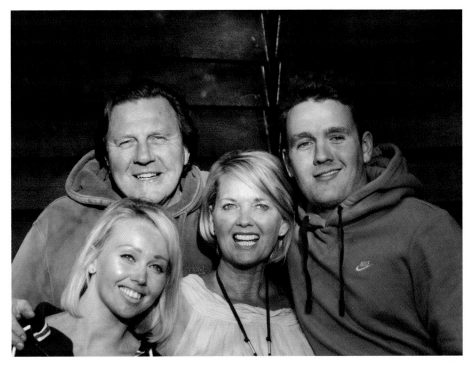

Happy families 3. Peter and Alison with Charlotte and
Oliver during a break at Center Parcs, April 2011.

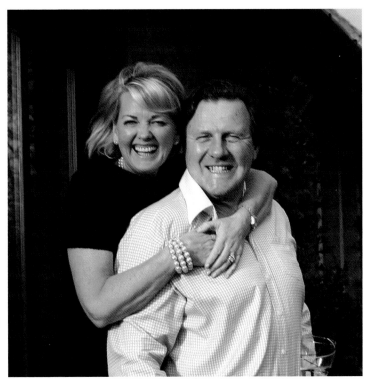

Two's company.
Party mood as
Peter and Alison
join the
celebrations for
their close friend
Christine
Deegan's
birthday.

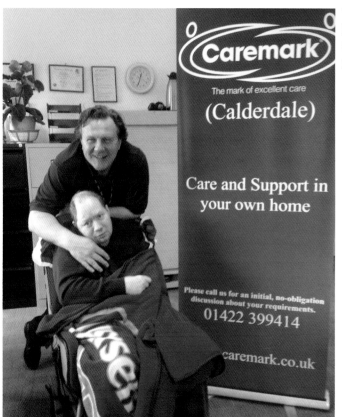

The Dean and me: Peter on duty at Caremark with his pal Dean Cornwall.

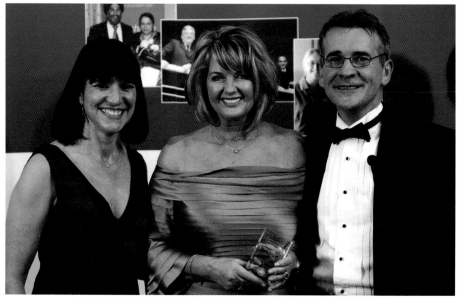

And the award goes to… Alison, with fellow winners Karen Pennington and Sean Cragg collects the Caremark north regional award at the company's annual conference in January 2012. (Caremark)

a team of five who would be looking after us. She ran through everything meticulously. We already knew what we were facing, but she asked if we had any further questions.

As part of the treatment, she handed Peter some aqueous cream to use at least twice a day throughout the next month. The radiotherapy will leave the skin as badly burnt on the outside as it is on the inside and the cream is to moisturize the skin around the throat area.

We were given the treatment schedule for what will be the next 20 appointments. The times vary every day, so it will be difficult to adopt any kind of routine. Today will be the longest time Peter will spend in his mask, with the final scans carried out, the areas and dose carefully planned and the mask marked.

He emerged after 20 minutes and said the only frustrating thing was a tickle on his nose which he couldn't scratch as his arms had to be kept by his side. Also, when he takes his two front teeth out, he discovers that he needs to swallow more which, again, is difficult as you really cannot move when you are pinned down to the table.

Strangely, they asked him to confirm his name and date of birth with the mask on. He said he was able to mutter something, which knowing him as well as I do, I'm sure they were all glad they couldn't understand!

The radiographers said he did very well; I was pleased about that as Peter's boredom threshold is unbelievably short. And they can stop the treatment at any time if he feels claustrophobic when he's strapped down with a mask on and can't move.

Peter never lets the anxiety and stress show. Indeed, his sense of humour is razor sharp. The nurses told him he looks well after his holiday and his response was that he'd show them his white bits if they wanted. They politely declined the offer.

As we were walking out of the main oncology reception, Peter's brother, Gerard, was waiting for us. He is doing some demolition work at another building in the hospital and was wearing his yellow high visibility jacket.

It was touching for him to be there, but it was just a usual male conversation. Football, a laugh and a joke, you know, a typical lads' discussion. They did not discuss the illness, but then again men never discuss a lot of the important things in life do they? But just seeing Gerard taking the time to see Peter was actually a very tender moment and meant more than any words.

I have certainly felt a little strange today. Not upset, just glad that it's out of the way. Peter was told he had cancer on January 15; the treatment finally began today. It seems to have taken an eternity with what seemed to be a lifetime of appointments, letters and other correspondence.

Once you get over the shock and devastation of being told the news that nobody ever wants to hear, you want to start treatment immediately. You feel to be wasting valuable time. But now a weight seems to have been lifted.

We are prepared for whatever this month will bring and I'm sure we will cope in a very positive and optimistic way. There is nothing more to wait for, treatment has started.

Friday, March 14: Day One
His first treatment. We had to be at St James' at 1pm and decided to go straight off afterwards to our little weekend retreat on the coast near Bridlington. We had to collect a large cappuccino at the cafe on our way up to the treatment waiting area. Peter is still drinking it red hot - against advice – because scalding the area before treatment is not recommended.

All went well in the treatment room with just a couple of minutes given on each side of the throat. Peter was absolutely fine, although he did have a worse tickle than yesterday. Not in the nose, the groin area! They all laughed when he explained the problem and said they'd seen much worse. He's tanned, looks far too well to be poorly, thinks this is going to be a doddle and cannot see what all the fuss is about! He insists he won't have any adverse effects throughout his treatment. We shall see.

Saturday, March 15
Bridlington is no Tenerife, but who cares? The sun is shining, the birds are singing and this wonderful, quaint seaside town is a beautiful place to be. What makes it even better, is Peter's health is almost as glorious as the weather. Apart from his voice being hoarse, he is my normal, bubbly, cheeky husband, whose sense of humour is as sharp as the sea air.

Perhaps, on any other occasion, I would never do this, but I actually spent the day giving Peter a pedicure. As you would expect from a professional footballer and manager, his feet have seen a lot of action over the years but this isn't some attempt at a makeover - it's actually an important exercise. He has a cracked heel and, as the immune system can sometimes be affected by the treatment, I don't want it to turn nasty. Prevention is better than a cure.

Sunday, March 16
Another lovely day…and nobody has rung since we've been here. When you are married to a football manager, you also become married to his mobile phone. Sad, but true. Sometimes, it just never stops. Chairmen, assistants, players, journalists and other managers all ring at some point. So it's nice when it stops.

We made the most of the weather and embarked on a long walk down the beach. The sweeping noise of the waves was very calming and I wish the tide could just have taken our problems and dumped them out in the North Sea.

Peter seems fine, although I've noticed that if he doesn't want to do something, or if he can't be bothered, he will use his Dr Dooker excuse. The doctor in question is actually Dr Dyker, the oncology consultant at St James's.

She is in charge of Peter's care and he really likes her. She has explained everything very clearly, making sure he understands every detail of his treatment. Having worked as a nurse, I know how the medical jargon can become extremely confusing and sometimes I've had to explain to Peter just what some of the doctors are saying.

But Dr Dyker is different. She keeps it very simple and seems to like Peter's cheeky personality. But since his first consultation, if I want to go somewhere and he doesn't fancy it, he'll say, "Dr Dooker has told me this is not good for my health."

He's now decided to take this to the extreme and the words Dr Dooker are uttered around 20 times a day, like a stuck record. But anybody who knows Peter will tell you this is what he can be like.

He refuses to do chores like taking out the rubbish; Dr Dooker has advised him not to. There's lots of homemade lasagne left and I ask Peter if he'll have some for his lunch. No, Dr Dooker says he can't have it two days running. Can he put some pebbles in the garden? No, Dr Dooker says they are too heavy. It's driving me up the wall. But I suppose when he stops muttering, "Dr Dooker says", I will begin to worry.

Monday, March 17: Day Two
He's still eating and drinking OK. It's something I have to constantly monitor, especially if he starts to feel pain swallowing. If so, he'll need painkillers.

On our way back from treatment, we called into Huddersfield to look at a table I'd seen earlier in the month. I couldn't find the shop as Peter was being very impatient, telling me it was too far to go. It was only a two-minute walk, but Peter said he was too tired and Dr Dooker wouldn't be happy with it.

I'm not really sure how tired he is, but it seems early days to me. I bet if we'd been looking for a new suit it would have been a different story, although when we got back home, he did sleep for 90 minutes.

It's clear that he's already getting frustrated at not being able to work. He says he feels too well not to be at his office. Perhaps he is missing the banter and the camaraderie. He enjoys all the interaction with the players and he has taken to the Lincoln job like a duck to water.

He loves working there but I have to tell him that he just cannot go back. If he was working nearby, then perhaps he could get away with it. But when he's tired, a 90-minute drive to Lincoln would be impossible. It's eating away at him, but it's for his own good.

And his mood isn't helped because he's had some acid reflux today. A couple of Gaviscon tablets. His voice is particularly bad at the moment but the throat is only sore down the right-hand side and not too bad. Only a couple of paracetamol are needed.

I could tell he was a little touchy today, which I guess is all down to a combination of not being able to work, having a bad day with his voice and other little factors that are building up. Not wanting to upset him any further, I just agreed with everything he had to say. I know he must be feeling some emotion and I just wish he would open up.

If he did, then perhaps I could help him with his problems. Has he never heard of a problem shared is a problem halved? But that's typical Peter. He is not forthcoming about discussing any feelings he may have. It's an impenetrable fortress to break into.

He's not a robot, though, and I know he has worries, just like everybody else. He won't lose any face by telling me so every time I ask if he's OK, I just get the same old response. "Yes, I'm fine."

Tuesday, March 18: Day Three

A lovely sunny morning and the perfect opportunity for Peter to cut the grass and trim some bushes. He's a bit of a green fingers, an Alan Titchmarsh in the making. When we bought the house, the garden was his project. Every tree, every bush was planned like some military exercise. It's his pride and joy and it's beautiful to look at.

He caused me some concern though, because when I peered out of the bedroom window to see how he was getting on, he'd clambered up to the top of a large wall, with an electric hedge-cutter in his hand. One foot was on the wall, the other on a bush. Thankfully he survived. I don't want another trip to the hospital if I can help it!

We arrived at the hospital in good time and have now developed a routine. We park the car in the multi-storey car park, go into the shop to pick up a copy of The Sun - it's good for sport, but not much else - and a red hot cappuccino with brown sugar sprinkled on top.

We then head into the lift down to floor minus 2. It's a bit like Groundhog Day as, every day, we seem to pass the same people, all having treatment of some kind. We had to wait 45 minutes as one of the machines had broken in the morning so there was a backlog of patients.

Peter said he felt tired but I think he just meant he was bored. He said he might just have a little nap on the floor while waiting and complained that beds should be provided. I hoped he was joking - you never can tell!

Since suffering problems with his throat, Peter has become very intolerant of smokers, despite having been one himself. He now hates everyone who puffs on a cigarette. He blames the fags for making him ill and cannot hide his disgust for the cancer sticks, which, in effect, is what they are. In Tenerife last week, if anyone was smoking nearby, even outside a restaurant, he gave them a filthy look and complained about the smoke if it wafted into our area. It used to be the other way around.

What does amaze him, though, is when we walk into the main reception entrance to the oncology unit there are always two or three patients in dressing gowns and slippers standing with a chemotherapy drip stand in one hand and a cigarette in the other.

This is in temperatures of three degrees. Walking from the car park to the main door is just like being in a wind tunnel. I'm fully clothed and really cold so they must be desperate. They probably think they are getting a breath of fresh air! Don't they realise what they are doing to their bodies? It's just unbelievable. Nicotine has to be most the addictive drug ever.

I went to see our own GP today to get Peter some medication for the gastric reflux, which seems to be getting worse. He needs a lot of Gaviscon, which doesn't really help any more. This condition can be aggravated by stress and he told me today that he had vomited some bile yesterday teatime.

That's not too worrying at the moment but it will be difficult to vomit in the next couple of weeks when his throat gets sore. The doctor prescribed Mepradec, which reduces the amount of acid produced in the stomach, and it seems to be working already.

He's tired tonight as he hasn't slept all day. But he's eating and drinking normally and I'm still applying lots of cream to his neck, three to four times a day. There's no redness yet.

And me? I spoke to work today and told them that I could return on May 1. They are all very understanding and keep in regular contact. I really don't know where the time goes. How did I ever work full-time? Life does seem a bit unreal at the moment.

Wednesday, March 19: Day Four

My boss Chris came to see me for a chat. My colleagues have been fantastic and are so supportive. I confirmed that I hoped to be back on May 1, but it all very much depends on how Peter is feeling. I intend to keep them all updated every couple of weeks.

Peter had a meeting with Steff Wright, the Lincoln chairman, and looked incredibly smart. He was tanned, his hair was slicked back and he looked the business. He looked far too healthy and I sometimes think he feels a bit of a fraud because he thinks he should be very ill. He was home at 3.30, just in time to set off for 5pm treatment.

On our way in, we were stopped by a Huddersfield Town supporter who had just been diagnosed with bowel cancer. His treatment was to be chemotherapy, radiation for seven weeks then surgery. He wore his Huddersfield sweatshirt in case he bumped into Peter.

Since Peter was diagnosed, the amount of cards and e-mails has been astounding, but there are also tales from people whose lives have been hit by cancer. Iffy Onuora, his assistant at Lincoln, called this morning and brought another stack of goodwill messages. I had a quick glance through, and noticed one was from a girl I know, Jean. Her husband had just completed his radiotherapy treatment for a brain tumour.

Thursday, March 20: Day Five

That's a quarter of the treatment done. Peter slept fine last night but his mouth is getting very dry and he sleeps with a bottle of water at the side of the bed. His throat still just feels sore and no worse than before the treatment started. There are no sign of redness on the neck area as yet and he is still applying the cream religiously, at least five times a day.

Although he feels OK, he's still trying his luck with me. We were getting ready for hospital when he asked if I could iron his jeans. Oliver instantly told him to stop milking it and then posed the ultimate question: "Can't you iron your own?"

Now Peter, being Peter, has never ironed anything in his life. Men just don't like ironing full stop. When it comes to tinkering with the garden or a bit of DIY that's not a problem. Ironing, however, is a big no-no.

But Oliver was just trying to point out that he could do something for himself if he put his mind to it. I've run about non-stop after him today and must have clocked up more miles than a marathon runner. I know he's ill, but when he's like this, he'd test the patience of Job.

This morning, it was: Can I make him a boiled egg? Followed by two cups of coffee (not quite strong enough). Where is his white T shirt (no, not that one, you know which one I mean). He has about 25 white T shirts.

It's been one of those days where I have to grit my teeth, wear a smile and simply get on with it. Yesterday he wasn't tired at all as the whole day was football-related and he was busy doing something he loves. Today, however, he cannot do anything, mainly because Dr Dooker says it would be bad for his health. Dr Dooker has a lot to answer for and we've only seen her once.

While we were waiting for his treatment, two old men checked into reception. One was pushing the other in a wheelchair. They both looked ancient and, to be honest, we were not really too sure who the poorly one was. When the receptionist asked him his name and date of birth, we couldn't help overhearing.

"How old does that make him?" Peter asked.

"Exactly 20 years older than me, and 23 years older than you."

"Jesus. Let's just blow all our money and really enjoy ourselves while we're young enough."

I sat and pondered. Will we be like that in 20 years' time? Seeing them made us realise how time is running out for everybody. Present situation excluded, we have really enjoyed our life and neither of us has anything to go back for. But it makes you think: is there anything else we really want to do?

It seems there's never a right time. The children are too young, the children are at school, we're putting them through university, saving up for them to get married, looking after the grandchildren. Then we're too old and ill and it's too late! But I'm certainly not complaining.

Having left the two old men, our next move was to see the nurse, Ellen. Peter said he didn't want to waste her time as surely she had some really ill people to see. He told her that we had to rush off to make our next appointment…what he didn't say was that we were going to meet his brother Anthony in Ilkley and it really wouldn't matter if we were late.

She asked him to sit down. She has to assess his health at the start of the treatment so she can closely regulate and record it throughout. He said he was fine and didn't plan on any side effects.

Anthony is the loveliest man you could ever meet and he's always there for Peter. They are very close and speak at least three times a week. Cath, his wife, has a wicked sense of humour. If ever you need cheering up then this is the couple you turn to.

Anthony has his own demolition and stone business and has done very well for himself and his family, although he has worked extremely hard over the years. He is now 53 and slightly overweight - well probably a few stone!

He has never been ill in his life then last week he woke up in the morning and felt numbness and tingling in his arm and down the side of his face. He was admitted to hospital and discharged the next day with appointments for various tests.

Thankfully he is OK and everything is back to normal. Apart from being slightly tired there are no other effects. He stopped smoking immediately, went on a diet and must drink in moderation and do more exercise. Let's just hope he heeds the warning.

Another question pops into my head: are we now at that age when everyone is starting to be ill?

Friday, March 21: No treatment

Good Friday. I needed to buy Peter an electric shaver as he is now not allowed to wet shave his neck and throat because it will cause irritation. In time, the area will become very sensitive.

But Peter is a well-manicured man. He likes his suits, his nice ties and keeps himself in pristine condition. So I don't know how he will react to not being able to have a wet shave. He says the electric shaver is a load of rubbish and he doesn't need it. I wasn't going to let him win. I bought it anyway.

When we arrived home, the first thing he did was have a shower and a shave. Yes, a wet shave. A wet shave that included his throat area. Is he ever going to listen? He was tired afterwards and went to bed for two hours in the afternoon. Radiation does make you very tired and that side effect is certainly kicking in.

Then we had some chicken for tea, which was really tasty. Charlotte and Oliver agreed but Peter said it didn't taste of anything. So maybe his taste is being affected now.

In the evening, the home phone starts to ring, family and friends checking if Peter is OK. All football calls usually come through on the mobile. It can be tiring repeating the same thing over and over again, but it's lovely that lots of people are so concerned.

Sometimes I bump into people in the supermarket or in town and they ask how Peter is. They say they haven't phoned as they don't know what to say. But why don't they just phone and say they are sorry to hear of his illness and how is he? Some people are frightened that you may burst into tears. Mind you, if they had asked me a couple of weeks ago that's probably what I would have done.

Saturday, March 22: Day Six

Easter Saturday and a layer of snow on the ground! As we are travelling straight to Bridlington for the weekend, Peter is wearing his comfortable training gear and looks more like he's about to go training with his players than undergo his sixth treatment of radiotherapy.

On the way out, he asks if the doctors have got the results, the biopsies, scans and diagnosis wrong as he feels too well to be ill. He thinks they have him mixed up with somebody else. We're only on day six and he's bored now.

Lincoln had a match against Barnet and he felt he should have been there. He doesn't realise he's feeling so well because he's sleeping when he wants to and is completely stress free. If he was working and travelling, it would not be a breeze. However any hopes of relaxing were soon dashed as Peter watched the football on TV all afternoon. When the half-time score came in, Lincoln were losing 3-0 and were beaten 5-2. Peter was desperate to know just what had been going on and afterwards, he was on the phone, finding out who played well, who didn't.

Monday, March 24: No Treatment

Still a lot of snow on the ground, which made for some lovely walks. Peter's mood was also lifted because Lincoln beat Hereford…and with only 10 men. It was a great result against one of the better teams in the league. He is particularly delighted for Iffy after the defeat at Barnet. His throat is now sounding very sore, but he says it's OK. He's still managing to eat and drink normally and sleeping well at night. But his mouth is feeling very dry during the night.

Tuesday, March 25: Day Seven

Went for a walk on the beach for an hour. It's only five minutes' away. This is a place where you can forget all your troubles, relax, chill out, take in the sea air and just find a few moments' peace. Peter was a little quiet and that is not like him. Maybe he gets fed up of having to repeat himself every time he speaks.

We passed about six people walking their dogs and they all said good morning, Peter greets them back but I don't think they can hear him. They probably think he's a miserable git with such a lovely cheerful wife!

We arrived in Leeds in time for our 2.12 appointment. Both the quiet rooms were in use so we sat in the reception waiting area. Peter drank his normal hot cappuccino, still insisting there is nothing wrong with him apart from a sore throat.

We waited with some frail and ill-looking patients. People just nod at each other and sit down and wait their turn, reading magazines and doing the crossword. There was a young girl waiting with her parents and wearing a headscarf, obviously because she's having chemotherapy as well as radiotherapy.

"There's always somebody more ill than you," Peter says. There is, but it still feels very strange that the only person you are really bothered about is your loved one. I'm sure they all feel the same.

Leaving the car park, we waved to the man who lifts the automatic barrier for us. He sits in a little box behind a window and he can see on his monitor who is leaving. He must start to recognise people who are daily patients. But each time he just lifts the barrier and looks very frostily at us.

We always wave and smile but his mean expression never changes. Still, we'll carry on waving and smiling for the next 13 treatments and see if we get a smile. We're probably wasting our time but persistence usually pays off. Why are some people so miserable?

After lunch, Peter said it is now very painful to swallow. But he's still refusing analgesia and that frustrates me because he is clearly in pain. You can tell by the look on his face that he is finding it difficult. His voice is now very quiet and it's really difficult to hear if I'm not actually looking at him. His dad, who is nearly 80, can hardly hear him at all on the phone…but he is slightly deaf anyway.

Peter's tired but he keeps fighting it. I sent him for a lie down upstairs away from the telephone and he had an hour's sleep before the children arrived home from work. He says we'll go back to Bridlington on Saturday night but I'm not really sure if he will be well enough.

I suggest he may be finding it more uncomfortable to swallow and he may be feeling more tired with the effects of radiation by then. But he says he'll be fine and it's not going to affect him like it affects everyone else. No point arguing. If he wants to go and he's well enough, which I hope he is, then that's fine with me.

At 9pm, he wanted some pâté on toast and ate it watching TV. He didn't know I was watching him but it looked pretty painful to me. I suggested he had some paracetamol and he said it might be a good idea.

In fact, he could hardly talk at all this evening and was speaking in a very frustrated whisper. Charlotte thinks he is much worse than he was a couple of days ago. I decided that ice cream may help…and remembered that he had to eat it with a small spoon not a big one. I was told off about that last time. Dr Dooker said so.

When my dad was ill with prostate cancer a few years ago, Mum served him a yoghurt as a dessert after his tea. He looked at her in disgust because she had served it in the pot. She had to go back into the kitchen and put the yoghurt into a dish. I couldn't believe she had done as he asked, but now I completely understand – anything to make life easier.

Peter ate very quietly but I could tell he was in pain when he swallowed. He decided to call it a day and went to bed at 10pm. I applied lots of cream to his throat, which still does not look red. He needs a shave tomorrow so let's see which razor he'll use. I think I can guess.

Wednesday, March 26: Day Eight
His voice has totally gone. I have been able to hear a faint whisper trying to shout "Ali" from which ever room in the house he is in, but hearing him is nigh on impossible. I have suggested he claps his hands when he needs me then I can stand in front of him and lip-read.

We started the new system at 9am and he got the hang of it pretty quickly. An hour later and the house sounded like the bloody London Palladium. I can see this suggestion may not have been a good idea. It's OK if he really needs me, but not for, "Can I have another cup of coffee?" I think to myself that the treatment is for his throat and not his legs but I still make him one with a loving smile. As only a devoted wife would do!

Steff rang to make arrangements for tonight when Lincoln reserves play at Elland Road. Peter thought he'd be OK to go so after his treatment, I dropped him off in Leeds to meet Steff and Iffy. It was probably the quietest meeting they have ever had.

Thursday, March 27: Day Nine
Peter had some eggs for breakfast but insisted on toast as well. As usual he refused any pain control. Does he believe that I'll think he's a soft touch for having painkillers? It's hardly a sign of male weakness!

He told me that it's just as painful to swallow water as toast, there's no point taking anything. How brave. Perhaps he used to have Sinitta's "So Macho" as his theme tune! He says it's like swallowing razor blades. In the end, I couldn't watch him struggle any further and I reached into the cupboard for two paracetamol. I put them in his hand with a glass of water. He took them without saying a word.

What's the point in not taking them regularly? Why would you want to suffer in pain when simple regular pain control every four hours would alleviate the stress? Hopefully Doctor Dyker can convince him it would be a good idea.

We actually went to see the doctor while we were waiting for treatment. It wasn't Dr Dyker so Peter was very disappointed. But the doctor insisted that he took something regularly for the pain. He prescribed soluble paracetamol, soluble Diclofenac and Mucaine, a local anaesthetic gel to be taken 10-20 minutes before eating and drinking to anaesthetize the throat.

I heard the radiotherapist ask Peter to confirm his date of birth. He answered with January 1, 1983, which would make him 25 years old. She then asked him to confirm his address and he answered Rampton High Security Hospital! He gives her a different date of birth and address each time. She just shakes her head in disbelief.

Most of the journey home was spent with Peter trying to talk, me turning the radio down and saying pardon, Peter repeating himself and turning the radio back up…only to repeat the process about another 15 times before giving up. But you wouldn't know there was anything wrong with him until he tries to speak.

Friday, March 28: Day Ten

At 2am, Peter asked me for some painkillers so the pain must have been bad. I gave him a Diclofac tablet that I already had in the medicine cabinet. Not sure where they came from or even how old they were, but they did the trick and he slept fine.

I gave Peter porridge for breakfast as he couldn't go through the torture of toast like yesterday. I also gave him two paracetamol, which he took without arguing. He finally seems to realise it's a waste of time. If he does reject them, I'll put them in his food or his coffee.

We waited in our quiet room, read the paper and did the crossword together. He always buys the Sun, which I absolutely hate, then gives me a couple of pages out of the middle while he reads the sports pages.

The daily cappuccino has now stopped and is replaced by a bottle of water. Before we set off I always make sure there are at least three bottles of water in the car and one in my handbag. His neck cream is also in my handbag along with painkillers, my diary and his treatment schedule. When we arrived today, he gave me the car keys, the newspaper and a magazine I had brought with me just in case.

Then when we sat down he asked me for his lip cream. I'm not a bloody octopus. Yes I had some - at the bottom of my handbag. I smiled sweetly and, after five minutes' rooting around, I found it for him. Then he decided he wanted some chewing gum. Oh what fun we are having!

Work colleagues have mentioned how well I'm looking and how much weight I've lost. Must be from all the running about after Peter and also the weight of lifting the handbag. Who needs the gym membership he gave me?

As they called Peter in for treatment, a little toddler aged about 18 months was just coming out. It's bad enough when it's your husband having treatment. How on earth must you feel when it's your child? Let's just hope and pray the prognosis is good for them.

Saturday, March 29: Day 11

Past the halfway mark. I don't think he slept very well as normally he starts snoring straight away and that keeps me awake. Although he can only whisper now, the snoring is extremely loud.

He asked me for some more analgesia at 5am but I wanted him to wait until 7am as he really had more than he should yesterday. I had decided to give him paracetamol separately from Diclofenac so he can have some kind of analgesia at 7am, 10.30am, 2pm, 5.30pm, 9pm 12am and 3.30am.

But this regime is not working either so I went to the pharmacy for something stronger than soluble paracetamol. I bought some paracetamol and codeine Soluble so let's see if that works. He doesn't complain, but you can see he is in pain when swallowing and eating is extremely painful now. It's time for a softer diet I think.

At treatment, we chatted to an elderly man whose appointment was for 10.20, two hours after us. He was so early because he has to rely on hospital transport. He has to be ready at 8am and after treatment has to wait to be collected, which can mean sitting around for three to four hours.

I asked him if there was anywhere he could lie down and rest while waiting but there isn't. We felt really dreadful as he lives about four miles from us and normally we would have offered to give him a lift home. But we were going to Bridlington.

We went for a long two-hour walk on the beach and then Peter rested all afternoon in front of the television watching football. Although he has been in denial up to this stage, I think realisation has now kicked in. It is very, very strange to see him so quiet. Not the usual cheeky husband I know.

I have tried to explain that this is what would happen, this is how he would feel and this is about normal at this stage of his treatment. He hasn't listened before because he didn't want to know. Unfortunately there is nothing he can do about it, it's out of his control.

After all the football results came in, with Lincoln losing 4-0 at Peterborough, he snuggled up and had a sleep. Normally he would have been on the phone to everybody at the football club, but he just seems too tired.

Today is my best friend Christine's 50th birthday and we were invited to go out for a meal with her to celebrate. But I knew it wouldn't be possible as Peter cannot talk and has great difficulty in eating…he tried a pint of Guinness this afternoon in the pub after our walk but only managed a mouthful and then resorted to water. A first.

So instead, Christine and I are going to a health farm for the day on Monday, which will be a lovely treat for her and a relaxing time for me. Charlotte will take Peter and it will be nice for her to feel involved. But she absolutely hates hospitals so I am not sure who will be helping who on the day.

Tonight, he looks pale and tired, his throat is very painful and he is now actually asking when his next painkillers are due. He did try his normal glass of white wine but it's like pouring acid on an open wound. So he has come to terms that it was his last glass of wine for a while. And if the look on his face was anything to go by, there can't have been much pleasure in that last one.

Sunday, March 30

My sister Lizzy phoned at about 11am to say that she was on her way over to Bridlington for the day and we arranged to meet her and her boyfriend outside a coffee bar on the harbour at 1pm.

I knew it might be difficult for Peter as he can only speak in a whisper and Lizzy was upset to see him so quiet. As she thought it was really painful for Peter to speak, we only stayed with them for about an hour. But Peter managed to eat a fish on our way back to the car so his new pain regime is working.

When we got back, I discovered I'd lost the key and we couldn't get in. I'd left an electric fire on in the bedroom so we'll have to come back over on Monday for the night. Peter would normally have gone mad about losing a key, but he was very calm and said not to worry, there are worse things in life. He seems very chilled at the moment so I hope I'm not giving him too many painkillers!

As Charlotte is in charge tomorrow, I have written down the times for her to give Peter his analgesia and run through it with her. Peter can't be bothered with remembering anything so trivial.

Monday, March 31: Day 12

I've been feeling very guilty about going to the health farm but Peter insisted and said he would be absolutely fine. The treatment was scheduled for 3pm with an appointment to see Dr Dyker, too. Peter and Charlotte don't often spend much time just the two of them together so it was nice for them to have a catch-up.

They saw the nurse and Dr Dyker first and he explained how sore his throat was feeling. He still insists on calling her Dr Dooker and admitted that every time he couldn't be bothered to do something at home, he says, "Dr Dooker says I can't do that."

On the way out they saw Warwick, the elderly gentleman we had been speaking to on Saturday morning. He was waiting for the hospital transport to take him home and had already been waiting for a couple of hours.

Peter offered him a lift home and when he got into the back of the car, he said, "Peter, there's a key here. Is it important?" It was the key I lost yesterday. We'd searched the car from top to bottom so how on earth it had turned up on the back seat I haven't got a clue.

I had a lovely relaxing day at the health farm in Huddersfield. I phoned Charlotte a couple of times but she said she was managing absolutely fine and not to fuss. We set off back to Bridlington in the evening and luckily everything was OK…although it did feel lovely and warm!

Tuesday, April 1: Day 13

Peter needed pain control in the middle of the night so the oral morphine prescribed by Dr Dyker at his treatment yesterday hadn't seemed to work any better than any other medication. I'd given him a 5ml dose at 11pm.

The journey to Leeds took about one and a half hours, a long time trying to listen and hear what Peter is saying when he is whispering all the time. I am getting into the habit of whispering back and it's giving me a sore throat. So it may well be making his a lot worse.

At the end of treatment they often refer patients for voice coaching but Peter says he won't need it. But as his voice is important to his job I think he will. I told him it would be like physiotherapy for his vocal chords. If a player strains a hamstring he needs physio to speed recovery so why should it be any different for his vocal chords?

On our way out after treatment we looked for Warwick but couldn't see him. We stopped off at Marks and Spencer to pick up soft food and drinks, such as smoothies, yoghurt and ice cream. Had a fairly pain free day apart from a bout of hiccoughs which went on for about 15 minutes and looked extremely painful. Let's try the Morphine again at bedtime and hope it works.

Wednesday, April 2 – Day 14

A dreadful night. He went to bed at about 10.30pm suffering from hiccoughs, which kept getting worse. He was in absolute agony. When he has an attack, I just feel so helpless and he just has to bear it for however long an episode lasts.

Unfortunately, they continued for most of the night and he sat at the side of the bed going absolutely mad and swearing at the hiccoughs. There was nothing I could do, nothing I could say and I'm not sure if just being there stroking his back every now and again helped at all.

I really think this must be a side effect of the morphine as he has only had it for the past two nights. I hope it's not a side effect of the codeine as that is the only thing really helping the pain. Codeine can also make you constipated. I'm not supposed to mention that but I will anyway!

At about 5am I was exhausted and went into Charlotte's bed as she was sleeping at her friend Sadie's house. I gave him paracetamol and codeine before I went. Poor thing. He was exhausted when he got up at 9am. He managed porridge for breakfast. I am trying the Mucaine 20 minutes before eating but he says it doesn't help. I think it does. He says anything he eats feels like swallowing a boiled egg whole, even drinking water.

We were in and out of treatment in no time at all and guess what, we even got a smile from the car park man as we left. Don't know why but I wish it would happen more often. Peter hiccoughed all the way home.

After an afternoon nap, Peter mowed his lawn. It always has to be perfect and in lines. He loves his garden and it's a great way for him to relieve stress and relax during the football season. I sat and watched for a while with a cup of coffee and wondered what he must be thinking. I imagine it was football-related but he did look in a world of his own.

One of our cats, Rudderford, followed him around the garden. We have two beautiful white fluffy pedigree cats, Rudderford and Lucca. They both love loads of attention and are delighted we're both at home with them for so long at the moment.

Rudderford is a Cream Point Burman and he loves Peter to bits. He follows him absolutely everywhere and is more like a dog in some ways. Lucca is a Seal Point Burman, a few years older and a little bit more aloof.

The hiccoughs continued and he continued to swear each time a bout started. He will be swearing in public before long as it's now habit. People will think he has Tourette's Syndrome, where people can't stop themselves swearing.

We now have a scoring system to explain how much pain he is in. When he hiccoughs it is a 10; when he eats, it's anywhere between four and eight. Analgesia is still divided into seven doses per day, but unfortunately we don't now have the morphine to fall back on.

We are seeing the nurse tomorrow to find out if there is anything else that can be prescribed that won't make him hiccough. Although the pain is manageable at the moment, I'm sure it will get worse and we'll need something stronger. Probably this weekend.

On the plus side, I've scored one major success. Peter has made me promise not to mention his bowels but I will anyway. They are definitely not as regular as they should be due to the codeine. He has refused to take anything to help so I keep slipping Syrup of Figs into his medication. It turns the medication to a different colour so I have to pretend it's a liquid vitamin. He asks, "Are you sure you aren't trying to poison me?"

But tonight at 7pm he sloped off to the bathroom. Voila! The "vitamin syrup" seems to have had the desired effect and he is none the wiser. "I told you I didn't need anything," he said triumphantly. If only he knew!

Thursday, April 3: Day 15

Another bad night, but not with the hiccoughs this time. So that was obviously due to the morphine. Now his breathing is a concern. There is lots of mucous gathering at the back of his throat and I keep having to push him over on his side. At one point I had to wake him up so he could go and spit it out.

I'm not bothered about the noise as this can't be helped but at one point it sounded as if he may be close to inhaling it and I didn't want him to choke. I think some steam inhalations will be needed to break down the mucous and hopefully it will not be as sticky.

On the way to Leeds, Peter said it would be nice to go to Cornwall for a few days when his treatment finishes; a lovely idea, but I really think we should wait and see how he is before we book anything. I keep telling him that he will get worse for two weeks after the treatment before he even begins to get better but he chooses to ignore that. I always get the same response: "I'll be fine."

The radiographer popped her head out of the treatment room to ask if I am enjoying the peace and quiet at home. Actually it's a great excuse for selective hearing. After the postman had been this morning, Peter asked, "What bits are yours on the credit card?" I didn't hear him. I definitely got away with it.

After his treatment has finished, I'll try and wangle a new Chloe handbag out of all of this. Mine is ruined. It's the biggest handbag I possess and the only one that fits all his things for daily hospital treatment. Medication, bottle of water, treatment schedule, diary, newspaper, chewing gum, cream for his neck, car keys, two mobile phones and a little bit of room left for my lip-gloss! How do men cope without a handbag?

The nurse prescribed more medications and a nebulizer. Peter asked if it could be his birthday present. He will be 47 on Sunday. I can guess how many times this will actually be used because Peter, predictable as ever, couldn't be bothered to wait at the pharmacy. We'll collect the prescription in the morning.

When the nurse looked down his throat with her torch, she said it did look sore and inflamed as you would expect. She asked if he was still doing his mouth care routine. He is. She asked if he was doing his Saline mouthwashes after each meal. He is not. She asked him if he was using an electric shaver on his neck area. He is not. His skin is only slightly red though and not looking too bad at the moment. But one out of three isn't good enough.

Peter's pain is eight out of 10 this evening so I'm not sure what kind of night we will have. But at least he had another steam inhalation before bed. Let's see what additional pain relief we collect from the pharmacy in the morning. We may just need it for the weekend.

Friday, April 4: Day 16.
Peter was gurgling away most of the night and I was constantly conscious that he may choke on the mucous at the back of his throat. It sounded dreadful. I kept turning him on his side and, the first few times, he would nip to the toilet to spit it out.

This was soon going to exhaust him so I grabbed the kitchen roll and told him to use that instead of getting up every hour. Painkillers were needed at 3.30am and then I heard him gurgling really loudly at about 5.30am.

I daren't wake him again because I thought he would go mad. In hindsight, I should have done because, at about 6am, I think he must have inhaled some of the mucous. I had been frightened of that all night.

He woke with a shock and was making a dreadful noise in the bathroom to bring it up. The pain in his throat became much worse and all the retching eventually made his throat bleed. It was absolutely awful for him and he looked shocking. I got up at 7am. My eyes were stinging and I felt jet-lagged. Peter must feel even worse than me, poor thing. He does look pale and washed out this morning. I left him in bed an extra half an hour but he only managed a bit of his porridge and then we were caught in morning rush hour traffic.

Peter missed his usual girls but he was in no mood for joking anyway. Yesterday he had been James Bond of Rodeo Drive, Beverley Hills. Today it was Peter Jackson from Brighouse. Hasn't quite got the same ring to it.

The nurse gave him a nebulizer. It's very compact and light and about as big as a large handbag. Like my Chloe, in fact! It can be used as often as needed to break down the secretions and make them more fluid. Then it was up to the pharmacy to collect saline solution for the nebulizer, some sachets of Movacol for the bowels, morphine in tablet form which will hopefully not cause hiccoughs and more Mucaine to take before meals.

On our way to Bridlington I offered Peter a milkshake, which he refused. As he had only managed two mouthfuls of porridge this morning I said he wouldn't be able to take his 10am medicine on an empty stomach. Vomiting will be the next thing if he stops eating.

There is nothing worse than taking lots of fizzy medications on an unlined stomach. He refused his milkshake until I said, "Bloody well drink it!" But he's getting fed up of all the tablets; he says they are making him poorly. He drank the milkshake and then had the medication at 10am.

On the way to Brid we passed a sandwich van at the side of the road where we used to stop and have a bacon butty. He said he needed a bacon sandwich, well done and crispy. I carried on driving!

Charlotte phoned; she phones from work a couple of times a day. She hates any kind of illness and is very dramatic even if she has a spot on her face. She is very upset and weepy and left work at 1pm today as she burst into tears in front of her boss, Nicki, who has been very supportive. Although it hasn't affected Charlotte's work she is very emotional at the moment. She heard the coughing episode at 6am this morning and is very worried.

Me? I really hate to see him like this and all I can do is make things as easy as possible for him. It really is a full-time job. It's awful to see him looking ill. It's best to keep busy and devote my whole time to him, which I am sure he does appreciate.

It's also about knowing when to be there and when to back off...but always being there for when he needs me. The balance has to be right between pampering to his every whim and being a bit bossy when necessary.

When you know someone so well, you are able to read them. I can tell when he's feeling absolutely dreadful, when he just wants a bit of love and attention and when he just wants to be left alone. I can tell when he is in pain and when he is not.

I know when he's tired but will not give in. When I gently put him to bed - just for an hour – I know it will be longer. Sleep and rest is the body's way of recovery. You cannot fight it and sometimes even such a strong person as Peter just has to be told.

You need to maintain your sense of humour, be flexible, be supportive, and make it as easy as possible. I suppose it helps being an ex-nurse, although knowing when to be a little bit bossy and not take any nonsense may be nursing or it may be just a womanly nurturing instinct.

It's like nursing a baby bird back to health until it is well enough to fly back into nature. It won't be too long now before Peter is back managing his football club in Lincoln. That will be fantastic for him and then my job will be done.

Life will go back to normal and Peter will be the strong one in the family again. I will go back to work and I will see Peter just a couple of days a week again. That's life, full of ups and downs. We do just take "normal" for granted but I wonder if being so ill really does change the way you think long-term or is it just temporary and then soon forgotten when you are well again?

After his nap we went for a very short walk on the harbour, just to get a breath of fresh air. This normally makes him feel much better but today he looks very grey and tired. Still he is trying to battle on. His appetite has also gone, probably due to the unmentionable "bowel problem" and too much medication. He says not being able to taste anything anymore makes eating a totally pointless exercise and he doesn't feel hungry either.

This is when it is important to get nutrition in any way possible. He managed a milkshake and some white fish this afternoon all washed down with a Movicol Sachet to help with the "bowel problem". When we got back, he tried his nebulizer but got bored after about two minutes and said it wasn't doing anything. "Keep it on and stop being a baby," I told him. He kept it on.

Saturday, April 5

Our friends Christine and Peter Deegan have come across and will stay the night if Peter feels up to it. They understand what the evening may be like. Peter certainly cannot entertain but it's just nice to have some company and hear about someone else's week.

At 3.30pm, I decided we needed a bit more decking outside our Bridlington retreat so while Christine and I went to B&Q, the boys watched football. Now B&Q was a completely new experience for me so we went and found a store person and told him what we intended to do and ask what we needed to do it. He pointed us in the direction of the decking, some nails and a drill. Easy. We can do that, no problem. It should only take us an hour!

Peter couldn't stop laughing when we pulled up with our new "patio". We laid the decking down on the railway sleepers which were in place...

then discovered we didn't have the long metal thing (it's called a bit apparently) we needed to attach to the drill.

Back to B&Q. Then the long metal drill thing was too wide for the screws. Back to B&Q. Then the metal thing snapped when drilling. Back to B&Q. This is really a man's job I think. Peter usually goes mad with me when I make these rash decisions, but today he didn't even argue. He just said, "OK darling, you do some decking."

We ate around 9pm for Peter's birthday meal. He insisted on having chicken, the same as us, and managed it quite well, a small portion with lots of mashed potato and cauliflower cheese.

After having his nebulizer and morphine he retired to bed at about 10.15pm. He does look very grey and tired, he looks ill. Lots of love and nursing care is all I can do. The pain when swallowing was still about seven tonight, but apart from giving him morphine during the day, which would make him sleep most of the day, there's not a lot more I can do. He is OK when he is not swallowing though.

Christine, Peter and I stayed up for another hour or so and Deegs said Peter was much worse than when he saw him last weekend. That's the way it will continue.

Sunday, April 6: Peter's 47th birthday

Peter was expectorating all night. He woke up at 8am to "Happy Birthday, darling!" followed quickly by, "Here are your tablets." He opened his presents and cards, trying to show some enthusiasm for our sake rather than his own.

After breakfast we decided to screw the decking into the railway sleepers. It was a joint effort and it did only take one hour with all four of us helping. When Peter looked a bit grey, he sat and watched with a coffee and directed operations from his chair in the sunshine…mainly with hand movements.

I was really pleased with it - and also pleased I hadn't broken a nail. My first effort at DIY and it looked amazing. Happy Birthday, Peter - a new patio! So in the afternoon, Peter and I popped to B&Q again. My fifth visit in 24 hours and the fifth of my life. Peter's first…although he denies this. He says he once popped in to buy a light bulb.

We bought some bamboo fencing, a herb garden and a couple of big plaster balls for ornaments. Anyone would think we didn't have a garden at home. But this one is cute and cosy.

The nightmare started at 6pm.

He said he felt very cold. Ten minutes later, he looked very pale and was shivering uncontrollably. I wrapped him in lots of blankets and said I was going to phone an ambulance. I didn't like the look of this.

He refused and said if he could just get warm he'd be fine. I said, "Let's get you to the hospital to be checked out." I wrapped him up and got him into the car. His fingernails were turning blue. He started to vomit.

I thought he was going into shock and really didn't know why. I just knew I had to get him to hospital as quickly as possible. We arrived at Bridlington Hospital in about 10 minutes. All the way I was telling him to keep his eyes open, to hang on, we were nearly there.

I didn't realise that it wasn't an Accident & Emergency hospital. I ran inside, told them I had an emergency patient in the car just outside the main entrance and asked if a doctor could assess him.

I grabbed a wheelchair and ran back to the car with a staff nurse in tow. By this time he was vomiting with the car door open. We got him into the wheelchair and took him inside to keep him warm.

They phoned for a 999 emergency ambulance to take him to the nearest A&E hospital, 20 miles away at Scarborough. I was very calm and working on autopilot. Peter was very frightened and ill. He had gone into shock. The ambulance arrived quickly and we were on our way in sleet and snow with the blue light flashing.

After arriving at A&E, I gave the doctor a full medical history and the nurse did his observations. His temperature was 39.2, extremely high. Much higher and he would have started fitting. His other observations – blood pressure etc were fine. Very quickly a drip was put into his arm and a saline drip started. Blood samples were taken and sent to the lab. A chest X-ray was arranged to see if he had developed an infection.

He was given Intravenous (IV) paracetamol to reduce his temperature. He needed to be cooled down as much as possible. I bathed him with cold towels on his head and chest and the fan was switched on. He was admitted to the Acute Assessment ward where I gave two more doctors his medical history. He was still very ill and in a lot of pain in his throat. Medication was given for the vomiting.

His blood results came back; full blood count and white cell count normal. Blood cultures were sent to the pathology lab to see which bacteria was causing the infection and temperature. But that would take a few days.

I rang Christine and Deegs to tell them what had happened and they said they would come straight over to collect me. All the way from Brighouse in sleet and snow and terrible road conditions. What amazing friends. I didn't want to tell Charlotte and Oliver so late at night as there was nothing they could do and they would be really upset.

Christine and Peter arrived on the ward at 12.30am. Peter's temperature was still very high, but he was in good hands and there wasn't anything else I could do tonight. But I made it very clear to the registrar in charge that Peter had to be at St James' hospital tomorrow for his radiotherapy.

I would drive him myself if I had to. It was imperative that he should have his treatment because he cannot have any longer than a two-day break in treatment for this type of cancer. I kissed him goodnight and said that if he wanted me to come back through the night I would. We arrived back in Bridlington at 1am.

Christine and Peter set off for home as they were both working on Monday. It was now snowing heavily. They got to bed at around 3.15am. I phoned the ward before I climbed into bed and he was sleeping. His temperature was 38.9 so still extremely high. I had a couple of hours' sleep. I was worried sick. What on earth was going on?

Monday, April 7: Day 17

The weather was dreadful. Sleet was driving down and the roads were very icy. The fuel gauge showed nearly empty so I stopped to get some petrol. I knew we should have done that yesterday. The main road from Scarborough to Whitby was closed.

At 8.45am, I was just parking the car in the car park at Scarborough Hospital when Peter rang to see where I was. The doctors were on their ward round. I raced from the main entrance to the ward, which was at the other side of the hospital.

I got there just in time to see the consultant who was looking after him. He told me the ambulance had been arranged to transfer him to St James's. A huge relief. His chest x-ray had come back clear and they had no idea where the infection was. Peter just looked so pleased to see me. He looked so ill.

His IV fluids and antibiotics had been continued overnight. He was still in a lot of pain even though I had left him his tablets to take overnight. But the nurses had also given him extra morphine in liquid form and he had suffered with hiccoughs most of the night. Agony and exhausting.

He was in too much pain to eat and or even drink his water. I gave him a bed bath and cleaned his teeth and did his mouthwashes. He was very weak and kept drifting in and out of sleep.

I was so worried, just seeing him lying there, devoid of any colour. It was extremely upsetting. He kept waking up to clear all the mucous from the back of his throat. I just sat at the side of his bed, cooling his forehead with a cold cloth to try and reduce his temperature. Every now and again he would wake up just to check I was still there.

At midday the ambulance arrived and I followed in the car to Leeds. I parked the car and made my way to the department. He was sitting in a chair in the waiting room with a vomit bowl.

The nurse came and we took him through immediately to see Dr Saunders, the registrar who is in charge of Peter's treatment. He just looked at him and asked what on earth had happened since Thursday when he saw him last. I don't think he could quite believe how Peter's health had declined so much in just a few days.

He explained that there wasn't a bed in the Oncology unit but agreed he needed to be admitted as soon as a bed became available. I left it with him and wheeled Peter down for his treatment.

The little child was in before Peter and they were taking longer than usual. We went into our quiet room. Peter just wanted to sleep. I told him to lie on the floor and put my coat under his head. He was asleep in seconds. It had been a long journey but at least we were there. I had phoned the children at 9am to say that Dad wasn't very well and to meet us at St James's in the afternoon.

Fran, one of the team of five radiotherapists in charge of Peter's treatment, came in to get him. She was really upset to see him looking so ill. She found him a trolley and a pillow to sleep on until a bed became available.

Charlotte and Oliver arrived with an overnight bag. Although I had explained how poorly he was, it still came as a shock to them but they tried desperately not to show it. He is their dad, the strong man of the house, their rock. But here he was, weak, in pain and completely out of it.

I gave him his tablets for pain. He was really struggling to swallow and also very dehydrated. Finally, a bed became available in the late afternoon and a porter took him to the ward.

Peter was too tired to be bothered about anything. I was just hugely relieved that he was now in the right place. Oliver looked very distressed and Charlotte made herself busy unpacking towels and wash bags and arranging the bedside locker.

Peter slept and we sat very quietly at the side of the bed, watching, waiting, hardly saying a word. When the nurse came to set up his IV, the children made themselves scarce and went downstairs for a coffee.

I said I would join them asap. When Peter was comfortable and drifting off I told him I would leave him to sleep for a while. I went to the café, joined the kids and told them everything that had happened…and everything that would happen next. As they headed for the rush hour traffic I told them to drive carefully and get home safe.

I made Peter comfortable for the night and told him to ring or text me if he needed me at all. I got home at 8pm, shattered. Charlotte ran me a lovely bath, poured a glass of wine and made me something to eat.

I reassured the children that Dad would be fine. But added that unfortunately he will get worse still before he gets better. Treatment finishes on Thursday and then he will get worse in the following two weeks. Peter says he cannot possibly feel any worse than he does now, but I reckon this is just the beginning.

I phoned the ward and spoke and texted Peter. We told one another how much we loved each other. I made some phone calls to relatives to explain how Peter was. His brothers and dad asked if they could visit him tomorrow but he is probably going to be too weak and tired.

Peter managed to text a lovely message before I went to bed.

Tuesday, April 8: Day 18

I awoke at 7.30am and phoned the ward. Still in incredible pain and hiccoughing most of the night. Visiting hours are supposed to be 2pm-8pm but I got a phone call from Peter at 8am to say I had to come in to be with him this morning. He'd checked with the nurse and they said it was fine.

I went into the ward and I could have cried. He looked so alone, so poorly. I couldn't quite believe how my husband's health had disintegrated so easily. I sat on the side of his bed, cuddled him for a while.

His IV had stopped a couple of hours ago so this was a perfect time to get practical and I got him out of bed and into the shower. He felt too tired, too ill and simply couldn't be bothered. He was exhausted after his shower and shave but admitted it was worth it to put on a clean t-shirt and pyjama bottoms.

I brushed his hair and gave him his mouthwashes. I covered him in talc (whoever wears talc these days?) and tucked him in bed. He instantly fell fast asleep as I just sat and stared while he drifted off into never-never land.

The doctors were convinced Peter had an infection but the chest x-ray came back normal and they still had no idea where the infection was. Dr Saunders said that it could also be a virus and he would need a naso-gastric tube passing at some point today to get some nutrients into him. At this stage of the treatment it is crucial for him to have lots of calories to help the healthy cells build and repair themselves after being damaged by the radiotherapy. He cannot afford to lose weight.

He went down for radiotherapy, knowing that he has only two more treatments to go. His neck is looking very red and sore. It's starting to blister and the skin is breaking down pretty quickly. It looks worse by the hour. He's having aspirin mouthwashes as a gargle, Corsodyl mouthwashes four times a day, IV fluids and antibiotics, the morphine dose has been increased along with medication given to stop the hiccoughs. He's now only sipping water.

In the afternoon, Peter's brothers, Anthony and Gerard, called. They popped their heads between the curtains and were truly shocked at how ill he looks. He is still very pale, asleep on his side and making dreadful breathing noises with all the mucous gathering at the back of his throat. They both looked enormous, fit and healthy.

Peter must have heard them whispering and roused from his sleep. He was confused and disorientated when he woke and didn't know where he was. He came around after a minute or so and Anthony asked him how he was feeling. Incredibly, despite being so ill, and being in and out of consciousness, Peter answered, "I feel like shit. And to make it worse, I haven't had a hard-on for three days, so there's definitely something wrong with me."

Everyone burst out laughing and then Peter turned over and fell straight back asleep. It was a surreal moment, but it was comforting to know that behind all the tubes, pain and worry, my husband's character is still there.

In the afternoon, the doctor came to pass the naso-gastric tube through his nose and down into his stomach so that a liquid loaded with calories and nutrients can be given. Passing the tube past the throat was not only uncomfortable, it was agony because his throat is so painful.

I held his hand and gave him lots of reassurance. The doctor did a great job but if he hadn't managed to get it down the first time he would have to do it again and again until it had gone in.

Each time you try it becomes more distressing so I kept telling him this over and over again. It went in the first time thankfully. He did really well. An x-ray was arranged to check it was in his stomach and not his lungs before feeding could commence.

Charlotte and Oliver came into the ward. Charlotte was heartbroken to see her dad with all the tubes in. We sat in a television lounge and over in the corner was a very attractive girl around Charlotte's age, mid- 20s, with a chemotherapy drip in her arm.

Charlotte asked me where her cancer was. How on earth would I know that? Then she asked if the girl would be OK. I could only reply that she is young and having treatment so let's hope so.

A bed became available on the oncology head and neck unit and the kids helped to pack up Peter's bags and we helped the porter move him to Dr Dyker's ward. He has his own room, a television and a view over the city. He is not too interested in any of this at the moment though. I stayed until they collected him for x-ray at 7pm but even though I was very tired, I couldn't get to sleep until well after midnight.

Wednesday, April 9: Day 19
I put a bag of things together to take to hospital, clean towels etc, then realised I had forgotten to tumble dry his Calvin Klein cotton bottoms. He only has two pairs and doesn't possess any pyjamas.

I nipped to Tesco and got four pairs for £20. What great value. Let's hope Peter is too drowsy to check the label. From Armani suits to Tesco pyjama bottoms. What next? I was absolutely delighted when I saw him. He looked so much better and managed a big smile. Certainly not well, but a 100 per cent improvement. His temperature was normal, he had completed his course of IV antibiotics and they had done the trick. But we still don't know where the infection has been.

He had been seen by Dr Dyker and Dr Saunders who were both really pleased how he was responding to treatment and thankfully, he is more or less back on track to where he should be for day 19 after such a huge setback.

He felt well enough to sit in his chair, had a look out of the window and then read the Sun and I read the Daily Mail. After half-an-hour he was tired and I sat at the side of the bed very quietly reading my book. But he kept opening one eye just to check if I was still there.

His dad and Gerard arrived to visit in the afternoon. His dad looked really sweet in his collar and tie and jacket. Peter was pleased to see them but because he was whispering and his dad was deaf, Gerard and I had to repeat everything. In the end, Peter looked pale and tired with the effort. So did Gerard and I!

We sent each other a couple of goodnight texts and the good news is…I think I got away with the Tesco pyjama bottoms!

Thursday, April 10: Day 20

The day we've been waiting for. The last one, the final treatment. Let's pray it has worked and the cancer has been completely burnt out.

The radiation will continue to work for the next couple of weeks so the side effects will get worse before they start to subside. Then the road to recovery will begin. Even so, Peter says he's sure he cannot possibly feel any worse than he has done these past four days. Let's hope not.

As I was getting ready for hospital I reflected on the last few days. As a trained nurse, I understood the urgency of getting him to hospital as quickly and as calmly as possible, ignoring his pleas of, "No, I'll be OK." In a similar situation, a 'non-medical' person would need to dial 999 immediately.

The condition of a patient with a virus or infection can deteriorate very quickly. Speed and medical attention are crucial. Do not hesitate and do not think you are wasting anybody's time.

The other thing that struck me was the number of times I had to repeat to a doctor Peter's full medical history and an account of what happened on Sunday. First to the paramedics in the ambulance from Bridlington to Scarborough, then to the doctor at Scarborough A&E, then to the Acute Medical Assessment Ward, then a junior doctor, then a senior house officer and then the registrar.

They all took notes…but do they actually read each other's notes? I was exhausted repeating the same story over and over again. Three times is fine but five is not necessary.

I stressed to each doctor the importance of getting Peter to St James' for his radiotherapy treatment on Monday…but one of them actually mentioned that he might be able to have his radiotherapy at Scarborough. So not to worry.

What! All those weeks of measuring for a mask, marking the mask and working out the dose of radiation needed, making sure it was accurately targeting the right areas. All the preparation.

Where exactly did the Scarborough doctor think they were going to zap? How would they possibly know? Again, I hope any relative would push and insist that their loved one was taken to the right hospital for their treatment.

Anyway. Back to today. Peter rang me about 8.30. He'd coughed up blood in the night. I told him he must mention it to the doctors this morning and if it happens again to show the nursing staff. I am so excited that it is the final day of treatment. I know we still have to wait a couple of weeks for the all-clear, but after today, his treatment will be finished. Over.

On my way to Leeds to give Peter his midday shower, I called in at Tesco to buy chocolates for the staff on treatment room number nine. The radiographers, including Sarah, Fran, Lucy, Julie and Mike, the two receptionists, Patricia and Jenna, who showed us to our quiet room every day.

They have been so lovely and caring for the past month. They are always so pleasant and cheerful. I decided to give them all individual boxes and put them in a gift bag, with their names on the tag and a big bow.

When I arrived, I discovered they had put Peter's mask in a plastic bag as he told them he wants to take it home. If it were me, I'd just want to burn it. But he wants to put it in the garden as a feature and grow flowers in it. Is he mad?

I normally never interfere with his beloved garden, but I really must say no to that one. Who on earth needs a constant reminder? I just want to put it all behind us and move forward. I want it to be a distant memory not to sit and sunbathe staring at it.

When I arrived Peter had been down for his last radiotherapy treatment but didn't seem as excited as I am about it. He is still expectorating a lot but is now nearly pain free in his throat.

He has begun to accept a certain amount of pain even though he is still on a lot of morphine and Voltarol, which will continue for the next three or four weeks. His naso-gastric feeds have been increased slightly from 30 ml per hour yesterday to 75ml today. When he can tolerate 150ml he will be allowed home.

The dietician called in to explain the equipment he will be sent home with. He will go home on 1500mls of feed per day, which will take 10 hours per day to administer. This can be done overnight, which will allow him to move about during the day. All medications will also be given down the tube. If he can manage a bit of water orally this would be good as it helps maintain the swallowing reflex and muscles. All being well he should be allowed home on Monday

Peter asked one of the nurses if they had a television with Sky so he could watch his football. Apparently, Lily who is 92 and a couple of doors away, has Sky and hates football. She doesn't really know what Sky is, bless her, and as long as she can watch her soaps in the afternoon, she's happy. So is Peter now they have swapped tellies!

Christine and Peter visited for 20 minutes, Charlotte for one hour and Oliver and his girlfriend Stacey called in after work. These are all the people closest to him but it was still too much. We left him to rest.

I also took a box of chocolates for the man on the car park exit, the one who never smiles. I bet nobody ever brings him chocolates. I just needed to see him smile once before I stopped daily visits to this car park. But he wasn't there today.

Anyway, treatment done. We can move forward. And the mask? I chucked it in the garage.

Friday, April 11: Recovery Day One

The dietician met us to talk about the feeding pump, amount of feed and everything we will need at home. It should all be delivered on Monday. They will send him home on Monday with two weeks' supply of feed, a pump and a table top stand to hang the feed on.

He will need the feed to run for 12 hours so overnight would be the best time, 8pm to 8am. Between now and Monday, the feed will be increased to 1500mls and up to 125mls per hour.

There will be two kinds of feed, one high energy, one high fibre, supplying all the nutrients and calories and vitamins he needs. Extra water will also be put down the tube as he needs 2000mls of water as well.

The night feeds will leave him free during the day to potter around the house and garden. I am not sure he will want to be seen out and about, although people know he is overcoming throat cancer anyway.

Lots of people are wandering around St James's with naso gastric tubes. It's a sight you just get used to but it's different outside the hospital environment and I'm sure he'd get some very strange looks. Charlotte was horrified the first time she saw a patient with one in the lift so I suppose that's what some people out of a hospital environment will think.

I think Peter is very conscious about how much time I am spending at the hospital and feels guilty. He has told me that on Saturday I should do something for myself and go shopping in Manchester or Leeds. I say there is plenty of time for that when he is well.

This is becoming a difficult stage. I know he wants me there so I take it as a personal rejection when he says go shopping. Conversely, he will also see it as a rejection if I actually do go.

We are trying to read each other's minds, I suppose. Putting ourselves in the other person's shoes. How would I be feeling if it was me? I would be saying, "You go to football and do something for yourself." And I would mean it. But then I would be watching the clock and be really excited when he walked through the door.

Iffy had arranged to travel up from Lincoln after training but with bad weather and heavy traffic, he didn't arrive on the ward until 8pm. Peter had asked him to bring his Manager of the Month trophy, which is in a box, and when he passed the nurse's station he asked which room Peter was in. The nurse must have thought he was a parcel delivery man and said she wasn't going to sign for anything at this time of night. Iffy wasn't too happy about that.

Neither was Peter when they told him he would have to move into a room with four beds again. Another patient is very confused and they will need to keep a close eye on him. So Peter won't have control of the television remote control any more.

Iffy decided to sleep at our house. It was too late to travel back to Lincoln and they are playing at Chester tomorrow. The spare bed is in the office and I had to change the "Forever Friends" duvet cover, which would not be too appropriate for Iffy. If you've seen Iffy, you will know what I mean. He's massive. Over 6 foot tall, solid muscle. He looks more like a bouncer at a nightclub than a footballer. But he's a gentle giant and has always been a good friend of Peter's.

They played together at Huddersfield and then, when Peter was manager, Iffy was one of his players. The only time they fell out was when Peter left him out of the Division Three play-off final against Mansfield at Cardiff in 2005.

In football you meet a lot of acquaintances, but not many good friends. You always need somebody you can rely on as it can be a ruthless business, which is why Iffy is now Peter's coach at Lincoln and is in charge at the moment.

Charlotte and I quizzed him about his love life and girlfriends. He is 40 now and like most men separated from their wives, his girlfriend's ages start with a two. I asked if he has a lot in common with them and if they manage to hold a good conversation. He assures me he does…and bursts out laughing.

But we soon get into the flow and it's nice to know that men do talk sometimes, but not very often, about something other than football! We all went to bed about midnight and Peter texted me to tell me he has just moved rooms. He will not be happy.

Saturday, April 12: Recovery Day Two

I was woken by a florist who delivered a huge bunch of flowers for Peter from everyone at my work. Lovely but work is still the last thing on my mind at the moment. I had planned on taking leave until the beginning of May but Peter will have his feeding tube in for about four weeks, which will take us until May 10. It's still too early to make any decisions but I'm contemplating taking the summer off and going back in September.

Peter has been moved into the four-bed room. He said he slept well but I'm not too sure about the other three if Peter was snoring! Maybe if he snores loud enough they will move him back into single room tonight. Which would be worse? A confused patient or Peter's snoring? It's like water slowly dripping on your forehead – torture. In fact, I might decide to bring the confused patient home instead of Peter on Monday!

When I spoke to Peter this morning, I suggested he should ask the nurse in charge if he could come home for the day. I could give him his analgesia via his tube. He rang me back in less than two minutes and yes, I could pick him up.

Charlotte and I arrived at hospital at 10.45am. Peter was in his dressing gown and slippers and started to charge towards the lift. I told him to slow down, we couldn't keep up with him. When we reached the car, which I'd parked just outside the main entrance, Peter said he'd drive. I thought he was joking, but he was absolutely serious. He had enough morphine in him to sedate a donkey. I gently pushed him into the passenger seat.

When we arrived home he went straight into the garage. I just stood there, amazed. Is he confused from all the drugs? Is he going to cut the lawn? No, he was only going to check the newly delivered garden furniture. He had me worried for the moment.

He had a nap, took a shower, put on a clean dressing gown and made himself comfortable in front of Sky Sports to watch an afternoon of football. It was lovely to have him home even for a few hours.

He managed a small bowl of ice cream and a tiny piece of bread and butter but said he feels neither hungry nor full. He doesn't feel anything at all. It must be strange but at least he's trying to keep the swallowing muscles going.

When we arrived back on the ward, I gave Peter his 6pm analgesia and a staff nurse came to supervise me putting up the feed and setting up the pump. There's only Peter and one other gentleman now in the four-bed ward. I didn't ask where the other two had gone; neither did Peter.

What a lovely day! He does look so much better when he is in his home environment. Not long to go before we have him home. When I arrived back, Charlotte had set the table with lots of candles and lots of chilled wine and her chicken stir fry was a winner. The best I have ever tasted!

Even though Charlotte is 24, she still thinks it a treat if she can sleep with me. While we were chatting in bed, she said that, as she didn't feel too squeamish when I was giving dad his medication via his tube with a syringe, maybe she would like to be a nurse.

I think she was being serious…so I told her that maybe she should stick to her glamorous world of advertising as there is a little bit more to nursing than a syringe and a naso gastric tube.

Sunday, April 13: Recovery Day Three

I slept really well last night. Maybe it was the wine…maybe because it was finally mission accomplished with the car park attendant yesterday. Yes, I actually got a smile! I have seen him nearly every day for month and smiled and waved even though sometimes I have felt more like crying.

I've been trying desperately to get some kind of response…but nothing. Until now! OK, it wasn't the biggest smile I've ever seen but he did lift the corner of his lips and showed his teeth.

I gave him his box of chocolates and said: "Thank you for being so cheerful for the past month. I may not see you again quite as often but thank you." He was speechless and said thank you, nobody had ever given him chocolates at work. I thought, "I'm not bloody surprised," as I sped off.

I phoned Peter to ask what time he wanted me to pick him up. Inevitably, he said, "Now." He had a big smile to greet me and had told the nurses he wanted to get home for a Sunday morning sleep in.

We snuggled up and soon fell fast asleep. The phone woke me at lunchtime. Peter soon drifted back off again. Sleep will do him the world of good from now on and there really is nothing like your own clean bed.

I woke Peter for his 2pm medication and he seemed a bit spaced out during the afternoon. Better that way than being in pain, I suppose. He managed three slices of bread with cream cheese, followed by a piece of soft sponge cake, which he admitted was very tasty.

If he carries on like this, I'm sure he won't need his tube in for the full month. But it's early days. I gave him his three different mouthwashes and gargles but he was horrified that I gave them in the wrong order. It really doesn't matter but I just bit my tongue and said: "Sorry darling, I will try harder next time!"

After a shower, he applied loads of body creams and face creams…he laughs at the amount I put on but he's just as bad if not worse. His neck is looking very red, like bad sunburn. It is cracking. Where he has a natural crease in his neck, the skin is wet and breaking down badly.

The wet areas need to be kept dry and clean and we applied some scent-free aloe-vera cream to the dry areas. It is not recommended by the hospital but we tried it anyway. It certainly cannot do any harm. He wanted to use my Crème De La Mer so I'll have to hide that.

We arrived back on the ward at 7.30pm and the nurse hovered in the background, watching as I set up the feed. I got top marks and all being well we should have him home tomorrow.

Monday, April 14: Recovery Day Four
I had to be at the hospital at 11am as Neil, the nurse from the feed manufacturer, was bringing the pump and drip stand for us to use at home. He ran through everything to make sure we are OK with the pump and how it works.

I suppose if you are a layperson with no nursing training, as most people will be, this could be a bit daunting. But it wouldn't be difficult to learn and there's a full instruction book. The drip stand, the pump and the bags of feed arrived in big boxes, the tubing in a big bag.

The pharmacist brought a huge holdall of medication and the nurse all the mouthwashes and gargles. The amount of equipment is unbelievable and it's a good job we still have the Volvo estate.

On the way to the hospital, I'd stopped off in Leeds to collect some new bedding for the spare bed…I can imagine I may have to spend a couple of hours a night in there. In fact, though, the snoring is actually better while the tube is in Peter's throat but when I tell him this, he says he's not keeping the tube down his throat for the rest of his life just so that I can get a good night's sleep. But at least the Forever Friends bedding can now go in the bin. Iffy will be pleased.

We saw the parking attendant on the way out and he thanked me again for the chocolates, waved and wished us all the best. I said we'd see him again on Monday when we come to outpatients. It took about eight trips to unload the car.

Peter was really tired and went to lie down. I woke him after three hours and I'm really not sure how long he would have slept if I had left him be. He was very startled and didn't know where he was. He really is dosed up with analgesia.

He managed a sandwich and can swallow this better than he can swallow a cup of tea. But we have to get two litres of fluid down on top of the 1.5 litres of food. It takes some doing, time-wise as much as anything.

I haven't been in too much trouble today as I managed to get his mouthwashes and gargles in the right order. But I was told off for wearing a comfortable tracksuit. What on earth does he want me to wear? I ignored the "skirt would be nice" remark and carried on regardless. What a shame I gave all my nurse's uniforms back all those years ago, although I'm not sure they would still fit.

Peter was spark out after his morphine but while the snoring has stopped with the tube in his throat, it has been replaced by bubbling noises. It was like trying to sleep in the bottom of a fish tank. I stuck it for 10 minutes and then went in to sample the new cotton sheets in the next room. I left both doors open in case the bleep on the feed pump alerted me that something was wrong.

First, I couldn't sleep because I was worrying what I should wear tomorrow. Then I couldn't sleep because of the new £50 shape-to-the-head type pillow I'd bought with the bedding. It was like a boulder. I threw it on the floor and resorted to my old one.

And after all that, I simply lay awake listening for the bleep.

Peter's thoughts: When I was first diagnosed with throat cancer and told I'd need radiotherapy, I thought I'd breeze through it. Twenty-one radiation treatments? Nothing to it. After ten treatments, I went to Elland Road to watch Lincoln Reserves against Leeds. But the bad times started after that, gradually at first. The neck, burning and blistered then scabbing over. The retching, the vomiting, the constant nausea, the pain. I didn't feel I needed painkillers at first, even though they were prescribed. "Why do I need these? I'm not even poorly." If Alison hadn't insisted I would have been in a bit of a mess.

I never really let on how I was feeling but I cried a few times. Alison and the kids were probably looking for me to show some emotion, to let it all out, but I was never going to do that. I thought it would upset them. I just wanted them to think I was getting on with it in my own way and I'd be fine. But I cried in hospital when Alison left me to go home at night.

It's taken me five years to start thinking about little bits of what I actually went through. It was a strange situation. I was there suffering from cancer but somehow it wasn't really me at all. It was somebody else. It was as if someone else was inside my body, really bizarre.

When we went to see the doctor in hospital I never listened. I just blanked it and thought about football. Alison took it all in. She was the one who took everything on board. I didn't have a clue. It was as if I wasn't actually going through it. Alison was with me all the time: every visit to the hospital, the doctor, the pharmacy. When I needed medication, Alison was there to give it.

Was I upset and frightened? Of course I was. Particularly when I was rushed into hospital in Scarborough and then taken to St James' in Leeds next day. That was really frightening. An ambulance with flashing lights all the way from Scarborough to Leeds. Just me and a paramedic and Alison following behind in the car. It hit me then that this was really, really serious.

When we arrived at St James's I was wheeled on a trolley to the x-ray department. That meant going from the old part of the hospital to the new part through a tunnel, like being in a dungeon. I was just looking up at the ceiling as they wheeled me away and I remember thinking, "This could be it. I might not make it here." I really felt that bad. It was the darkest time.

I was in hospital for a week and at first, I was genuinely frightened that it might be the end for me. I felt really dreadful and for the first time, it hit home how poorly I was. Before that I'd thought, "Yes, I'm poorly but I'm not that bad." And if it was that hard for me, imagine what it was like for Alison, Charlotte and Oliver. It must have been twice as bad seeing me lying there in that state. They took the brunt of it because I was on medication and out of it half the time.

At one stage I was in a ward with three other people and one of them, a lad who was younger than me, died while I was in there. That makes me feel so humble to have recovered and grateful for the treatment I received.

Tuesday, April 15: Recovery Day Five

As I lay awake last night, I wondered what Peter must be thinking. Is he angry? Is he thinking, "Why me?" Is he wondering if the radiotherapy has worked? Is he wondering, "What next if it hasn't? How long am I going to feel so ill? When will I start to feel better? When will I be well enough to go back to work?"

Maybe he is just too dosed up with morphine to even be thinking anything like that. I don't know what he is thinking as he finds it really difficult to speak to any of us about it. He probably thinks it will upset us so he keeps it to himself.

I think there will be lots of emotional issues to come in the next week or so. I know he's strong and always in control, but this is something he cannot control. A positive mental attitude really helps and I know he is fighter. But he must have some thoughts on his condition.

I am also aware that when patients are angry about their condition, they do tend to take it out on the person nearest to them. That will be me. I will have to remember not to take it personally.

However he has spent a long time in silence, by himself in hospital. Even in the four-bed ward he never spoke to the other patients. Some of them were too ill, some of them were too old and because it was the head and neck cancer ward, lots of them were undergoing the same treatment as Peter and could also only speak in a whisper. They said good morning and good evening to each other and that was it. It really is a very quiet ward and quiet is something Peter is definitely not used to.

Although yesterday was tiring, I'm sure we will get into our own little routine. But the day seems to revolve totally around giving medications, giving 200mls water every hour for 10 hours and lots of mouthwashes and gargles. I seem to be constantly sitting by Peter's right ear putting liquid into his tube and moving away huge bags of nasty tissues.

I'm not quite sure when last night ended and today started. I put his eight-hour feed up at 11pm. Then he needed the loo at midnight, 2am and 4am, so I got up to help him. He had a coughing episode at 3am.

His feed drip ran out at 6.45 so I got up to take it down, flush it with water and then give him his 7am MST, which I have reduced to 20mgs this morning to see if we can wake him up a little today. If he is in more pain I can give him the other 10mgs later.

I then slipped back into bed. The phone rang at 8.45: the pharmacy checking if all this feed they have on prescription is right. They say it is a large amount and I say unfortunately it is. I can pick it up tomorrow. The interruptions are never ending. I gave Peter his Voltarol, paracetamol, Losec and Movicol and flushed it down. Great. I decided I might as well get up. I feel as if I am taking morphine, too: pain-free and zombified.

Peter got up at 10.30 and took a shower. It was a real effort and he was exhausted. I decided to pop to Halifax to buy a new printer for my laptop. Peter came with me and sat in the car, reading his newspaper.

We arrived home an hour later and he looked grey again. I can tell when he is tired...he goes a funny colour and feels very cold. I checked his temperature. Normal. I gave him his medicines, he climbed back into bed at 12.30pm and woke up two hours later. I checked him regularly and he was fast asleep. His neck looks absolutely dreadful from the outside. It is purple, red and very sore.

It has crusted scabs and the areas where he has a natural crease are very wet. We will need to try and dry out that area and make sure he doesn't touch it, which is difficult when it is tickling. I am applying cream to the very dry and cracked areas only. He refuses a dressing.

My boss from work called for a coffee to discuss the not too pleasant situation in the office, where there are going to be redundancies. It sounds dreadful, although my job is apparently safe. I do feel sorry for everyone concerned though as many of them have families and mortgages to look after.

After Peter woke, I cleaned his neck with saline solution and applied a dry dressing. He hated it and took it straight off. He was very agitated and did seem very down today. He is really fed up now and can hardly be bothered to talk.

I hate to see him like this and he will get worse over the next five days before he starts to get better. I try to chat to him and carry on as normal but he doesn't seem to listen. Dreadful.

I can't blame him but it won't be for much longer. I keep telling him just another five days and then he should start to feel better. I bathed his neck with saline again, but it is very wet and seeping in the deepest crease in his neck. I really do need to keep an eye on that as it will get infected. That's all we need.

At 10pm he demanded his medicine as he was going to bed. Oliver helped us up the stairs. Peter cannot be bothered to carry anything. He cleaned his teeth and I stood at the side and watched him. I can't wait to have my husband back to normal. It is really difficult to see him like this.

When his morphine kicked in, he had the startled look in his eyes again. He asked if I was coming to bed with him. I said I would be just downstairs if he needed me. He asked how I would know. I told him I'd leave the doors open and he could clap loudly.

I called in to see him every 15 minutes as he seemed scared to be left alone. He was fast asleep but making very loud gurgling noises. He will have a very restless night. I had a coffee with Charlotte because I felt too tired to sleep. What a horrible day. Unfortunately, I can't see tomorrow being much better.

Wednesday, April 16: Recovery Day Six

I woke at 3.30am when Peter was having a loud coughing episode, 5am to take the feed down and 7am to give him morphine. His throat looked as if it had been seeping and bleeding a bit (on the outside) during the night. I think it dries out better in bed as his neck is in a different position.

At 10am, the routine began. Shower, mouthcare, gargles and mouthwashes, fluids down tube, medications every two hours down tube, water down tube hourly. I absolutely insisted on dressing his neck otherwise that is going to be a major problem.

I changed all the plasters around the nose and forehead area as we need to keep the tube securely in place. It hadn't moved. It is also important to draw back some gastric secretions and test them with litmus paper to make sure the tube is still in the stomach and not the lungs. It looks fine but I must get into a routine of checking daily.

Bob, our gardener, popped in to see Peter. He received radiotherapy for mouth and jaw cancer two years ago and called to reassure Peter that he knows exactly how he must be feeling. He said this was the worst time for him; he experienced a lot of pain and extreme tiredness. He reassured Peter he would feel better and just to rest when he needed to and continue with the painkillers. But he said it took him weeks to feel better.

I knew that at some point, I would have to fit in a trip to Tesco, which would give me something to look forward to. Look forward to? I can't believe I could ever think that. I used to hate going to Tesco. With a passion. It's the most boring thing in the world. I used to dash in and literally run around in my lunch hour. When my life was normal.

Now I look forward to Tesco and wander round. I think, "How marvellous, they have brought out a new yoghurt. And guess what's on a three for two offer today?" What on earth is happening? I cannot wait to find Tesco a real chore again. That will mean Peter is healthy and fit and life is back to how it was.

Peter was in bed when I said I was going. He looked shocked and asked how long I would be. What if he needed something when I was gone? I reassured him I would only be 45 minutes and put his mobile by the bed.

This was the first time for a couple of weeks that he'd been left alone. I kept my mobile in my hand all the time, dashed round the store and was only away for 45 minutes. At least four people stopped me to ask about Peter.

In the afternoon, Peter's dad came with our niece Victoria, who has just arrived back from a 12-month around the world trip. Then my brother Jonathan arrived on his motorbike. After cups of coffee and biscuits for the visitors and a syringe of Paracetamol and Sterile water for Peter they left us to peace and quiet and Peter managed mince and mashed potatoes with tons of gravy. It looked painful to swallow but he did really well.

He also kept the dry dressing on his neck in place, although it was wet through at 5.30 but when I changed it, his neck was looking clean and a little dryer. Peter said he was not going to sleep in it, but I insisted. He listened and gave in. I usually get my own way in the end and with this one I'm not backing off. He realises there's no point arguing.

By the time the kids came home, Peter was tired and everything just seemed too much for him. When you feel so ill you just want peace and quiet. This is a typical example of when our Bridlington retreat comes in really handy but we know that isn't an option for a while.

Thursday, April 17: Recovery Day Seven

I knew he would get worse before he got better but I don't think I ever envisaged him being this bad and needing so much nursing care. Last night was absolutely dreadful. I went to bed at midnight and checked on him before getting into the spare bed. I left both doors open as normal so I could hear if he needed me during the night.

It's amazing how quickly you get used to the noises and coughing and can manage to sleep through, although I am only half asleep anyway. At about 1am he started having a coughing fit, which made his throat very painful. I sat with him until it subsided.

Then at 3am he started to vomit, only a small amount but very painful for him and painful to watch. I sat him up as it seems that when he lies down the feed starts to make him feel sick. But as soon as he drops off to sleep again he slips down the bed.

At 4.30am, with his feed nearly finished, he started to vomit and wretch again. I took the feed down, gave him some analgesia and he went off to sleep. But as he wakes up every 20 minutes to expectorate, it's no surprise he's so exhausted during the day.

I got up at 7am and gave him the full dose of morphine allowed. I then climbed back into bed and we both woke up at 10. His neck looks absolutely dreadful and he says it feels as if he has been burnt with a blow torch.

If the same is happening inside his throat, which I imagine it is, then it really must be agony. I'm not surprised he needs so much analgesia. I'm just not bothered how drowsy he is during the day, he definitely needs everything I'm giving him for the pain.

I irrigate his neck on the outside with saline and apply a dry dressing. It's clean but the amount of serious fluid leaking from his neck is awful and it's also bleeding slightly. I phoned the district nurse and she will call tomorrow morning. I asked her to bring some clean dressings.

I decided to start his 12-hour feeding regime at 2pm this afternoon. His pump is battery operated, fully charged and he can move around the house freely if he needs to. But he couldn't be bothered to move at all today and didn't have anything to eat or drink.

There were no cheeky comments or witty one-liners; there haven't been for a while. He can't even be bothered to talk. I absolutely hate seeing him like this. All I can do is the practical things, give him a little kiss every now and again and tell him it's not much longer now before he'll start to feel better. I keep telling him he's nearly over the worst. Soon we can have a holiday, perhaps in a lovely cottage in Cornwall. We haven't been on a holiday in England for years.

He just sits in front of the TV dosed up on the morphine. He seems to just stare at it. I'm not sure he is really watching it. Golf today, not football, which makes a change. This is like running a marathon that you haven't trained for. It's exhausting and repetitive. It is not expected to be fun and fun it certainly is not.

How on earth do people manage when they have to do this for a really long period? Or even a lifetime? At least this is only temporary. I keep thinking it won't be for long. Just until Peter can eat and drink normally again. On Monday, if the recovery period goes to plan, he should be at his worst. He will then start to get better. Soon all this will be behind us.

The local pharmacy stopped by with eight more boxes of feed. I have never been less excited about a delivery of boxes. Usually boxes are exciting to open. Not this lot. I store them with the others, out of sight in the dining hall. Not too warm, not too cold, room temperature and out of direct sunlight.

Iffy rang at 5pm to check if it is OK for him and chief scout Jeff Lee to visit Peter tomorrow as arranged. Who arranged this and when? I check with Peter exactly what they are meeting for. Are they just going to call in for five minutes to see how he is?

No, they are going to discuss players' contracts and pre-season matches and signings. Plan for next season. Now this may not be a very good idea. Peter is not well enough to hold a rational conversation, never mind make Football League club decisions.

He may suggest they sign David Beckham or Ronaldo. He is very ill and dosed up with morphine. It would be like making major decisions after drinking a full bottle of vodka. I told Iffy it really is not a good idea.

Peter was also complaining about the pain. I have given him everything he can have but if the pain continues, I'll have to give him extra morphine in the form of Oromorph, the medication which gives him hiccoughs. I suppose as a last resort I may have to.

It will help with the pain but will also cause more pain and discomfort with hours of hiccoughing. Swings and roundabouts.

A dreadful day. Let's hope we have a better night than last night, but I really can't see it. I'll sleep in my velour tracksuit as I know I'll be up and down all night.

Friday, April 18: Recovery Day Eight

I took Peter up to bed at 10.30 and when he was in the bathroom, he started to wretch over the sink. It sounded awful and must have been agony. To stand and watch was heartbreaking.

I opened the window for some fresh air, kept mopping his forehead with a damp cloth, reassuring him, trying to keep him calm and telling him to take deep breaths. Then he started to vomit. I was just about to go and get a syringe to aspirate his tube when he vomited his naso gastric tube out of his mouth.

It was unpleasant, distressing and he was panicking. His first instinct was to grab the tube from the mouth end and pull. I stopped him immediately and, very calmly but as fast as possible, took the plaster off his forehead and nose and pulled the tube out via the nose. It only took a few seconds but must have felt an eternity to Peter.

I got him into bed and calmed him down but Charlotte had heard all the noise. She popped her head around the door and promptly ran away. I didn't have time to attend to her but when the drama was over, I nipped downstairs to find Charlotte.

She was sitting on the kitchen floor crying her eyes out. I sat and comforted her for a while and told her to put the kettle on. Putting the kettle on always seems to work at times like this. It does on TV anyway.

I ran back upstairs to check on Peter, who was looking very pale. I ran downstairs to check on Charlotte, who was laid on the kitchen floor looking very pale. I decided not to look in the mirror at myself! I tidied up all the mess while Charlotte lay on the bed with her dad. She looked like a ghost with mascara running down her white face.

Peter slept upright and I lay in bed next to him until he was asleep. I knew it wouldn't be for long as he would be expectorating all night. He managed his usual restless sleep and I popped in every hour to check he was OK. Well, as OK as possible.

At 7am I gave him his morphine by mouth. He tolerated it. Just. It was very painful for him to swallow. Then I weighed Peter on my scales. He's lost over a stone in two weeks. This should not be happening.

The feed he is on should provide all the calories he needs to maintain his weight. I did leave a message for the dietician yesterday and I'm waiting for her to call back. I also phoned our GP and asked him to call to review his analgesics as the morphine is not controlling his pain.

I don't believe anyone should suffer with pain. It is unnecessary and sometimes badly managed and thankfully the GP arrived soon after my call and wrote a new prescription. The district nurse also came and had to fill in a form with questions like: have you got smoke alarms fitted in the house? I know it's procedure, but honestly smoke alarms are the last thing on my mind at the moment.

I phoned the hospital in Halifax to ask when a doctor would be able to replace the NG tube. But when we arrived at the ward, we bumped into Michelle, the Macmillan nurse, and she said she would do it. When we got home, I put up his feed and he lay down in bed for a couple of hours.

That gave me a chance to catch up on my alternative life as a sports reporter! While Peter is ill, I am writing his column in the Lincolnshire Echo, updating all his loyal fans on his condition and progress.

It also lets a lot of friends and acquaintances know how he is, both in the newspaper and on the Internet. When they read he has had a bad week they all ring to check how he is. Not good at the moment is the honest answer!

Saturday, April 19 – Recovery Day Nine

Peter was clapping his hands at 7am. I must remember to get a bell from somewhere. I don't want him getting sore hands as well as sore everything else. While Oliver, his girlfriend Stacey and I were having breakfast, Peter came down and said he fancied some scrambled egg. He only managed a couple of mouthfuls, but at least he tried. His neck still looks dreadfully sore but it's healing from the outside corners in. He's also managing to keep his dressing on now and actually says it feels better with the dressing on.

Oliver went off to meet his cousin Anthony, who is getting married in June. He needs to be measured up for a suit. Let's hope Peter is strong enough to enjoy the day... and we can stay long enough to get my money's worth from my outfit.

Stacey went to the chemist to collect the increased doses of medication only to be told that the wholesaler had sent the wrong order. She said that wasn't good enough, that we have a very ill patient who has been waiting since yesterday for this medication. They phoned around frantically and she had to drive to Boots in Halifax town centre. They had it all in stock.

Then, as she was walking past a charity shop she saw a little porcelain bell in the window. The assistant gave her a strange look when she bought it, probably wondering why a trendy 20-year-old should want an old-fashioned porcelain bell.

It was probably once used by a sweet old lady ringing to say it was time for afternoon tea. Now it is going to be used frantically for "Get me some more tissues!" or "Is it time for my medication?" I hope he doesn't break it as it's very delicate.

At 2pm I asked Peter how much pain he was in on a scale of 0-10. He said five. OK, time to try the Oromorph again - the hiccough medicine. Five minutes later, I heard the bell ringing.

He asked if I'd given him something different as he felt sick. I sat with him and it wore off. He felt tired but would not go to bed, lying on the settee instead. No hiccoughs though but no pain reduction either. At 6pm, it was still at level five.

He had a football afternoon, watching the scores and getting very excited as Lincoln were winning. He must feel better as he is getting enthusiastic about football again. And the bell was in constant use.

I spent the afternoon in the other room, reading the paper, and every time the ball rang it was to show me a football score. I jumped up and down each time just to humour him but eventually he looked at me as if I was stupid. So no point in wasting any more energy then.

But apart from the football scores, a peaceful and uneventful day, thank goodness. All the kids' friends arrived and they went off for a big night out; we had another Saturday night in.

Sunday, April 20: Recovery, Day Ten

Ten days after treatment finished. Peter should be at his worst today. He woke at 8am and felt a bit sick. The pain did seem better to me yesterday and I think he now automatically says five on the threshold when I ask him. I am not too sure.

I jumped into bed next to him. "How much pain are you in?"

"Five."

"Are you sure?"

"Stop quizzing me, it's fucking agony."

Stacey and Oli were sitting at the bottom of the bed when he answered and we all just started laughing. He did sound funny. Have you ever tried to shout when all you can do is whisper? I think he is getting his sense of humour back...but he said it wasn't supposed to be funny.

Oliver has been the light-hearted one through all this dreadful time. Although he has been terribly upset in private, he always puts on a brave face in front of his dad. He has a witty sense of humour. Very dry. Sometimes he comes out with something that I can laugh at for hours.

No one else will find it funny but Oliver and I just laugh at the same things. Tears can roll down our faces and we make each other worse. By the time we stop laughing we've forgotten what it was we were laughing at in the first place.

Oliver will come home from work in the evening and just carry on as normal. He quickly asks how Dad is and then elaborates on the day's events. He paints a great picture. Even when Peter has been too ill to listen, he tells his stories anyway.

He works long hours in sales for a Mini dealership in Bradford. It's a perfect role for him as he's very smart, young and handsome. He cares about people and is very good at building relationships. He is well liked by his customers and colleagues and always looks on the bright side of things.

When Charlotte rang from her cousin's house, she sounded worse than Peter so she had a good night. She rang again about one hour later and said she thinks it's more than a hangover as she can't keep even a sip of water down. I reassured her it is a hangover!

While I was tidying up when Peter was having a lie-down, I decided I'm having withdrawal symptoms from no shopping. I decided to resort to the Internet...and immediately the bell rang upstairs. So he must have known what I was doing. Never mind, will try again later!

Peter was ready for his shower. Teeth regime done, gargles and mouthwashes done, cream applied to drier bits on neck, cream applied to lips, dry dressing applied to wet bit on neck. More medication. Lots of water via the tube as he's still not managing to drink any water at all.

The feed regime started at 1pm. Peter now hates it and seems a bit agitated and annoyed with it all. It pins him down, he says. I told him he would only be watching football on TV anyway.

He has to have it some time, there's no escaping it. He doesn't like it overnight now as he thinks he may choke so it has to be during the day, which makes him less mobile. What can you do? He is still too poorly and tired to do anything anyway.

He read the paper for a while but could not seem to concentrate for long. Then he watched the TV but I'm not sure if he was really watching or not. Visitors arrived in a steady flow. It was far too noisy for him and he got up with his feed and took a couple of walks around the house.

It was much too cold to go outside. He stood at the door for a breath of fresh air. He seemed agitated and snappy with me and with himself, although he put on a bit of a smile for everyone else.

He just didn't know what to do with himself. At one time in the lounge there was Peter, me, Charlotte, Oliver, Stacey, Amanda, Francine, Anthony and Cath. Peter and Christine had just left. Everyone was talking and it was just too much for him. He looked like a caged animal. I really felt for him. He just wanted everyone to go home.

He says he only likes it when it's me and him, nice and quiet. Now I know he doesn't really mean that as they are all family and people he loves, but it did seem a bit overpowering. Normally it's the noisier the better but he just cannot cope at the moment.

He just wants to be looked after and pampered. He just wants to be stress free. He just wants to be quiet and relaxed. When everyone had left he just sat with his head in his hands.

I didn't speak. Just gave him a cuddle. He must just be so fed up with everything. He feels ill and tired and always has a degree of pain. He was shattered by the end of the afternoon. He said he'd try a bit of bread and cream cheese, had one mouthful, which looked agony, and threw it to one side. I threw it away.

He asked if we could go to Bridlington this week, just the two of us. I said it would be lovely and we'd see how he feels. But I know it's extremely doubtful and I think he knows it, too. He decided to go to bed at 9pm, just to lie in the dark and quiet.

I took him up and did his feet for him then went up every half an hour to see him. He was OK but still not asleep. Just nodding and enjoying the peace. Then I got all his overnight and early morning medicines ready to take upstairs with me.

At 10.30 I checked on him before climbing into the spare bed. I gave him a little kiss on the forehead like you would a poorly child. He was asleep. I lay in bed waiting for the buzzer to go at 1am when his feed will be finished for the day.

Monday, April 21: Recovery Day 11

Review clinic at St James's. His neck is looking much better. It has stopped weeping so there was no need for a dressing today. In fact, when I look closely at his throat, it looks wrinkle and crease free. This is what women pay a fortune for - a chemical peel! It has taken ten years off his neck. Not worth the pain, of course, but I manage to look at it as a slight bonus!

In the reception area, we spoke to a man who has had operations to his mouth and jaw and chemotherapy. He is now following all of this with 35 treatments of radiotherapy. He's on treatment 20 today and has not lost his voice at all.

He was diagnosed with throat cancer after 18 months' going to the doctor with a cough. The doctor had told him it was an infection or a virus and kept giving him antibiotics. Then he said maybe it was asthma.

Eventually he stormed into the doctor and demanded a second opinion. He was diagnosed with throat and mouth cancer. If he had not insisted on a second opinion he would only have had about two years to live.

He was funny and very matter of fact about his illness. He said he'd seen Peter a couple of weeks ago on a trolley. He'd thought, "Well, it's got the big guy down after all." He guessed Peter had lost about three stones in weight but actually it's 19lbs since he started his treatment.

The majority of this has been lost in the past couple of weeks while having his NG feeds. He is beginning to look too thin and certainly doesn't want to lose any more. We are called through to see Dr Dyker.

She asks how he is. He says fine. I say he has been really ill.

She asks him how he is tolerating his feed. He says fine. I say he is on Maxalon as he feels sick.

She asks him if his bowels are OK. He says fine. I say he has intermittent diarrhoea.

She asks him how his pain is. He says fine. I say it is still five on the 0-10 scale.

She asks if he's sleeping OK. He says fine. I say he is not and has the occasional night cold sweats.

She asks him how much he is expectorating. He says not a lot. I say about four kitchen rolls a day.

She asks him if he can swallow anything. He says he tries. I say he cannot even swallow water at the moment.

She asks him if he has lost any weight. He says a couple of pounds. I say 19lbs.

What planet is he on? Why doesn't he tell her the truth? She can see how ill he is by just looking at him.

She decides to send him for some blood tests and will need to see him again next week. She increases his MST to 50mgs morning and night. I ask how much it could safely be increased to. She says a lot more than that.

Peter asks can it go up to 200mgs morning and night. She laughs and says that would not be a good idea. He asks has anybody ever done that. She says no. He says he wants to do it for charity. She says there are perhaps other things he could do which would be much safer!

Iffy phoned to see if he could visit. I looked at Peter and he was turning that shade of grey again and his eyes were nearly closing. I told Iffy he just wasn't up to it. I felt really awful but he would just be wasting his time.

Peter fell asleep on the settee as soon as we arrived home. He looks exhausted, his eyes dark and sunken. Surely he should be feeling and looking better soon. I fear it will be a long and slow climb back to health and he was very fed up this evening. I think it's because everyone he has spoken to at the hospital always seem to have had more than one cancer. They are always worse than Peter and all very matter of fact.

He went to bed at 9.30 with his increased dose of morphine (not the 200mgs he had mentioned to Dr Dyker). He asked me to check on him in 15 minutes but I got engrossed in something on TV…and soon the bell was ringing from upstairs.

I dashed up, thinking something must be wrong. But no, just that it's 20 minutes since I left him and I said I'd be back in 15. I must remember to set my alarm next time! He said he was sorry and asked if I'm getting fed up of him. I lay in bed with him until he started coughing and spluttering, by which time I'd missed my programme. Never mind. I'm sure it will be repeated some time.

Tuesday, April 22: Recovery Day 12

The choking and vomiting started at 3am. I grabbed the syringe and started to aspirate. Nothing came up. I gave him 10mgs of Maxalon very slowly in a little water, told him to keep it down for 20 minutes and he should feel better.

I took the feed down – it still had a couple of hours to run. I threw it in the bag at the side of the bed, which is already full of kitchen roll. I sat at the side of the bed with him, mopping him down with a face cloth. I opened the window for some fresh air.

His throat was very painful with the wretching. He said it was the new stuff I had given him and asked me if I know what I'm doing. Am I trying to poison him? OK sweetheart, go back to sleep now. I propped his pillows up, made him comfortable and sloped off back to the spare room.

In the morning I cleared up around the bed and went to tidy up downstairs. I looked at myself in the mirror. I look shocking. Absolutely knackered. At 10am, I decided that, as he was still asleep, I could pop to M&S in Halifax.

It takes about 15 minutes each way and I told him I would be back at midday and no later. He nodded his head and I left a note downstairs to remind him where I'd gone. I rushed into M&S for some food, thinking what he could manage to eat at the moment. I got some crème caramel, which normally he loves…but I know they will end up in the bin on the expiry date.

Then I got the urge to shop – withdrawal symptoms kicking in. I was conscious of the time but fortunately it's only a tiny store with not many clothes so there wasn't too much damage to the credit card.

A bit of retail therapy normally cheers me up but this time it didn't work. But at least I didn't waste a fortune and the pink shoes with the just right size heel will look fab with my black tight jeans.

When I get home, bang on midday, Peter was waiting for me. Where have I been and why didn't I tell him I was going out? I showed him my few goodies and he said I already have all of those upstairs. He said I'll never wear those shoes and I probably won't.

I got him his medication and asked what time he wanted to start his feed. "Now, let's get it over with." He refused to have any Calogen. I gave him it anyway. Again he asked me if I know what I am doing.

He says the feed is making him sick; I say he will be even sicker if he doesn't have it. He says he is not getting better because he is having 2250 calories in and he is vomiting 8000 calories out. It's my fault he's vomiting, I must be putting it up wrong.

I give in. I've had enough. I tell him to give his own medication and put his own feed up so he knows exactly what he is giving himself. I give him the medicine chart, the syringe, the sterile water, the box of medication, the giving set, the feed and I go and put the kettle on. I feel like telling him where to stick the drip stand. I sit down and have a lovely cup of coffee.

I was sitting reading the paper and drinking my coffee when he came to find me. He said I'm not looking after him properly. I didn't say anything, just gave him "the look". I very calmly put my coffee and newspaper down. I put up his feed and gave him his medication. Nothing else was said.

As it was a lovely sunny day we sat outside on the patio for a while. I suggested getting out the new patio set but he said it was too cold. It's 18 degrees. He wandered up and down the garden with his drip stand in his hand and Fergie, our next door neighbour, offered to cut the grass.

They had a discussion about how many millimetres short it should be and what blade setting it should be on. All very boring stuff but at least he was showing an interest in something, which must be a good sign.

His lie-down had to be timed in between more medications and I had to shake him awake before I gave him any more. He complained, why had I woken him up? I can't win. Whatever I do is wrong so I carry on regardless. I will continue trying my utmost to make him better. I will not get down about this. I will just "bat on" as the saying goes.

Loads of people phoned to ask when they could visit. I have been very honest with them and told them not at the moment. He is still not well enough, but next week hopefully he will be a lot better. When I put the phone down after one of the calls, Peter said I was "short" with them. I wasn't, but perhaps I could let him plan his own visitors as well as doing his own medication.

When I gave him his night's fix of morphine, his eyes glazed. That's when he gets impatient and snappy. He shouted at the cats to move out of his way. He says he can't touch them as they have germs. Oh dear! I haven't bothered asking him about his pain all day as I know what the answer would be. Yep, you guessed it a five.

After I put Peter to bed I gave Charlotte the pink shoes.

Wednesday, April 23: Recovery Day 13

I think we are turning the corner. Peter said he'd had a bad night but not as bad as some. He just longs to sleep all the way through. I keep telling him that not too much longer and he will be sleeping like a baby.

He managed a soft-boiled egg and a crème caramel but he still cannot swallow water. I poured him a cup of tea, which I have done every morning. He took two sips and I threw it away, as I have done every morning. But he looks much better in himself. He actually grabbed my bottom and gave me a little kiss so things are definitely looking more positive!

After lunch, he decided he needed to weigh himself. He has put on one pound since Monday. Great news, I'm delighted. I have been slipping in more Calogen than the 30mls three times a day. More like 50mls…but it has worked.

His dad phoned to say it was raining where he lives so he wouldn't be coming over to trim the bushes in the garden. Peter was really mad and said he'd do them himself. I had visions of him hanging off the wall with his electric garden shears in one hand and his drip stand in the other. I told him that would be impossible. At least wait until his backpack arrives.

It will be delivered tomorrow. It means he can carry the feed and pump around on his back and can use it any time of day. Now Peter always thinks that people with backpacks are geeky so we will see. He thinks he'll look like Roy Cropper out of Coronation Street. But it might be OK in the garden or for a trip out in the car.

I kept looking at him and felt so happy that he looks so much better. I wondered if I dared ask him the question: "On a scale of 0-10, how is the pain?" I'm astounded at the answer. "Two."

While he was having a couple of hours' nap in the afternoon, I nipped to Tesco. I spent ages there and bought all sorts of things. I felt I had at least an hour where I could escape from the house.

I bought some balls that look like stone but they have a wick and you fill them with lantern oil for the garden. A couple of new vases, new pillows for Oliver's room, lots of magazines and newspapers, a Delia Smith Cookbook. You know, all the essential things in life…and a bit of food.

When I got home the sun was shining and it was lovely to sit out, have a coffee and read the magazines. Christine called on her way home from a meeting and we sat and had a girlie catch-up.

Peter appeared at about 4pm. "What's all that rubbish you've bought from Tesco's?" He didn't seem quite as excited as I am about the stone balls. But he then spent a while on the phone to Iffy and Steff. Another good sign.

He sat outside with us for an hour, reading the paper. Then he checked out the new cookbook. I told him I'd make him anything at all as they are all really easy recipes and cooking is something I don't normally have time to do.

He said the first thing he'll want to eat will be a Cornish pasty followed by a pizza. Neither is in the new cookbook so I'll have to resort to buying them. May as well put Delia on the shelf with the rest.

Talking about food must have given him an appetite and he managed a couple of spoonfuls of soup before telling Christine we might be going to Cornwall this weekend. He does live in a dream world sometimes. But at least he must be feeling much better to even think about it.

We may be able to make it to Bridlington for a day or two soon but we'll see how he feels in the next couple of days. He wouldn't be great company at the moment but I could always sit on the new decking if the weather was nice.

At 6pm, he fell fast asleep on the settee. He'd only been awake for two hours but I think he was building up the energy to watch whatever match was on Sky tonight. I was on the phone to Joanne when I heard him frantically ringing his bell in the lounge.

I threw the phone down and ran out of the kitchen through the hall into the lounge. He was standing there, bright red in the face and jumping up and down in pain. In his hand was a glass of orange squash! He said he'd fancied some and poured it himself.

The acid must have really stung his throat. I passed him his glass of water and phoned Joanne back. God knows what he would have done if I'd left him in charge of everything as I'd threatened yesterday. It doesn't bear thinking about!

Thursday April 24: Recovery Day 14

Two weeks since treatment finished; surely there should be some improvement today. It's like when you are having a baby, you expect to give birth on the day it's due. It doesn't often happen and then you get bored and frustrated when the baby doesn't arrive.

I leaped out of bed at 7am to give him his MST. I don't know what I was really expecting, sitting up smiling or something. No. He looked exactly the same as he did yesterday morning and the morning before and the morning before.

I went to bed for an hour and decided that if Peter was still not well enough to do anything, I'd clean a wardrobe or something. His dad arrived in his gardening gear but it was so wet outside he decided that electricity and water do not mix. So he'll have to trim the bushes another day.

He had some breakfast; Peter sipped iced water. He tried an egg but that didn't go down at all this morning. He got very angry and frustrated and threw it to one side. Nor did he have much patience about whispering to his dad, who couldn't hear him. Here we go again with the translation.

I ended up forgetting who the deaf one is and this time Peter shouted - by the look on his face he was trying to shout, "I'm not the bloody deaf one." Gerard arrived so there was more coffee and toast and an ice cube for Peter. I let him take over the translations for a while.

Caroline and Faye, my friends from work, came for lunch and Peter sloped off to bed as I don't really think he wanted to be seen with a big tube up his nose. After lunch I nipped out for a coffee in town with Joanne, another friend. We called in at a little boutique on the way home.

When I got back, Peter said I had been neglecting him. In fact, I'd been out of the house for less than two hours between his 2pm and 4pm medications. He's very frustrated now. He cannot talk, he cannot eat, he cannot drink, he cannot socialise, he is extremely tired all the time, his throat is still painful, he's still knocked out with massive doses of morphine, he looks pale and ill. He tells me to go out for a couple of hours, but hates it when I do. It is awful for him. He is even bored with his television.

I showed him the 'Roy Cropper' backpack that arrived this morning. He took one look at it and said, "As if…" I can understand, but it may be worth a try. I'll try again tomorrow, but I haven't got a clue how it's all supposed to fit together.

I asked him if there was anything at all he would like to try and eat. I said it wouldn't matter if he tries and we just have to throw it away. I said I could blend anything at all for him. He said he rather not eat blended mush, it would look like baby food. I tell him not to look, just to eat. He didn't answer.

At 7pm he leaped up and marched into the kitchen with his drip stand in tow. He came back with a piece of toast! Now this I have to see. Is he on some kind of kamikaze mission? He says anything is painful and he is going to ram it down. OK.

It took him about half an hour to swallow three mouthfuls but at least he tried. In the end, he gave up and just watched TV until bedtime. It has been very difficult today to jolly him along and I feel absolutely exhausted.

I also feel guilty that I haven't given him 100 per cent attention. He looks like a rejected puppy that has been left at home by himself for the day. Both kids arrived home looking fed up and tired.

They feel for their dad. They hate to see him like this and just want to see some sign of their old dad back again. Fit, healthy and full of life. We all look as washed out as each other. Where has our lively, upbeat, happy family gone?

Friday, April 25: Recovery Day 15
I decided today was going to be a much better day and we'd try the backpack. No arguments. He was not quite as enthusiastic about the idea and asked where, exactly, were we going? Anywhere. Just out.

He left a cup of tea and said he needed just a little more sleep. I left him until 10am and was not going to give in easily. Persistence pays - usually. I went downstairs and got out the backpack.

I laid it on the floor and looked at the pictures of how it all fits together. Easy. When it was all fitted up, I went upstairs and tried to enthuse Peter. He looked about as enthusiastic as he would if I was teaching him to knit a jumper.

He reluctantly went into the shower and got dressed. I then attached up the kitbag, slung it over his shoulder and dragged him into the car like a child going to his first day at school. I must say the bag doesn't match his designer jeans and jumper. Never mind, he isn't going to see anybody.

He asked where we were going and I said to see his dad, who lives about 12 miles away. Half a mile into our journey, he said he felt sick. I carried on.

Then I was going over too many bumps in the road. I carried on.

Then I was breaking too hard. I carried on.

Then, I was driving too fast. I carried on.

Then why did I come this way as it has too many bends? I slammed on the brakes. I stopped the car. I asked if he wanted to turn back as I was struggling to remain cheerful and could think of many other things I would rather be doing. He said no, we were nearly there now so we might as well carry on. He shut up moaning.

We arrived at his dad's house and he went and sat down and read the paper. He did look tired. His dad made him a cup of tea, which he left untouched as always. He made us feel very welcome and we had a walk around the garden to look at his fish pond.

Then home. A short visit but just enough. He went straight to bed when we get home and slept from two to four pm. Meanwhile I phoned Christine and we decided to try Bridlington for the night tomorrow. We'll see how he feels in the morning.

In the evening, he tried some mashed potato and cauliflower cheese. It looked very painful but he managed a few mouthfuls. He did look a bit more cheerful and I think his hour out of the house has done him good.

The backpack was a success, he managed a bit of food, he doesn't look quite so grey and he seems quite excited about Bridlington. He also made lots of football calls today so things are looking up. Let's take it step by step but at least everything is looking more positive.

Saturday, April 26: Recovery Day 16

I was really hoping he'd be well enough to travel to Bridlington. I took in his cup of tea, pulled the blinds up, opened the windows and turned on the shower. He said he wasn't well enough to travel. I had a lovely fluffy bath towel ready as he stepped out of the shower and had got him some clothes to travel in. He said he wasn't well enough.

I set his feed up and put on his Roy Cropper backpack. I had to make the decision; is he really not well enough or is it just that he really can't be bothered? Decision made. We're going. All he has to do is sit in the car.

He climbed in reluctantly and off we went. His face was a picture, like a spoilt child. When we arrived it was a lovely day; we phoned Charlotte at home…it was raining.

He helped to empty the car but his feed pump alarm was ringing, meaning there was a blockage somewhere in the tubing. He just carried on as if nothing was happening. The tubing was nearly wrapped around his neck but he wasn't bothered. I sat him down and sorted it out. He made himself comfortable on the sofa.

Christine and Deegs arrived soon afterwards and after the 2pm medication, I had two hours to escape for a while. The boys stayed in and watched football and me and Christine went into Bridlington for a wander around the shops.

And it made me wonder when I will be allowed to go to Leeds or Manchester again. It seems like an eternity since I did the normal things that women like to do, like looking for shoes or that really nice dress.

We arrived back in time for Peter's medications to discover Lincoln were winning at Morecambe. Great news and Peter was really pleased. We ordered a takeaway pizza from the little Italian Restaurant where we would normally eat on a Saturday night and when Christine and I went to collect it, all the staff asked how Peter is doing.

I told them he is now improving slowly but wouldn't be able to manage any of the pizza. Instead, they sent him a bowl of ice cream to try. On the way back, we passed the little village pub that has just been refurbished. They are having a live band tonight for the re-opening.

We have been invited and normally it would be our kind of thing. I just wish we were in a position to make the choice. Instead, we all stayed in and Peter must have felt guilty because he suggested that we should pop out for a drink, he would be OK by himself. We all said we'd rather not go.

Instead, Deegs said he'd have a cup of coffee. I gave him a bottle of red wine and told him not to be silly. I had one drink…I have to be completely sober when giving him all his medications.

Peter went to bed at 10pm, feeling sick. It must be really awful for him. How can anyone take so many medicines without feeling sick? Do you cut out a lot of the medication and be in pain or do you take the medication and feel sick?

Things have to get better soon. It's a very slow climb back and he's very fed up. I'm getting very fed up for him. He thinks he should be getting better much faster but no two patients' recoveries are the same.

Compared to last week he is a lot better. And I told him that this time next week he will probably have his tube out as he'll be able to eat and drink. Fingers crossed.

Sunday, April 27: Recovery Day 17

He managed a little bit of toast at breakfast. Toast was always good for children when they had their tonsils removed; toast and crunchy cornflakes to help remove the scabs at the back of the throat. This stopped the tonsil bed from getting infected and helped with healing. It sounds like being cruel to be kind but it worked. So it must be a good sign if he can manage it.

Normally, on a Sunday morning we'd all have a long walk on the beach, whatever the weather, and usually end up with a big bacon sandwich by the harbour. Not today though. Peter was too tired and at lunchtime he was ready to go home.

On the way back he kept whispering to me, thinking I could hear. I couldn't and couldn't face him to lip read because I was driving. It's the same on any journey. Eventually he stopped trying and I babbled on about anything and everything until I ran out of things to talk about. I turned the radio on. He turned it off. Too noisy. We sat in silence. He tried to talk again, I couldn't hear him.

We practised making noises – aah-eeh etc. Nothing worked. I said he is going to need some voice coaching when the time is right. He says he isn't. I said if a player breaks his leg, he needs a physiotherapist. A voice coach is just a physio for his vocal chords. He didn't answer.

When we arrived home he was tired. I was tired. I gave him his medicine, which he says makes him feel sick. I just accept that he feels sick as there is nothing else I can do. I have no idea why he feels sick, I can only do my best and it isn't good enough.

I have tried everything and I'm continually thinking, "Maybe if I give this with this, maybe if I try this with this, maybe if I give that 20 minutes earlier than this." I have tried every combination possible. Nothing works.

At 8.30 he decided to go to bed. I don't think he was tired, just annoyed that he is so restricted. Normally I would have gone upstairs to help him. Tonight I just sat and watched TV with Charlotte and felt just blank inside.

To be honest, I wasn't even watching TV, just staring at it. I usually keep all the doors open when he goes to bed so I can hear him. But tonight I couldn't even be bothered to open them. I sent Charlotte upstairs to see if he needed anything. He said no.

At 10pm I took his feed down and gave him his medication very slowly. He sat at the side of his bed with his head down, saying he felt sick. I asked him if he wanted me to continue. He said yes. I carried on very slowly. Soul destroying.

I tidied up around him and kissed him goodnight. As I went out of the door he said thank you and told me he loves me. I told him I love him too. Then I sat downstairs feeling helpless. I am doing absolutely everything I can for him, but feel as if I am getting absolutely nowhere.

I told myself not to be ridiculous and not to let it get me down. But I am only human. I just sat and cried; the cats just sat and looked at me. I waited for 30 minutes, hoping and praying he will be fast asleep when I go upstairs. Sleep is a great healer but it's just not working at the minute. I can't help but feel worried.

Monday, April 28: Recovery Day 18

An afternoon appointment at St James's. When we arrived, we waved to a few people we have met along the way. Some looking a lot worse than they did last week, some looking a lot better. All conversations finish with, "Good luck." Not goodbye, or see you later. Good luck.

Dr Saunders reviewed his medication, adding Gaviscon four times a day and changing the Losec to Lansoprazole to see if it will help with the gastric reflux and vomiting. He also increased the Maxalon to 10mgs four times a day.

The good news is that Peter has maintained his weight this week; the bad news is they still haven't discharged him and we have to be seen again next Tuesday, after the Bank Holiday Monday. They want to keep an eye on him until his NG tube is removed.

When we got home, I gave Peter his painkillers and then Iffy, Grant and Jeff arrived, Grant with a lovely big flower arrangement for me. I explained that one hour would be long enough and that I didn't want to sound bossy but any longer really would exhaust him. And I'd be left with an over-tired toddler to sort out. They stayed for just an hour.

When they had gone, Peter started to vomit acid reflux again. He also said his throat felt very sore from talking a lot. Whispering more like. It was the first time Oliver had witnessed this vomiting and retching.

I sat with him until it had passed off. If anything it's getting worse. I stopped the feed, gave him more Maxalon and also Gaviscon tablets to dissolve in his mouth. I really cannot think of anything else I can give him.

While we were having tea, Peter popped into the kitchen to see what we were having. It must be awful to smell food so we do try to keep out of the way. We also had a glass of wine, which Peter just looked at. I could tell he could murder a glass but there's no chance.

Then the phone calls started. Anthony and Cath from Portugal, where they are on holiday, staying with their friends at their villa. They invited us to stay whenever we can. I cannot imagine this will be for a while yet. A holiday in the sun seems a long way away.

He looked tired tonight, but he actually didn't have a sleep today, which is a huge move in the right direction. I am sure that when we get on top of this gastric reflux and vomiting he will feel so much better.

Tuesday, April 29: Recovery Day 19
Today was always going to be eventful because I had an appointment at the hairdresser's at midday. I gave Peter all his medication at 11.30 and I told him I would be home at around 2.30. Oliver was having a day off and Fergie and his son Dave were due to jet spray the patio so I was hopeful there wouldn't be a crisis.

At the hairdresser's, I enjoyed all the banter, caught up with all the girlie gossip and had just got myself comfortable on the uncomfortable backrest when Richard, who owns the salon with Sally, came over and said that Oliver was on the phone.

I dashed through the salon with my hair wet through. It was Peter and I could hear a faint whisper that his feed had got air in the tube and the alarm was ringing. I told him to stop it and detach the tubing.

He then needed to flush a syringe of water through the tube to stop it blocking. He has seen me do it countless times but has never done it himself. He said he would try. When my hair was finished I called in the local deli for a salad on my way to the car. That's when I got a call on my mobile telling me to rush home. I asked him if he was OK and he said, "Just rush home."

I drove like crazy and arrived to find him in the garden chatting to Fergie, his wife Pam and Dave. He looked OK to me. I asked him what all the rush was and he said he was missing me.

Oliver and Stacey have put in an offer for a little cottage and he wanted us to have a look while they are waiting to see if their offer has been accepted. We drove to take a look through the window and it looks lovely, perfect for a first-time buyer.

This has been Peter's best day by far. He looks so much better in himself. He managed some toast and ice cream tonight. The only problem is I had to endure another night of football on TV. Great!

Wednesday, April 30: Recovery Day 20

Twenty days since the radiotherapy was completed. I have to say it has been a far worse ride than I expected and has gone on far longer, too. I hadn't envisaged that the NG would still be in place. I hadn't expected the vomiting to be this bad or the pain to be still so severe. Sleepless nights? I hadn't believed they would ever be this much of a problem.

All in all, it's a bit of a shock. Even Christine and Deegs, who spent the day with us in Bridlington at the weekend, were shocked at how poorly he still was because when they have popped in twice a week he's put on a brave face. He cheers up when we have visitors.

I had planned on keeping this diary for 20 days of treatment and 20 days after treatment so today, when we were due to see Mr Sutton at Huddersfield General Infirmary for a check-up on his lip, should have been my last log. Good news on the lip: everything is fine.

On the way home we had a call from Oliver to say that the offer on the cottage has been accepted. They are so excited. I am so pleased for them but the house will be very quiet without him and his stories every night. We'll miss him and I feel a little bit tearful; must be the hormones!

In the evening, Peter managed some boiled fish in butter sauce and some mashed potatoes. He said it tasted lovely.

Thursday, May 1: Recovery Day 21

Peter is well enough to leave for short periods as the vomiting and gastric reflux seem to have settled down a lot. He ate a bit of fish at teatime but swallowing seemed worse than yesterday. His feed continues as normal and he still has great difficulty in tolerating fluids by mouth.

Lincoln had their player of the year awards this week and they sent the DVD through to Peter. We sat and watched it this afternoon. It was lovely to watch shots of him before the illness, the big strong man we know and love, the big strong manager the fans know and love. It was also strange to hear him talk as all we hear at the moment is him whisper.

We may go to Bridlington tomorrow, we'll see how he feels in the morning. He seems to have been worse today than yesterday but he is staying awake for much longer periods and went to bed at 10.30 tonight. After watching the football, of course.

Friday, May 2: Recovery Day 22
We set off for Bridlington at midday. The usual drive: Peter can still only whisper and I can only guess at what he's saying, although I am now quite an expert. We both expected, or certainly hoped, that the tube might be down by now, but he could certainly not eat or drink enough or swallow his medications. So there is no chance yet.

Today he told me that although he is fed up of feeling ill, being in pain, having his NG tube in and not being able to do normal things, he really thought he was going to die when he was struck down by the virus or infection four weeks ago.

I said there was never any question of that. But he insisted that he really did think it was going to happen. He felt so ill that he really didn't think he was going to pull through.

In the afternoon we drove to B&Q for some varnish for the new decking and he came into the store with me, the first time he has been out in public with the NG tube in and his backpack.

He received a couple of strange looks but didn't seem to mind or pretended not to notice. He certainly didn't want any sympathetic looks. I was very proud of him as I certainly wouldn't have been seen out in public if it was me.

But he seems to be getting very frustrated about not improving fast enough although I keep telling him to be patient. He is improving although he still gets tired very easily and looks extremely pale. I suggested some Lancaster self-tan for his face. He refused and gave me 'the look!'

And today, he ate scrambled egg on toast, a small piece of cheese and some tiny soft cheese biscuits. He asked if I thought he'd be able to manage them and I said just to try anything he feels like now. He was also able to drink half a glass of water.

Saturday, May 3: Recovery Day 23
More scrambled egg and toast and then he started to vomit again. This time it was a bad one and he vomited out his NG tube. He felt much better afterwards and decided to mow the lawn while I varnished the new decking.

But the tube has to be replaced within 24 hours. As the replacement tube is at home, we decided we'd go to Halifax Infirmary tomorrow to have it put back in. First, though, we would see how he goes on with his eating and drinking because it is essential for him to keep hydrated and receive his medications.

He actually looks a lot better in his face…maybe because he doesn't have a tube dangling out of his nose and tucked behind his ear. But when Christine arrived at 2pm, she said, "Wow, that's amazing. You look so much better."

Is that because he actually feels so much better? Or it is psychological? Either way, he insists he's going to drink and eat enough to make sure the tube doesn't go back in. He has eaten all sorts of things today…and drunk water, too. Little and often is the order of the day so he does not overload his stomach but he ate a full carbonara from M&S for tea and asked if he could have a glass of wine with us this evening. The answer to that was a definite no.

I'm trying not to get too excited.

Sunday, May 4: Recovery Day 24
Peter said he fancied a bacon sandwich for breakfast; we thought he was joking. He wanted to try anyway. Christine and I went for the papers so we brought back some bacon. He managed a full bacon sandwich…but it didn't stay down for long. All vomited back within 10 minutes.

So he trundled back to bed for a sleep, looking tired and pale, and got mad when I woke him for a drink to stop him becoming dehydrated, telling me to stop nattering about him drinking. I explained how important it is to get at least one and a half litres of water down him or else he will end up being ill again.

An intake of calories to help build and repair the damaged cells from the radiation treatment is also vital and this will now be harder. All he has had for over three weeks is milk nutrients so it's difficult not to overload his stomach and he soon feels sick

It's Bank Holiday weekend and I really do not fancy battling with tourists up the East Coast to Scarborough hospital. We've been there once before. So when he refused his water, I packed up the car. We're going home. End of story.

He got the message and drank 500ml of water on the return journey. Good. And when we reached home I told him not to overload his stomach and just eat little and often. I gave him his medication and told him to take it before 2pm. I gave him a litre bottle of water and told him to drink it all before 8pm…if not, the tube would go back in.

I am not going to argue any more, it's down to him. Having to help Peter when he is not in the mood to be helped is very tiring so I decided to take myself out of the way and went to bed.

When I awoke an hour later, he was watching his football. He'd eaten a slice of bread with cheese and a Kit Kat and was well on with his water. It was pouring down outside and I wondered what the weather would be like in Bridlington. Still, never mind. Better to err on the side of caution because we're not out of the woods yet.

Yesterday, I bought some mini Cornish Pasties, which he has been longing for. He managed to eat two, with lots of gravy…not both at the same time but with a couple of hours in-between. He kept them down.

By the time he went to bed he had probably eaten about 900 calories all day, which is nowhere near enough to maintain his weight. We'll see what happens tomorrow and then we have an appointment at St James's on Tuesday. He could go rapidly downhill so it is essential to keep a close eye on him and if necessary, I will need to insist that the tube goes back in tomorrow. We will see.

Monday, May 5: Recovery Day 25
I measured out two litres of water and told him only once that he must drink this throughout the day. He is an adult and I am not going to fall out with him. He can either drink it or dehydrate. I have explained in detail why he needs to drink this amount and I left it to him.

By 1pm he had mowed the lawn in a temperature of 70 degrees and drunk about 200mls, which is not good. I tried not to get too annoyed and really bit my tongue. But he looked pale and ill again and I suggested it was because he had not drunk enough.

I really cannot understand the reluctance to drink. I will be the one who has to take him to hospital when he collapses. At the same point, I had drunk about five or six times more than him.

By 6pm, he'd got the message and had drunk one and a half litres. He has eaten little but often and tolerated it really well. No vomiting at all today. All in all a really good day and he managed without a sleep.

Tonight we were looking through some photographs I have been taking along the way and compared to this time last week he looks so much better. Keeping photos is a really good reminder because when you think the progress is very slow, it's possible to look back and see the improvement.

Tuesday, May 6: Recovery Day 26
I finally slept in our bed again last night. The expectorating is not unbearable and he used only about 20 pieces of kitchen roll all night. More improvements.

And later, when he was whispering to me, a croaky sound came through. It was the start of his voice coming back. It was then intermittent throughout the day and it was really strange to hear him talk.

We cancelled his appointment at St James' as they said that if he was OK, he didn't need to attend. We'll now wait for an appointment in outpatients at our local hospital.

Wednesday, May 7: Recovery Day 27

Gerard came for coffee and toast and Martin Booty also visited. He has just been released as a coach from Huddersfield Town. That's football. He was upset but I don't think it had properly sunk in that he was out of a job.

Peter looks as if he is thinking a lot at the moment and I can tell football is on his mind. Who can he sign and who can Lincoln afford, I should imagine. He has been making lots of football calls this week. Steff is coming to see him tomorrow so budgets will certainly be on his mind.

He is so much better. His morphine has been reduced to 80mgs today and paracetamol and Diclofenac twice a day. The pain is between one and two. I think we should soon be able to reduce it by 5-10mgs a day, but I will assess each day and see.

There's no rush but I know he's desperate to get off it and feel completely rational and fully awake again. He thinks he can just stop it but I suggest this would not be a very good idea. It will make him ill.

The dietician phoned to see how he was doing and was surprised he can eat Cornish pasties. She's going to call again next week but I have cancelled the next delivery of his feed.

They won't take away the unused stock in the house, though; we just have to throw it away. What a waste of money! But she told us to hang on to it anyway for a while longer. "You just never know," she said.

And today we booked to go to St Mawes in Cornwall. It's far too early to holiday abroad and at the moment I feel much safer knowing I am close to a British hospital. We're going to stay in a lovely beach house overlooking the sea. I haven't been to Cornwall since I was a child.

As I'm the only one who can drive – because Peter is still on his morphine – we'll probably set off tomorrow and break up the trip. The weather forecast for all next week is fantastic. Let's hope we can eat in some nice restaurants when we're down there; if not, I'm sure he'll manage a cream tea.

Thursday, May 8: Recovery Day 28

Exactly one month today since the radiotherapy finished. This morning we reduced the Morphine to 35mgs.

Football club business was on the agenda as Iffy and Steff came to discuss budgets and players for next season. They sat outside in the sunshine and I served lunch and lots of cold drinks on the patio.

The weather was so good I sat in the garden and sunbathed while they were having their meeting. At 3pm we set off for our long drive to Cornwall. The sun was still blazing down as we set off but after a couple of hours we drove into thick fog and rain. To make things worse it was still sunny and hot when we phoned the kids at home.

Never mind. We reached a Travelodge not far from our destination and talk about a healthy diet! McDonalds for evening meal and Peter managed to eat chicken nuggets and a few chips. I wondered what the dietician would say to that.

His pain ranked at two for most of the day but he still struggles to swallow without pain. Expectorating has eased a lot too and he only needs one kitchen roll a day.

Friday, May 9: Recovery Day 29

I gave Peter 40mgs Morphine and left him to sleep, went downstairs for a cappuccino and brought Peter a croissant for breakfast. Travelodges aren't the easiest of places if you want to eat healthy.

We arrived at Portscatho, near St Mawes in mid-afternoon. The house was delightful and overlooked the harbour. Very modern inside and decorated by an interior designer. Lots of lovely soft furnishings in light blues, white and pale yellows. Fabulous paintings and decorations. Amazing sea views.

It's beautiful, peaceful and certainly worth the long drive. We stopped at the local supermarket for stocks of fish, fruit, bread and a proper Cornish pasty for Peter from the local bakery. It's what he's been longing for so mission accomplished.

We drove into St Mawes for a wander around and a Cornish Cream tea and in the evening, took a walk on the beach. Peter was in bed by 9.30 and insisted I went, too. He says he can't go to sleep until I am in bed with him. I think this theory has been proved wrong over the past few weeks…but who am I to argue?

The lovely thing about this house is that there is no reception on either of our mobile phones.

Saturday, May 10: Recovery Day 30

We caught the ferry from St Mawes to Falmouth to visit the National Maritime Museum, something Peter was keen to see. Fish and chips for lunch and they seemed to go down very well. However, he seemed to be in more pain today and said it's been at level three on the scale.

It was a long day and he looked tired when we got back at 5pm. He's difficult to judge as I know he's pushing himself. But when I ask him if he is OK he goes mad and says to stop asking. While he slept for 90 minutes, I looked back at today's photographs and then read my book. I've brought lots of new CDs, tranquil music because Peter's is rubbish and far too noisy.

For some reason, he seems more cheerful in the evening than during the day. Not sure why. And I try to ignore it when he doesn't look too happy. I hope he is enjoying himself and I am sure he is in his own way.

Normally we would be going out for meals and sitting in pubs a bit more often and I think he is missing having a drink. He does still seem to be impatient about his recovery and I think that is the problem. This is something he really cannot rush.

I also think he is worried about his football. I think he feels under pressure to get back before he is ready and that is worrying him. Although he has been spending a lot of time on the phone, it's not the same as being in the office and at meetings most of the day. He will need to pace himself if he wants to be fit for pre-season.

Still it's a change of scenery and I think he's trying to enjoy it for my sake. The house and the area are beautiful even though the weather is awful and it will do him the world of good. I just wish he could relax and enjoy it but that's what life is like as a football manager. I don't think you can ever relax.

Sunday, May 11: Recovery Day 31

A car ferry to Truro today and a look around the shops. It's lovely. Then a short drive to Loe beach at Feock, near Truro, for the afternoon, reading the papers in the hot sun. But Peter hasn't looked very happy today and I'm not sure if he is in pain or not.

He still goes bonkers if I ask. He makes me feel as if I have done something wrong. I try not to let it bother me but he just seems very down and I know he is trying hard not to let it show.

He is very short-tempered and I never know what he's thinking. But I know something is bothering him. I can only guess, but who knows how I would be feeling if it was me? He may be worried whether the treatment has worked, if he will make a full recovery.

He does keep his feelings to himself. These are all normal feelings I am sure, but if he won't discuss anything then I cannot offer any reassurance. I just sit and look at him sometimes and he looks so sad. I just wonder what is ticking over in his head.

Who knows? Peter is not one, and never has been, for discussing anything apart from trivial things. Anything with any depth or seriousness is a definite no. Part of being his wife is also being his mind reader! But he will be absolutely fine, I know.

He is also probably thinking about football. He needs to sign some players and is always in his own world at this time of the season. Who he wants to sign and who he can afford are two different things. Players and managers are all away on holiday for the first couple of weeks after the season finishes but he is making a lot of calls even though we are away.

Football, Football, Football.

Monday, May 12, Tuesday, May 13, Wednesday, May 14: Recovery Days 32, 33, 34

We've visited lots of different places around the Roseland Peninsula. The weather has been either scorching hot or drizzling rain but who cares because Peter is eating everything and anything and enjoying his food again.

We can even eat out in restaurants. Alcohol is still very painful but he can manage a couple of lager-tops. It's not a good idea to be drinking alcohol while on morphine anyway. His pain is always around a two and he seems to have got used to that.

His voice is great, better than before his treatment started and he can even be heard on the other end of the phone. Everyone says it's great to be able to hear him again. He's sleeping really well at night and doesn't even need a sleep during the day.

The expectorating has more or less stopped and he now only needs a couple of tissues during the night. Gone are the days of two kitchen rolls.

His throat on the outside looks absolutely fine and I keep reminding him to apply suntan lotion so as not to burn it. But when he has a few days' beard growth it looks really strange as you can see clearly the shape of the mask. The hair will never grow where the radiotherapy mask has been. All the hair follicles have been destroyed. By the way - he never did use the dry electric razor!

He also seems much more cheerful and relaxed and looks much more healthy with a suntan. His mood seems to have lifted. It's good to visibly see him improving each day. And now he can speak it's not so frustrating for him.

He's getting his good old sense of humour back again and is shouting at people down the phone, which is a good sign. In fact, people who know him well are delighted to be shouted at.

Thursday, May 15: Recovery Day 35
We were supposed to be going home tomorrow but decided to stay in Padstow, in an apartment overlooking the harbour, for the next five nights… even though the forecast is not good.

Friday, May 16: Recovery Day 36
The apartment is lovely, very modern and new. It overlooks all the harbour and has a sweet little patio with chairs and planters at the back. All decorated in a yachting type of way but far more minimal than the house in Portscatho. Shame about the weather though.

Peter is enjoying everything he is eating and drinking and making up for lost time. He still says it feels like swallowing a boiled egg whole so there is still some inflammation but the pain seems much easier.

All in all he's progressing really well now, spending a lot of time on his mobile with football matters, speaking to Iffy and Steff and lots of football agents, trying to sign players. I'm sure he will be down in Lincoln for a couple of days when we return. I just hope he doesn't try to do too much too soon.

Saturday, May 17: Recovery Day 37
All through last night, I kept waking up with hot flushes throughout the night; age problems I would imagine! I tried to open the bedroom window

at about 2.30am but they were not easy to work out. I tried and tried and got hotter and hotter!

Peter woke up and asked me what I was doing? I asked him if he could open the window for me; he said I was extremely selfish for waking him up. He opened the window, moaning while he was doing it.

He promptly went back to sleep and I lay awake in disbelief at what he had just said. "Selfish for waking him up!" I thought about the sleepless nights, how many times had I jumped out of bed during the night to attend to his pain, vomiting, expectorating, choking and generally worrying about him?

Giving him his painkillers and anti-sickness drugs, changing his feed throughout the night. Sitting with him until he felt a little bit better, changing the bed when he had vomited, propping his pillows up and staying with him until he fell back asleep. And yet how selfish of me to ask him to open the window!

We decided first thing that we can't do anything about the weather so we hired two bikes and went on the Camel trail. It's supposed to be the most beautiful bike ride in England and runs along a disused railway line alongside the Camel estuary.

We just did the five miles from Padstow to Wadebridge and five miles back. It's a long time since I've ridden a bike and I suggested to Peter that, as he is not fully fit, that may be just enough for the both of us.

It was actually really enjoyable despite the weather. It was warm and dry when we set off and we stopped off for lunch at Wadebridge. The heavens absolutely opened on the way back and we got drenched. Let's see if I can walk tomorrow.

Peter then watched football while I did a bit of shopping. I can't get enough shopping at the moment and I can browse around the shops for ages making up for lost time when my limit was a 45-minute trip to Tesco.

Sunday , May 18: Recovery Day 38
We had a great night out in the pub last night. We only called in for one drink after we'd eaten in an Italian on the harbour but it turned into a long night. It was so lovely to enjoy a meal out together again.

Today was much better weather-wise and an opportunity to board the ferry over to Rock, where we had lunch. Plenty of walking on the beach in the sunshine and then we sat by the harbour most of the afternoon. We couldn't get into Rick Stein's restaurant so decided to eat in his fish and chip shop instead.

Monday, May 19: Recovery Day 39
Took a drive to Newquay but wished we hadn't bothered. It wasn't really our scene and certainly not as we remembered it from many years ago. We drove straight through, found a little cove and spent the rest of the afternoon

sunbathing and walking on the beach.

Tuesday, May 20: Recovery Day 40

Our last day and we decided to visit Tintagel Castle, we thought for a gentle stroll around. But the climb to the castle is not for the faint-hearted and once we were there, there wasn't a lot to do apart from climb it.

There were hundreds of steep steps and we took it very slowly all the way to the top. We were both worn out but even the 100 French exchange students aged about 14 were stopping to rest so we didn't feel too bad…or too old!

In the afternoon, we went to Boscastle and at night we were both shattered, Peter more so than me. A gentle reminder that he should not do too much as he still tires very quickly.

Wednesday, May 21: Recovery Day 41

Time to go home. This time we shared the driving.

Peter's thoughts: It isn't that I don't want to remember; I just can't. I was on morphine and all sorts of medication and I slept a lot. I'd just wake up, take my medication and then go back to sleep knowing it was going to be a long, hard road. In the space of a month, I went from a fit football manager to a bed-ridden invalid.

It was only when we went down to Cornwall, originally for a week, that things started to come together again. Before that our only respite had been our little place near Bridlington. That was our bolthole. Away from it all, no telephone, no people asking how I was, no funny looks when we went out. Just the two of us, an escape.

But eventually Alison decided I needed a complete change, not to be waking up in the same bedroom in the same house every morning. So she booked a place in Portscatho, near St Mawes, and we set off. The journey is just a blur but I know we stopped off for a night on the way down. I must have been asleep most of the time and I suppose Alison was absolutely knackered with the driving. It was my club car from Lincoln, a Volvo Estate. Like a tank. I can remember driving away from home and next thing I knew we were in Cornwall and me saying, "Cornwall already? That hasn't taken long."

Yet it was in Cornwall that things suddenly started to improve, so much so that we booked in for a second week, this time at Padstow, where I had my first half of lager for around seven weeks. It took me about three hours to drink it. Normally I can sup a pint in ten minutes, no problem. So that was my big test…in a beautiful pub by the harbour. I was on the way back at last!

I sometimes look back on my football career and reflect on the good times and the not so good times. I like to find some good in everything, to be positive, but with the cancer I can only look back and think how awful it was for everybody, what they all went through. It seems such a negative time. The only good thing is that I survived it, thanks to Alison and all those wonderful people in the NHS who helped look after me. They were special people and I couldn't have received better treatment. And having an ex-ward sister alongside me twenty-four/seven meant I couldn't have been in better hands.

I went back to Lincoln a different man. Football had always been my life but the illness taught me there's far more to life than that.

Thursday, May 22: The End Of The Road

We have reached a huge milestone: six weeks since Peter's treatment finished. The break has done us both the world of good. And it has pushed Peter to do a little more fitness-wise than he may have done.

We've had lovely walks and lots of fresh sea air. He has rested when he needed to but when you are visiting new, exciting places every day you do a lot more than you would if you were resting at home. Peter looks 100 per cent better than he did this time last week.

He is eating and drinking really well and is back to a normal diet. His throat is still a little bit sore but probably feels like a normal sore throat. His morphine is reduced to just 10mgs and within the next two days he should be off it completely. His mood is much more positive and he is much more alert. No more zombified look.

The expectorating has completely stopped so we don't have to buy kitchen roll by the bucket-load. There is no more gurgling in the night…and the great news is that he has stopped snoring completely.

His voice is doing well and I can hear him clearly. In fact, it's so good that he's going to be on Soccer Night on TV on Tuesday. That's a huge step in the right direction and a really positive sign that he is feeling well enough and confident enough to do it.

He is doing a lot of football business over the phone every day and is planning on spending maybe one day a week in Lincoln over the next couple of weeks. But he does need to step back into work slowly rather than rushing things.

It's too early to consider going back to work full on. He would be exhausted pretty quickly and I think it's very important both for himself and the football club that he is fit and well for the first match of the season in August.

We are still waiting for his next appointment from hospital. This will be to pass a tube into his throat and hopefully give us the good news that the treatment has worked and the tumour has been completely burnt away.

To hear that news will have made this all worthwhile. It has been a long and difficult journey, much worse than I had anticipated and something that you cannot prepare yourself for. You manage on a day-to-day basis.

When friends used to say how well I was coping I never thought about it. I was just on autopilot. Looking back it was absolutely exhausting, both physically and mentally. And I don't think anyone really thinks about the person who is caring for the sick patient.

I really take my hat off and respect anyone who has to do it long-term. It really is not the real world they live in. It is not what life is all about.

Life should be lived and enjoyed and appreciated. Long-term carers must learn how to cope somehow and receive their strength from somewhere. I suppose when you love someone so much you just do it.

It will be interesting to see how much Peter remembers about his journey. When I show him photographs I have taken along the way, he cannot remember an awful lot about it. I suppose that's good in a way. I really do not know if he realises just how ill he has been. It is something you quickly want to put behind you, move on and forget.

I am going to take the rest of the summer off work and enjoy some me time. Back to lots of shopping and back to enjoying going out with our friends and family. Doing normal things again, things we all normally take for granted.

I am delighted to have my husband back to his nearly normal self and we can put all this behind us. I feel my job is nearly done and he will soon be back to his beloved football.

I'm wondering if I will get my new Chloe handbag…and yes, the good news is that I hate going to Tesco again.

13. Picking up the pieces

Treatment and recovery over, Peter returned to Lincoln in time to supervise the club's pre-season programme. Business as usual, then. But for Alison, on the rebound from sixty days of round-the-clock care, business would be taking a back seat for the foreseeable future. "Instead I spent the next twelve months or so doing the things people usually take for granted."

Alison's Story

For a year after Peter went back to work, I thought I was in heaven, although it felt strange at first to be on my own after we'd been stuck together like glue during his illness and recovery. And I did think he went back to Lincoln too early…although he would never admit that. Anyway, I'd done my bit, he was fit and well again and ready to resume his football career. It was time for me to relax.

Throughout Peter's illness, MGMS had been very supportive and said my job would be there for me as soon as I felt ready. But I told them I wouldn't be going back, that I wasn't ready to start working again. They didn't want to take no for an answer, gave me a bit more time and then offered me the chance to work part-time. But I knew there was no way I could do that job in a half-hearted way.

So instead, I gradually learned to live a 'normal' life again, a life that featured shopping expeditions, going out for lunch with friends, devoting time to the house…and even creating my own vegetable plot. Oh dear, my vegetable plot! I've mentioned before that the garden has always been Peter's pride and joy and apart from what I considered to be a few well-chosen words of advice, I've more or less left it to him.

But one morning, when Peter was in Lincoln, I was sitting on the patio, running my eye over the garden while I enjoyed a cup of coffee, and I decided that the one thing we lacked was a vegetable patch. Flowers, shrubs, lawn were all very well but why not have a working garden, too, and grow some veg? But where? There was an area of lawn, beyond where I hung out the washing, and after weighing up the options carefully for all of fifteen seconds, I decided that was the place, the perfect spot for growing my veg.

"Easy," I thought, as I went into the shed and found a shovel…or should I say a spade? Easy it certainly was not; back-breaking more like. But I stuck at it and by late afternoon, when I reckoned Peter would be on his way home, I'd dug over a patch about three yards square bordered by a little wooden fence, that I'd nipped out and bought from the garden centre down the road. I was absolutely knackered by the time I sat down and surveyed my handiwork…and that's when it began to dawn on me for the first time that the veg patch was, perhaps, a bit intrusive. And maybe it didn't really enhance the overall effect after all.

But there was no going back now, although I suspected Peter would go absolutely mental when he arrived home. I decided that my best line of defence would be to try to convince him how good it would be for us to live off the land for a change, instead of spending all his hard-earned money in Tesco. And even if the worst came to the worst, he could soon re-turf it, couldn't he? I heard his car draw up in the drive, sat back and waited for the explosion. Instead, he took a long look at the patch and just laughed. Before long I was explaining my plans to grow carrots, potatoes, cabbages, the lot on what was once a corner of his beautifully manicured lawn. I hadn't thought that the garden would be part of the equation when Peter said after his illness that he'd be adopting a more laid-back approach but obviously it was.

First thing next morning, I was back at the garden centre buying packets of seeds. I placed them all in rows, as per the instructions, and then attached the packets to canes so I would know what was planted where. Peter seemed impressed and for a while, everything in my veg garden seemed rosy. Then one night the wind blew, the rain lashed down and when I inspected the patch in the morning, all the labels had blown away.

I decided that shouldn't be a massive problem and before long, green shoots started to appear that gradually grew into loads and loads of fully-fledged plants, far more than the family could hope to eat. It reached the stage where every time friends came round, they'd leave with piles of homegrown veg, with my cabbages the star of the show. We thought they were lovely and so did everyone else. "That was the most beautiful cabbage I've ever tasted," was a frequent response. "Gorgeous, a really different flavour." Then one day, white things started to appear in the middle of the leaves and I realised with horror that my prize cabbages were in fact cauliflowers. I consoled myself with the thought that the leaves must have been good for us all.

The veg plot lasted for just a single season, although it's still there to this day, boasting a solitary rhubarb plant. However it coincided with my change of role from full-on cancer nurse to vegetable gardener, cook, housekeeper and housewife. I started reading recipe books, planning elaborate menus and visiting farm shops and supermarkets for all the ingredients that I couldn't grow myself. I must have spent an absolute fortune and for the first time in my life, I was heavily into cooking and baking. The house was spotless. If the weather was nice, I might have lunch and a glass of wine on the patio with friends; if not we could always pop out to a local restaurant. And a slap-up meal would be waiting for Peter and the kids when they arrived home from work.

Apart from going to matches, I never spent any time in Lincoln. Peter usually stayed over at least one night a week and I sometimes suggested that it would be nice for me to have a couple of days there as well. Steff Wright, the chairman, and other people at the club used to tell me what a wonderful city it was and how I'd love things like the Christmas market, but Peter didn't want to know.

It was as if Lincoln was about football and, apart from my hostess role on match days, I didn't have a part to play in that world. I never really pressed him for a reason but it was unusual and it did upset me. I just wanted to have a look around the city where he worked and see the hotel where he stayed so, when I was back home on my own, I could at least visualise where he was. I wouldn't have been a nuisance or interfered with his football. Just a look around the shops and the sights and then out for a nice meal together in the evening.

But I suspect that's the way it is for the wife of a football manager, or player for that matter. When a manager's in a job or things are going well for a player, football is his life 120 per cent of the time and he doesn't need anyone outside his own little world. Then when they're out of football, they need their partner all the time and expect her to drop everything. That's life when you're married to a footballer and one of the reasons I'd always been determined to have a career of my own.

And, as the days shortened towards the end of my second summer at home, picking up my working life again began to occupy my thoughts. I'd started to become bored and restless and I realised it was time for a new challenge.

Peter's Story

The start of the new season was just a couple of weeks away. The players had done well pre-season and a 3-1 win over Aston Villa in a friendly at Sincil Bank showed we were moving in the right direction. A super performance. Afterwards, I said, "Thanks, lads. You've all worked really hard so I've got a treat for you."

There are loads of little waterways around Lincoln and boats leave the waterfront for pleasure cruises all through the summer. So I arranged to hire a boat for an afternoon cruise and fixed up an evening barbecue in the beer garden of a waterside pub. I told the players it was all set for the Thursday after the Villa match, with one condition…that they all wore sailors' hats. The one exception would be my skipper Scott Kerr, Captain Marvel. I gave him a peaked hat with a bit of gold braid round the brim. They all reported for duty at the quayside and bang on time, HMS Imps, complete with Admiral Jackson and his crew, weighed anchor and sailed off into the sunset. It was a great evening.

The cruise marked a landmark for me: confirmation that I could still hack it as a manager and finally turn my back on the nightmare of my three months' treatment, although I needed regular check-ups for the next four years. Even though I'd handed over the reins to Iffy Onuora, my number two, at the start of my radiotherapy, I talked to him and Steff Wright on a regular basis, although as my voice deteriorated it became more and more difficult. And gradually, as the treatment took its toll, I was less and less involved.

But there was one thing I could not leave to Iffy: the retained list, one of the most important jobs for a manager. Decisions about which players to keep and which to release can only be taken by him. I'd watched the DVDs of every Lincoln game during my treatment and I knew who I wanted to keep and let go. I talked it through with Iffy and Steff but unfortunately, as I was still away from the club, it was then down to Iffy to break the news to the players who were being released.

The most difficult decision concerned our keeper Alan Marriott, who'd been with the club for nine years and would have been due a testimonial at the end of the season. He was a bit of a legend with the fans so it was a tough one for me. But I felt it was time for a change and I wanted to bring in Rob Burch from Sheffield Wednesday. Alan wasn't happy but those are the kind of tough decisions any manager has to make and there's no way round them.

The retained list is always a bit of a balancing act because there will be players in contract, players coming out of contract that you want to keep, borderline players and then those coming out of contract that you don't want. A manager will try and tie up the players he wants before the end of the January transfer window, starting to negotiate around Christmas. As far as borderline players are concerned, he's happy to wait for as long as he can, knowing they will be able to do a job if he can't find anyone else. He keeps them hanging on, which is sad to say really, but that's how it works.

Then there are the players a manager knows he will be releasing, players who are nowhere near the first team. He'll say, "Look, there's nothing for you here but if you can go out and fix yourself up with another club, that's fine by me." Clubs like Lincoln would always be happy to do that kind of deal because it saved money on national insurance, tax and so on. The harsh facts of life in the bottom division. Over the years, I don't recall any players I released coming back to haunt me by going on to have a career higher up the ladder and experienced pros had been through it all before and know the score.

It's a different story when it's time to tell a YTS lad that after three years' living the dream, he doesn't have a future at your club. They signed on as starry-eyed kids with visions of reaching the top and there across the desk is a manager killing that dream. They are just children really and while some could tough it out, I had quite a few break down in tears. And I did feel for them. I always asked the academy coach or someone in a similar position to be with me because it helped them to have a familiar and friendly face around. Sometimes parents would ring up and ask why and there was no way of dodging the issue. I simply told them that in my view, their lad wasn't going to make it, adding that it was only my opinion and didn't mean he wouldn't be signed by another club. Failing that, the earlier he could get out there and find another job, the better.

I'd set a target of being back for the start of pre-season training in July. That was the very least I owed everybody at the club and the fans who had supported me so much. But after Alison and I had returned home from our break in Cornwall, I decided to pop over a couple of times a week and plan pre-season from my office rather than home, even though the doctors said I should really have another month off. But I was up and about again, after all…it wasn't as if I could only walk with the aid of a couple of sticks. I needed to be back in the swing of it before pre-season started.

Driving away for the last time three months earlier, not knowing if or when I'd be back, had been a truly emotional experience. But now I just felt glad to be back with a lot of people around me, all living lives of their own. It was good to rejoin the real world and focus on something other than treatment and hospitals. Since the treatment started, I hadn't seen too many people, apart from family and close friends, but now, finally, I could return to the job that I loved and I had a brilliant response from everyone, both inside and outside the club. They all seemed genuinely pleased to see me and I felt I was making a completely new start. There was a real buzz.

If anybody was a bit wary about how to approach me after the illness, it didn't show, particularly in the dressing room. Like me, the players were just glad to be back again and the new arrivals hadn't been around when I was taken ill anyway. On the first day, I just sat everybody down and said, "Right, I'm back. The cancer was the past, this is the future. We've got a squad here who are capable of winning promotion so we're looking forward, not back."

The only problem was my voice. A football manager is lost without his voice. He needs it to shout at his players in training and matches, speak to them individually or as a group; for talking to the media, directors and supporters. And although my voice was becoming stronger every day, I couldn't rant and rave again until I'd been to speech therapy sessions at Huddersfield Royal Infirmary.

It was something I'd resisted at first but Alison pushed me into it. There were no other patients, just me and my therapist in a tiny room and at first I dreaded going. But she was really patient with me and once the voice began to improve, I became more enthusiastic. I had to pull odd faces, make strange noises and repeat phrases like, "How now, brown cow?" or "The rain in Spain stays mainly on the plain." But after six weeks' therapy, my voice was probably stronger than before the cancer and looking back, without her, I might never have really got my voice back. People moan and groan about the NHS and everybody has a horror story to tell. But for every one horror story there must be a thousand tales of people receiving top-class treatment, just like I did all the way through my illness.

The pre-season programme went well and at our media call, I raised the bar by saying we'd top the division. I did it with my eyes wide open and with the backing of Steff and the board. I needed that because we all knew it could backfire and I wanted to be confident they would still be behind me if things didn't work out right away. I brought in senior players like Frank Sinclair, Stefan Oakes and Janos Kovacs, all good professionals, and we sold a record number of season tickets as the expectations mounted.

And that 3-1 win in the warm-up match against Aston Villa only seemed to confirm my forecast. They were due to meet Danish club FK Odense in the InterToto Cup four days later and Martin O'Neill, their manager at the time, fielded a strong side. But after going a goal down early on, we came back really well and fully deserved to win. It was tremendous, a lovely summer's evening for my first game back and afterwards, I thought, "Aye, aye, if we play like this in League Two, no one can stop us." And I knew everyone leaving Sincil Bank that night would have been thinking, "We've cracked it!"

But it just didn't work out and we never reached the levels I expected. We were never in the bottom half of the table but we didn't really threaten the top seven either. We finished ten points outside the play-offs. It would have been very different if we'd had a better home record because our away form wasn't bad: eight wins and six draws. But at home we finished with six wins, six defeats and a massive eleven draws. If only we'd turned four or five of those into wins, we'd have been in a challenging position. In the end, the players were a little bit frightened of playing at home so I tried things like having a pre-match meal at the training ground and then a coach drive to the ground, trying to copy our away routine. But nothing really worked.

It was so frustrating because in both my spells at Huddersfield we'd always been strong at home and for any side to succeed, their home ground has to be a fortress, a place other teams simply don't like going to. And a good home record is absolutely crucial for a manager's long-term prospects. A club like Lincoln might take three or four hundred fans to an away game compared with three thousand or more at home. So while only a few fans see a poor away performance, a team not winning at home is watched by ten times as many. Ten times as many people to get on the manager's back, ten times as many people to moan about the manager in the pubs and clubs and ten times as many people to voice their discontent on match days. The directors notice the fans are growing restless, the tension begins to mount and the pressure to produce results increases. A manager will always be on thin ice if his team is not producing the goods at home.

One of the turning points was our defeat by Conference side Kettering in the first round of the FA Cup in November. We'd started the season OK, both at home and away, and when we went to Kettering we were only three points outside the play-offs. We drew 1-1 but the match was soured by racist abuse by a Kettering fan directed at two of my players, Danny N'Guessan and Sinclair, who was on the bench, and Iffy Onuora.

I reported it to the referee, Simon Hooper, afterwards and he included my complaint in his match report. Even though it was a relatively unimportant match in front of a small crowd, the type of abuse was unacceptable and I was saying this on radio when their chairman, Imraan Ladak walked by and we started arguing on air. Good copy for the media but perhaps I should have kept my mouth shut really. But how was I supposed to react when monkey chants were directed at my players and my number two, who also happened to be my best friend? The Kick Racism Into Touch campaign had been launched 15 years earlier and it was something I felt very strongly about.

Lincoln also reported the incident to the FA and soon afterwards, the Northamptonshire police launched an inquiry. A man was charged with a racially aggravated public order offence in January 2009 and appeared before Northampton magistrates in July. We had evidence in the form of pictures and tapes and Iffy, Matt Carmichael, the Lincoln kit man, and I all gave evidence and so did another Kettering supporter. But I sensed fairly early in the proceedings that it was going to be a waste of time and he was acquitted after a three-day hearing. To this day, I still can't believe the verdict but who am I to argue with the British judicial system?

Even so, I had no regrets about pursuing the incident. Maybe it would have been easier to just forget about it but it became a bit of a crusade. Racism was something I felt strongly about – it still is - and I wasn't prepared to turn a deaf ear. In some ways, I was also the club's figurehead so I felt it was important for people to see that Lincoln City weren't prepared to take the abuse lying down and I have to say that the club backed me all the way.

Inevitably there was a lot of tension going into the replay and we ended up losing to a late goal. We were booed off afterwards, for the first time in my time at the club. I was due to sign a new contract the following day but Steff said that it might be better to delay the announcement and it wasn't until January that I actually put pen to paper. Just as when I first joined the club, Steff wanted me to move to Lincoln but again, I said, "No, not on a two-year deal. I can't commit Alison and the kids to that and then, six months into the contract, get sacked."

I knew how Steff felt. I'd been in the same position when I tried to sign players because Lincoln is off the beaten track and not on the motorway corridor. So compromises had to be made. Lincoln's wage structure was probably middle of the table in that division, which didn't mean a lot of money, so we could hardly offer a player a one-year deal and then expect him to uproot his family. Instead they would commute on a daily basis, like I did at Chester, setting up car schools where three or four of them would share the journeys. Sometimes, if two or three players lived a long distance away, they would share a flat during the week. But attracting players to what they saw as a backwater, even though it's one of the most beautiful cities in the country, was always a problem.

We finished the season in thirteenth place, a small improvement but nothing like I'd expected eight months earlier. However the build-up to the new season went well again although this time I decided against a river cruise for the players' night out and opted for something different: camping. Before a training session, I erected a tent in the middle of the pitch and said, "Right, there's your pre-season treat this time. Anybody know how to put up a tent?" In fact, our destination was more like a boot camp and the cover wasn't a tent, just a canvas sheet as a bivouac. I reckoned it would be a good bonding exercise, all lads together and all that. But they absolutely hated it, even though I laid on another barbecue. Soon afterwards I was sacked…so perhaps camping wasn't such a brilliant idea after all!

We made a reasonable start with six points from four matches, including a win at Bradford City. Not brilliant but not the worst start in the world either. Then in our fifth game on August 29, we lost 3-0 at Dagenham and Redbridge and for the first time, the fans turned on me, chanting, "Jackson out! Jackson out!" I spoke to Steff afterwards and he said, "Peter, we're at Darlington on Tuesday in the Associate Members Cup. We have to go through." He didn't need to spell it out: if we didn't win, I was out. He knew it, I knew it, the board knew it, the players knew it and so did just about everyone else in the city. I made a couple of changes, went for the win and we ended up losing 1-0 in front of 828 spectators.

There were four board members and Steff waiting for me outside the Darlington boardroom. I said, "We play these in the league on Saturday. We'll turn them over." But they'd already made up their minds. As we walked away, Steff said, "It isn't looking good, Peter. I'll give you a ring in the morning." Before leaving the coach, I shook every player's hand and also shook hands with the directors. Steff rang as arranged and told me, "Your journey at Lincoln has ended." I'll never forget those words.

It was a blow but not totally unexpected. I'd realised towards the end of the previous season that the pressure was building because of our home record and maybe I'd taken my eye off the ball a little. Because of everything I'd been through with the cancer? Perhaps. Or maybe the racism court case had been more of a distraction than I realised at the time. Either way, I was able to take my sacking on the chin and move on. I'd been through far worse things than being sacked as a football manager and this time I could put it into perspective. After all, I was still alive, wasn't I?

I went over next day and cleared out my office. Two days later, I picked up Dave Roberts, the chief exec, at Wakefield Westgate station and drove to Hartshead Moor service station on the M62 near Brighouse, where Alison was waiting. I climbed out, shook hands with Dave and handed him the car keys. It was over.

There was no way I was going to criticise anyone at Lincoln City because everyone connected with the club had backed me to the hilt when I most needed their support. And one little cameo illustrated the bond that had once existed between us. When I joined the club in 2007, Wii boards were the big thing and Alison was desperate to have one. So I put a note on the Lincoln website asking if anyone knew where I could get hold of one straight away. Within a couple of hours, there were five replies, all offering a Wii for nothing. That was typical of the Lincoln fans. They were fantastic.

I don't believe I failed at Lincoln. To take over a team at the bottom of the league, go through throat cancer, win two Manager of the Month awards, sell over half a million pounds' worth of players and consolidate their Football League status was a hell of an achievement. I raised the club's profile and left them in good shape. It was a settled, happy club and, more to the point, an established Football League club. We hadn't done as well as I'd wanted or expected but there was plenty to build on. Steff left the following March and before long the club was on the downward spiral into the Conference.

14. Back in business

When Peter lost his job at Lincoln at the beginning of September, 2009, it was decision time for Alison...and time to go back to work. "Instead of relying on Peter's salary, we faced the prospect of no regular income. Clearly, my days as a lady of leisure were numbered and I would have to find another job. But what, when and where?"

Alison's Story

We sat down for a team meeting and Peter set the ball rolling. "Right, what are we going to do?"

"We'll start a business."

"What kind of business? All I know anything about is football. I can't do anything else." That attitude has always worn a bit thin with me but it's something so many people in football say, usually as an excuse for sitting around doing nothing. Of course they can do something else if they put their minds to it.

"OK, if all you can do is football, leave it to me. I'll buy my own business."

"But what sort of business? We need something that we can live off until I get another job in football, not just any old business. And what are we going to use for money?"

"Wait there." Peter had always funded the house, paid the bills and saved a bit as well. Anything I earned was seen as extra income. And even though I'd spent a fair bit on myself and the kids over the years, I'd also salted quite a lot away into my own savings...without telling Peter. I collected together all my savings documents and we totted up the bits and pieces I'd put into various places. When we'd finished Peter looked a bit bewildered. "How have you done that without me knowing? I thought you'd spent all your money on handbags and clothes."

"I'm not that daft!"

My original plan was that we'd use my money for our retirement. We'd reach the age of 60 and I'd say, "Look, here's this money you've never known about, this is our old age." But now it wasn't going to work out that way and maybe we would be retiring a lot later than I'd planned. So we decided to live off Peter's savings for the time being and I'd invest my money into a business that would bring in some money whether or not Peter returned to football.

But the same question: what sort of business? Answer: a recession-proof industry and a business that was not going to fall flat. Preferably something that would be cushioned by a franchise, like my time with Rosemary Conley. As a franchisee you are protected to some extent because at the start you are given the right advice, guidance and support and all the legal and technical information you are likely to need. You aren't stepping into the unknown. A franchise had been the right thing for me before but once again, it had to be the right franchise and not just some kind of whim.

So what are the absolutely recession-proof businesses? Commodities that people cannot be without, no matter how rich or poor they are. I narrowed it down to three options. First, the sex industry. A few massage parlours dotted around the place might make a small fortune although obviously I wouldn't have been hands-on, if you'll pardon the phrase. Sharing a Jacuzzi with a punter and then powdering his bottom wouldn't really be me. Let alone Peter. Second, a funeral director's. That's one profession that is absolutely guaranteed to be always in demand. But again, would it really be me? No.

Or how about some kind of health-related business? Like home care. With my background in nursing and healthcare, that was always going to be the best option. Let's go for it! We looked at various companies who provided domiciliary care, met the people in charge and in the end, we opted for Caremark, a company based in Worthing. The reason we chose them was simple: Kevin Lewis, the chief executive, who had founded the company in 2005. We met Kevin and Chris Wandell, the Franchise Recruitment Manager, at Caremark's headquarters and we could see how passionate Kevin was about the issue of care; he'd worked in the industry since 1987 and like us, he was open and up front.

We told him we would be putting our life savings into the venture and that it could not afford to fail. We'd both worked extremely hard all our lives and would work equally hard now. Kevin did not seem like the kind of ruthless businessman who would set us up in a franchise that might not work just to earn money for himself. We felt that he had our interests at heart, that he wanted us to succeed and that he would support us in any way he could. On top of that, we both liked him as a person and he liked us. That's vital when you are investing a lot of money in a business.

We talked over the pros and cons and arranged to meet Kevin and Chris for lunch the next day at the Grand Hotel in Brighton, which had suffered a terrorist attack at the Tory Party Conference in 1984. Kevin stressed that we should take our time and impressed on us the need to do our research, to check everything out and be absolutely certain it was the right thing to spend our money on.

However I'd already made up my mind: we were going to go for it. "No," I said. "I want to buy the business now."

"Are you sure?"

"Yes."

"OK, the next training course starts in two weeks' time. Obviously you're going to miss that one so let's look at the one after that, which is…"

"What do you mean I'm going to miss it? I'll be on that one. Where do I stay? What time do I start?"

The following week, Chris drove up to Yorkshire with the contract and all the paperwork and ten days later I started the course with three more would-be franchisees. It was very hard, in depth and intensive, the toughest course I've ever taken. It went into completely new areas for me, about the Care Quality Commission, how health care is brokered, all the legislation involved with health and social care, how to research the need for care in any particular community. It is an enormous minefield but anyone planning to run a successful operation has to know their way through it backwards. The Caremark team guided us through it stage by stage but even so there were times when I thought, "Oh my God, what have I let myself in for here? Why didn't I go for something straightforward?" But I was going to make it work.

Peter was at a bit of a loose end back home so he came down to Brighton for the second week and joined me in the classroom, not as an active trainee but to gain an insight into what would be involved when the business was up and running. It was important for him to know exactly what we were letting ourselves in for and how we might be able to involve him in the future if he wasn't working in football.

Once I'd completed the course and passed all the written and oral exams it was down to the nuts and bolts of establishing the business: finding an office, buying and setting up the equipment, putting together a business plan for the bank and above all, a business plan for the Care Quality Commission in order to be registered as a home care provider. That was all about the logistics of the business: where we would be based, how many people we would be caring for and where they would be living, how many carers we would need, how we would finance and fund it and details of my own working background. Plus a fully-enhanced Criminal Records Bureau check, something I'd never had before.

I sent off the application by registered post to the CQC headquarters in Newcastle and once I was certain it had arrived, I was on the phone every day, checking on its progress through the system, asking if there was anyway it could be speeded up. "I don't want to seem pushy but…" I was so desperate to get started. It didn't take long before we'd fixed up for representatives of the CQC to come and inspect our premises in the Else Whiteley Innovation Centre, a state-of-the-art business complex housed in a renovated textile mill in Halifax. It was a gruelling four-hour interview. Were the premises fit for purpose? Was I fit to be the registered owner of a business? Was I fit to be the resident care manager of the business? When it was all over, I was physically and mentally drained. But a week later, it was all worth it; on April 19, 2010, we were registered with the CQC.

I started with just myself, as managing director, and a care manager, who left after two weeks because she felt happier on the operational side rather than management. My second care manager left after three months because the job was affecting her health. So I thought, "Right, there's only one way to really get this business moving forward: do everything myself." So I did, combining the two roles.

Deciding on the number of carers was a chicken and egg situation. Do we wait and see how many clients there will be and then train our carers? Or do we train the carers anyway so that we are ready to go as soon as the care is required. I decided to go for the second option and drip-fed a team of ten carers who would be ready to go as soon as we were up and running.

And our first major area of employment came soon afterwards when Age Concern needed extra care workers and we were on hand to provide them. Then we were accredited as carers by Calderdale and Kirklees Councils and started acquiring private clients, too. Two years down the line, we had fifty care and support workers, two field care supervisors, who managed the quality of care out in the field, and four office staff, and had built up our care hours from nought to over 1,000.

In any business venture, you have to give 100 per cent, 24/7 and I have always been fine with that. But I simply did not realise how difficult this venture was going to be. It's been the hardest work, the biggest eye opener, the most stressful thing I've ever done, apart from looking after Peter when he was ill. That was a completely different type of mental stress. Having said that, all the jobs I've done have been hard work, I've always stretched myself and tested myself and given 100 per cent. But during the first 18 months, I started at seven in the morning and rarely left before eight at night, and for the most part, our social life went out of the window. There were times when I wondered if I'd done the right thing, if it was going to be too hard for me.

Maybe I was grieving the life we'd had before, a life that had been fairly glitzy and eventful. Instead, here I was tied to the business day in and day out and working weekends as well because I didn't feel I had people I could really rely on. I felt the only way I could move the business forward was to keep my finger on the pulse absolutely all the time. I needed to know everything that was happening because everything was under my control. In the first couple of years I probably aged four or five years and piled on God knows how much weight because I was living an unhealthy, stressful lifestyle.

However I eventually had to accept that the only way I could grow the business was to step back and start to trust people and I now have some good key people in place. I don't usually start before eight, I try to get away around six and rarely work at weekends any more. In 2011, we won Caremark's Northern Franchisee of the Year award but I will need to make more appointments to make sure I can step back a little more and see how we can develop the business in the future.

Care is a huge issue. We're an ageing population with more elderly people staying healthy and living longer than ever before. But eventually a large percentage of those people will become vulnerable and need care and support. If this is the situation now, heaven knows what will happen in ten or twenty years.

But instead of putting money into such an important service, central and local government want to cut back on the cost of care and the care companies they use are expected to reduce their budgets accordingly. I worry that at some stage there will be no care companies at all because increasingly it seems they are being expected to operate as a charity rather than a business. But no company is going to continue if it is working at a loss.

On top of that, the length of time we are expected to spend with an elderly person is being cut. Instead of a 30-minute breakfast call, we are supposed to provide the same amount of care in fifteen minutes, which includes a written log of each visit. That is physically impossible for any carer and inevitably, they run over time and are late for their next call. This can have a knock-on effect right through the day and then before long, relatives are complaining about carers arriving late.

Yet any carer who does the job for the right reasons will be prepared to go above and beyond any arbitrary time limits to make sure an elderly person is comfortable by the time they leave. The government and councils are taking advantage of this good nature by imposing such unrealistic time limits.

I am always being told that if we cut a corner here or there, it would chip a bit off the price and make us more competitive. But I prefer to negotiate with the local authorities to be given more time with needy clients not less. I have to be strong, make tough decisions and not make our service cheaper at the expense of the care we provide. And I can't help but notice that the companies who come in with rock-bottom prices seem to be the ones who don't give the right level of care.

I'm in this for the long haul. But in any business, you have to know when it's time to get out, as I discovered with Rosemary Conley. There will come a time to go, when we have built up the business so that it is big enough and successful enough for someone to want to buy it. What would I do next? Maybe we could start thinking about the sex industry or funerals after all!

Peter's Story

It had always been my dream job: manager of Bradford City, my hometown club, the club where I learned my football and played over 400 games. It was a dream that came true in February 2011. A dream that turned into a nightmare in the space of six months.

The opportunity to return to Valley Parade came out of the blue. For nearly a year, I'd been working alongside Alison at Caremark. I had two roles, up front as the sales and marketing director and out on the road, working alongside her team of carers. It was an eye-opening experience and a million miles away from anything my career in football had prepared me for. Believe me, anyone who talks about pressure in football should spend a week on the front line of home care.

I was still keen to return to management, though, and on February 24, 2011, I saw the news flash that Bradford City manager Peter Taylor had been sacked. It wasn't a massive shock. City were 21st in League Two and in grave danger of slipping out of the Football League just ten years after playing in the Premier League. Taylor was a big name, a former England Under-21 manager who'd been in charge at six clubs and also managed the full England team for one match. But City had lost seven of their last nine matches and he'd been under pressure.

I had numbers for City's joint-chairmen, Julian Rhodes and Mark Lawn, on my mobile so rather than going through a third party or the Press, I decided to strike while the iron was still hot and ring direct. Julian had my number because I'd been on their shortlist when Taylor succeeded Stuart McCall a year earlier and he would have known who was calling. He answered immediately…a good sign.

I went straight to the point. I told him I knew they would be looking around for someone to succeed Taylor but in the short term I would go in for two games in the space of four days, against Gillingham away and Rotherham at home. Both sides were in the top six but I told him I'd win both games for him. I'd get rid of the doom and gloom around the place and give them a little bit of time to sift through what was sure to be a lengthy list of applicants. Julian said he'd talk it over with Mark and soon afterwards, came back and said I would be appointed interim manager, whatever that meant. I said I'd give it everything until they found the man they were looking for…knowing that if I did a good job, that man could be me.

Although Taylor had resigned by mutual consent, for some reason he stayed in charge for the home game against Stockport on the Saturday. Julian and Mark asked me to sit in the stand and have a look at the side I'd be taking over. The fans realised what was going on and I was given a reasonable reception, although I knew there was an element who didn't want me to have the job because of my Huddersfield connections.

They remembered that when I was manager at Huddersfield I always said that my blood ran blue and white. And given the rivalry between the two clubs they couldn't stomach the idea of me as City's manager. But they chose to forget that when I was manager of Lincoln, I said that my blood ran red and white! Isn't that how every manager should feel? What's he doing in the job if he doesn't think that? I could understand where they were coming from but when I said those things, when I kissed the Huddersfield shirt, I was doing it because I was the Town manager, not because I didn't love

Bradford City any more. And when I returned home to Valley Parade, my blood ran claret and amber.

Whenever I had a chance, I explained that to my critics and before long, most of them seemed to accept that I really was City through and through. Huddersfield was a huge part of my life, so was Lincoln. But Bradford City was going back home. There were pockets of resistance, of course, and I heard that one or two internet sites featured people sounding off about my appointment, complete with abusive remarks about my time at Huddersfield.

I have never read that stuff and I've always tried to prevent Alison and the family from being exposed to it as well. People don't seem to realise that managers have family and feelings, too. When I was manager at Huddersfield for the first time, I wanted my dad to sit in the directors' box but he never would. Instead he preferred to sit in the stand and sometimes, if there was a load of abuse directed at me, it upset him a lot. Eventually I told him it might be better if he didn't come if the personal stuff was going to upset him. And he never really came too often after that, which was a big shame for us both

People think they can get away with shouting the most horrible things at a manager, something truly hurtful, because he's a sitting target. Sometimes the abuse can be very personal and very nasty. During my second season at Lincoln, after I'd been treated for throat cancer, we played at Port Vale and early in the game, a fan behind the dugout stood up and shouted, "Jackson you're a w****r and you should have died of cancer." For any grown man to say that to another human being is appalling and nobody, inside or outside football, should receive that kind of abuse. How could my family have handled that if they'd been there and within earshot? It's an aspect of the job that people don't appreciate and that's why I've always tried to protect the kids and to pick and choose what games they come to.

I met the Bradford players for the first time the day after the Stockport match, a 3-2 win for City. I arrived early and spent an hour talking to Mark, Julian and Dave Baldwin, the financial director, about how I would approach the next ten days. We were due to play at Gillingham the following Saturday and then the Rotherham game was at Valley Parade on the Tuesday after that.

After our meeting, Mark spoke to the players for ten minutes and then introduced me as the new man in charge. I told them I was a manager who backed his players if they gave him 100 per cent and said, "This is my club, I want it to do well, I want us all to do well for Bradford City and the supporters. You know you've under-achieved and this is a massive challenge. But it's one we can win if we all stick together." I had to get the players onside quickly and as it happened one of them, Jon Worthington, had been my captain at Huddersfield when we'd won the League Two play-offs seven years earlier. I was pretty sure he'd back me in the dressing room. I appointed Dave Wetherall, the youth team manager, as my number two until

I could bring in my own man.

The players worked well in training and I picked up a lot of positives ahead of our trip to Gillingham. During the week, I took Damian Buck, the physio, John Duckworth, the kit man, and Mark Harrison, the media officer, to one side. I told them we had to make sure the preparations were absolutely spot-on, no last-minute glitches, nothing left to chance. We trained on the Friday morning and Mark, who was in charge of catering on the journey, said he was going to serve hot food, pre-packed pasta from the microwave, en route. Fine.

The coach left Valley Parade, headed for the M62 and M1 and the driver had just pointed us in the direction of London when the on-board fire alarm went off and smoke billowed into the main compartment of the coach. Mark had put the cartons of pasta into the microwave without removing the outer wrapping. The driver pulled on to the hard shoulder, we chucked away the burnt-out cartons of pasta, opened all the doors and windows to clear the air and when we'd made sure everything was all clear, we set off again. We stopped at the next motorway services and bought a load of sandwiches and I couldn't help thinking, "This isn't exactly the start I was looking for, is it? At least it can only get better!"

We had a real go at Gillingham but lost 2-0. For a team low on confidence it wasn't a bad performance and the fans who made the 500-mile round trip gave us a good reception. But after that defeat, beating Rotherham, who were fifth in the table, on the Tuesday was going to be vital for the team… and for me. It was an emotional night and I couldn't believe how proud I felt as I tied my Bradford City tie, slipped on my suit jacket and walked from the dressing room to the dug-out. Alison and the kids were in the stand and I was given a great reception.

We beat them 2-1 and when we won 1-0 at Morecambe on the Saturday, I joked to the lads, "We've got an outside chance of the play-offs here!" Realistically, we still had eleven games to go and our only priority was collecting enough points to be sure of staying in the Football League. We were living on a knife edge and when we were beaten 3-0 at Accrington on Easter Saturday, I feared the worst. We were four points above the drop zone with only three more matches, starting with an Easter Monday game against Aldershot at Valley Parade. After that it was Hereford away and Crewe at home on the final day. Unless the players came up with something better, we weren't going to pick up many points from that lot.

The Accrington performance seemed to have totally sapped morale and Colin Cooper, my number two, and I worked desperately to lift the players afterwards. We knew that if we lost to Aldershot, who were in mid-table, we would be in real danger of going out of the Football League. We won 2-1. Omar Daley, who I had recalled from a loan spell at Rotherham, scored perhaps City's goal of the season early on and although they equalised after 43 minutes, we snatched it with a late goal from David Syers.

I don't think I have ever been more relieved as a manager and now I knew we would stay up, even though technically we still needed one point. That arrived when we drew 1-1 at Hereford, where my own playing career had started 32 years earlier, the following Saturday. After the match, I was totally drained. I just sat back in the dugout and filled up with tears. Keeping Bradford City in the league had meant everything. I was born and bred in Bradford and had played for the club so how could I have handled being the manager who took them out of the league?

After the final match against Crewe, we arranged a match out on the pitch involving the sponsors and boxholders. Mark Lawn managed one team, I managed the other and my lot lost 3-1. It was just a bit of fun but I'd been desperate to win because I knew that from then on, Mark would forever be going on about how easy football management was, that a manager just turned up, shouted a few instructions, made a few gestures and that was it. If only!

Even though we'd survived, I was still the interim manager…if people asked me what that meant, I used to say, "I'm a very fit manager, in trim!" In limbo, more like. When the season ended, I still didn't know where I stood. Nor, for that matter, did Bradford City. There was talk of the club going into liquidation, of leaving Valley Parade because the overheads were so high and moving to Odsal Stadium, home of Bradford Bulls Rugby League club, where we'd played after the fire in 1985. And it seemed nothing would be sorted on the managerial front until those issues had been resolved.

Even so, I went ahead with planning for the new season and decided to release 13 players. I arranged to see each player individually to explain why before giving the details to the local media. There was a list of times on my notice board but by the time I'd seen two of them, the 13 names were out on Twitter. That simply could not have happened when I was a player but social networking has changed everything. The days when a manager could say that whatever went on in the dressing room stayed in the dressing room have gone completely out of the window.

Anything goes. Soon after I took over at Bradford someone set up a Facebook site for Peter Jackson, pretending to be me, and someone else was impersonating me on Twitter. The tweeting was pretty much tongue in cheek and fairly harmless fun but the Facebook site was more sinister. I wouldn't have known the first thing about it if one of Charlotte's friends hadn't mentioned that she didn't know I was on Facebook. Neither did Charlotte! She double-checked with me that it was a fake and managed to have it shut down but not before a load of false information about me and the job had been published.

With the retained list out of the way, I started working on the players I wanted to bring in and planning a pre-season programme, even though I was still only the interim manager. It was a strange situation and with hindsight, perhaps I should have gone off on holiday for a couple of weeks until something definite was sorted out. Instead, I went into the club every day, planning for the new season and talking to players I would sign if and when I became manager. Of course, none of them would commit themselves formally until they knew who their manager was going to be. It was a weird situation. Finally, three weeks after the season ended, City's future at Valley Parade was secured and I was called in to meet Julian and Mark. They gave me the job on a 12-month contract, with Colin Cooper as my number two.

Colin had joined us after watching our win over Rotherham from the stand. I'd sounded out one or two people about who I might bring in as number two and Adam Pearson, Hull City's chief executive at the time, strongly recommended Colin. I knew all about his record as a top-flight player with Middlesbrough and Nottingham Forest and his reputation as a coach, although I'd never met him. He'd just left a coaching job at Boro and came to Valley Parade with his eyes open: I didn't have a contract, he didn't have a contract so either of us could have been shown the door at a moment's notice. But he'd liked what he'd seen against Rotherham and was keen to give it a go. In the circumstances, it was vital that the two of us hit if off straight away and I have to say that as a man and as a coach, I couldn't speak too highly of him. I couldn't have wished for a better man by my side and really felt the two of us could turn things round.

But it was not to be. Soon after I was appointed manager, Archie Christie, a man I had never heard of, arrived as chief scout and head of player development, a new role. His arrival marked the start of my downfall. It was a bizarre appointment. It was hard to find anyone who knew him or anything about him. John Still, the manager of Dagenham and Redbridge, was one of the people Bradford interviewed for the job earlier and Christie had been chief scout at Dagenham. I was told that he came up with Still for the interview.

As far as I was aware, Christie had little coaching experience or long-term involvement in the professional game. People looked him up on the Internet but until he joined Bradford, there didn't seem to be anything. I don't know whether he was being serious or not but he used to claim Tiger Woods had taught him to play golf, Jamie Oliver taught him how to cook and the actor Denzel Washington was a good mate. I used to wonder who taught him to drive. Michael Schumacher?

As well as setting up a scouting system to look at possible signings, Christie was going to oversee the establishment of a development programme to find players in the 17-20 age group who would bridge the gap between the academy and the senior squad. But I had already recruited Wayne Allison, who later worked for the FA, to do that job. Wayne held a UEFA Pro Licence, the top coaching qualification in the game, and he'd played for me during my first spell at Huddersfield. He was a man I could trust.

I felt Christie's arrival undermined my position and I said as much to Alison when we went away for a break. But I decided to give it time, to try and make things work. I talked to Christie over the phone while I was on holiday and it was obvious it was going to be difficult for both of us. I tried to explain that to Mark and Julian when I returned but they wouldn't have it and more and more, I felt that they were taking his side rather than mine. Day by day, week by week I felt my authority was being undermined...and not only by Christie.

Mark also used to come down to the training ground while Colin and I were taking sessions, something none of my previous chairmen had done. Early in the season, he received a tip from a friend in South Africa about a young kid who he was told had a bit of potential. He arranged for the lad to fly over so that we could give him a trial. He was called Jay Jay, a striker, and I could tell straight away that he wasn't going to be good enough.

Mark asked me to arrange a practice match with the reserves and juniors to see how good Jay Jay was and as he'd paid his airfare, I agreed. The match hadn't been going many minutes when Mark started complaining that the pitch wasn't good enough, that the other players weren't passing the ball to Jay Jay and he wasn't getting a chance. He abandoned the game and said we had to re-arrange it for the following Sunday at Valley Parade. That was the final straw. I knew that the senior players were starting to ask questions about who was in charge and now the chairman was trying to arrange a practice match over my head. My standing as manager would have been terminally weakened if I'd rolled over and let other people run the football side of the club.

Two days later, I held the usual Thursday press conference in the morning and after lunch, I put my suit on and set off to Valley Parade for the monthly board meeting. There were four directors there and Christie. I was running through the list of injuries ahead of our game against Barnet on Saturday when Mark suddenly cut in, "We're no better than last year. The players aren't good enough, we're not going to score goals, we'll go down." Another director said something along the same lines.

OK, we'd taken only one point from four league matches and lost 1-0 at home to Dagenham the previous week. But I felt I was getting it right. We had youth, energy and spirit and had performed really well in a League Cup-tie against Leeds at Elland Road, losing 3-2. And with so many new players, we would need time to gel, time I was not going to be given.

I would have expected the directors to take a more sensible view and ask me how and where I thought we could improve things. Instead, it was, "We're shit, we're going down," and Christie talking about why we'd been beaten by Dagenham. He was wrong but I had a feeling I was the only person in the room who thought so.

So I said, "Right, in that case, if everyone feels the same way, I'll offer my resignation." I didn't quit, I offered to resign. It was something I felt I had to say even though I knew I was giving them the chance to get rid of me. But I hoped that it would bring things to a head and give me an opportunity to put my point of view. I was asked to leave the room so they could discuss the situation. I was outside for maybe twenty minutes and when they called me back in I was told that my resignation had been accepted unanimously. That was all. No chance to state my case.

When I got home, Alison asked if I had any regrets. I said no because I would have been compromising myself, my staff and my players if I'd worked under Christie, a man who had been brought in over my head, effectively as director of football. However I feared I might have serious misgivings when I woke up next morning. I didn't. So I knew then that I'd done the right thing. I may look back in five years' time and say it was the wrong decision but at the time it was the only way forward for me.

Even so, I was desperately upset. When I first arrived at Valley Parade, there was no spirit at the club at all, from top to bottom. My first priority was to bring the club back to life and raise morale and that's what I did. And I believed we would have been promoted, either that season or the following season. With the support of the fans and the spirit of the players, I would have done it, I'm convinced about that.

And the support I had from the people of Bradford was magnificent, during my stay in charge and in the immediate aftermath of my departure. They knew how much I felt about Bradford City and that walk down the touchline at Valley Parade before kick-off was something I will always cherish. I still fill up when I remember it.

I sorted out a month's pay-out with Julian Rhodes and the following Tuesday I had a call to say that someone would come and pick up my Mercedes the next day. It was driven away, along with my dreams of taking Bradford City out of the bottom division. Three days after I left, Phil Parkinson was appointed manager. Christie left nine weeks later.

Strangely, this wasn't the first time Phil and my paths had crossed. Four years earlier, when I left Huddersfield for the second time, he was lined up as my successor and a press conference was called to unveil him. But he had second thoughts at the last minute and stayed at Charlton, where he was assistant manager.

His first season at Valley Parade was unexceptional but the following year he achieved what no manager had done before by leading a club from the bottom flight to a major Wembley final, in this case the League Cup final. I was absolutely delighted for them. I didn't think they'd beat Wigan in a fourth round replay, Arsenal in the quarter-final and definitely not Aston Villa over two legs in the semi-final. But they did and if the final proved a game too far nothing can take away what they achieved. I can't see a club from the bottom tier ever doing it again.

I felt I had to go. Dad didn't feel up to it on the day but Anthony and Gerard were there, too. They had escaped from the burning stand at Valley Parade 28 years earlier, the darkest day in the club's history, and I thought it was important we should all be together for what was without a doubt

City's biggest day since winning the FA Cup in 1911. It had been a long time since we all used to go and watch Leeds United together when we were kids.

It was a great day out. We set off at quarter to ten with our packed lunches in the boot, had a couple of pints when we got to Wembley and then joined the rest of the fans in the stand. I was even waving a flag! It meant so much for us to be there and I could see how much it meant to the supporters, too. OK, a lot of the 30,000 fans might never have been to a match before and might not go again. But for the hard core of true supporters that was one of the greatest days of their lives.

When I started at City as a kid, a handful of people used to come and watch the juniors play their matches at our training ground at Apperley Bridge. One of them was a young girl who would be about three years older than me. She and her friend never missed a match. I spotted her at Wembley and when she saw me, she came over and said, "You don't remember me, do you?" I replied, "Oh I do, you and your friend used to come and watch me in the juniors when I was 16." I was so happy for her and so many more of what I call the old crowd, fans who have seen the club through thick and very thin ever since the fire.

And reaching Wembley didn't do the city of Bradford any harm either. There hasn't been much for people to get excited about recently and there is a lot of hardship in the city. But all of a sudden people here and around the world were sitting up and taking notice of Bradford and for a while a little bit of that feelgood factor rubbed off on everyone. OK the result, a 5-0 win for Swansea, was a huge letdown and City never really performed. But no one who followed them to Wembley will ever forget that day. Me included.

As the teams came out, one supporter said to me, "Just think, Peter, that could have been you leading City out at Wembley." I thought, "Yes, it might have been…but it isn't. It's Phil Parkinson and good luck to him." And I didn't feel any regrets at all. I hadn't regretted my decision to resign at the time and 19 months later I still felt the same, even though I had not been able to find my way back into management. It was still the right thing for me to do.

Above all, I like to think the day finally demonstrated that Bradford City fans have forgotten all about the bitter rivalry when I was manager at Huddersfield. People don't ask for autographs any more – they take a picture on their mobile instead. And that day I must have had mine taken around 300 times. Hopefully that proves City supporters now see me as a man who was born in the city, played nearly 400 games for the club, endured the tragedy of the fire alongside them and returned for a spell as manager of the club he loves.

15. The way we are

Peter didn't have to look far to find a new team to work with after leaving Bradford City in August, 2011, returning to Caremark Calderdale, the home care business set up by Alison sixteen months earlier. And a career swerve away from football's comfort zone. "People talk about the pressures of football management," he says. "They should try working on the front line as a carer. That's real pressure."

Alison's Story

Never in a million years did I imagine that one day Peter and I would work together. For nearly 30 years we had our own separate careers and there seemed no reason to suppose that anything would change until we retired. Then along came Caremark Calderdale in April, 2010 and all of a sudden we were working as a team. It must have been a real culture shock for Peter after 13 years in football management but he's been a tremendous support from the day I decided to set up the business.

At first, when there was a good chance he would be going back into football sooner rather than later, he took on the role of front man as head of marketing and sales. He did a fantastic job in marketing the company and helping to recruit staff.

However we were both aware that having a high-profile personality on board could be a two-edged sword. As a positive, his presence attracted interest and publicity and helped put Caremark on the map. But it was vital that we also established the company as, first and foremost, a professional operation in its own right...rather than a care company in which Peter Jackson, a football manager, was involved.

When we set up the business, I suggested that even though Peter was waiting to go back into football, he might as well do his NVQ Level Two in Health and Social Care. It was a six-week course that gave him all the necessary training in looking after people so that he could go out and provide hands-on care if necessary. It wasn't easy for him. He'd been on courses for football qualifications when he was surrounded by familiar faces and covering familiar ground. This was different, something completely new.

Can you imagine a footballer, let alone a football manager, taking part in an NVQ course for carers? They operate in a different world. Managers are used to buying players, taking training, picking a side, dealing with club directors and the media. Not setting off at seven o'clock in the morning to get an old lady out of bed or cook her breakfast. Of course there's no reason why a manager shouldn't become a carer but let's face it, it's not the kind of thing you would expect. So Peter was certainly jumping in at the deep end.

Part of the course took place in the office with a tutor from Calderdale College and there were also sessions at the college. There would be fifteen or twenty people on the course and most of them were also from Caremark. So to them, he was just another member of staff and not a football manager learning something new.

There have been many more days in the classroom since then in which Peter was totally out of his comfort zone – but he has passed each course with flying colours and has survived. A position in care means updating training every 12 months and there will be more courses to attend. When he first started he used to say that sometimes he felt like a fish up a tree but he got through it and for me that was a real achievement. And I'm very proud of him as I know classrooms are really not his thing!

Now, after his brief spell as manager of Bradford City, he's involved all the time. He does some after dinner speaking and still works as a football pundit on television but caring is his priority. And he's very good at it. His clients love him because he is a people person. He always has a smile for everyone. I really take my hat off to him. At first he had his doubts about whether he was equipped to do this kind of work. He used to say, "All I've ever done is football," which was true. And what he achieved in that niche market, as a player and as a manager, was fantastic. But he has proved to himself through his work at Caremark that there is a life for him outside football, even though that was and always will be his first love.

If he hadn't joined the business, he wouldn't be the person he is now. He would probably be one of those ex-professional footballers moaning and groaning about how the game has let them down and how they've nothing left to live for. That's a real danger for football people who have spent their lives in the public eye and have enjoyed all the glamour and the accolades.

But that all comes to an end one day and they have to realise there is a real world out there, too, and they can be a part of it if they try hard enough. That's what Peter has achieved and I genuinely believe that if and when he goes back into management, he will be better at the job because of the time he has spent with Caremark.

Like I say, though, I never thought the day would dawn when we'd be working alongside one another. But so far so good. We combine well and realise that in a work environment, it's all about getting on with the job first and foremost. So if there's something that needs doing urgently, whatever it may be, Peter will do it.

If he isn't out in the field with his care duties, marketing or networking, he'll come into the office to see how we are. He's a bit like a caged animal and he doesn't usually hang around for long. He'll come bursting in, everybody has their head down, busy, busy, busy and Peter will start causing a distraction. He can't keep quiet for long and soon gets bored so he'll make lots of coffee. But then if we ask him to do some filing he'll suddenly remember he has to dash.

For the first couple of years I assumed he'd be in and out of football for the rest of his working life and I wouldn't be able to rely on having him here. So I took on a lot of things myself that he might have done. But now I can safely hand over all sorts of things to him and I know my life would be a lot tougher and busier if he went back into football. Would I miss him if he did? Yes, we all would: his clients, the people he meets in his recruiting and marketing roles, the girls in the office, the other carers. I suppose all the other people who work in the Elsie Whiteley centre would miss him as well because he's such a big, cheerful personality about the place.

He's a big help, although sometimes he doesn't realise it. He may think that because he doesn't sit in the office doing the filing that he isn't valuable to us but believe me he is. Because of his football, he's a great motivator and he'll do anything if it will benefit the business. He goes round to job centres to let people know we're looking for staff, he drops off leaflets and post cards all over the place and he'll talk to anyone who's prepared to listen and tell them who we are and what we do. We couldn't have done anything like as much of that without him and he's been a great ambassador for the company.

Every night when I get home, whatever time it is, his first question will always be, "How's your day been?" Whether he's been in the office or out on the road. Sometimes I'm still trying to absorb something in my own head before I want to discuss it and he'll spot that straight away. Or sometimes, I'll go straight in at the deep end and say, "You won't believe what's happened…" And then he'll be ready to listen while I get everything off my chest. Either way, I'll eventually ask him for his opinion, to make sure we're singing from the same hymn sheet. And usually we are.

We certainly don't spend all our time at home talking about work but we can't pretend it doesn't exist just because Peter's finished his calls and I've left the office. We both know we're in this together. It's our future and the future of our children.

Peter's Story

There's an old saying that once a day, every day, we should do something that really frightens us. Well, I was frightened every day for months and months…and more than just once a day, believe me. When I started working for Caremark, I moved out of my comfort zone many, many times and tested myself up to and beyond what I thought was my limit. I had to push myself every day, getting up at six o'clock in the morning to set off on a round of breakfast calls to old and vulnerable people.

At first, I struggled to get through it and often, my old life at Huddersfield Town came to my rescue. Some of my calls were in the Dalton area of Huddersfield, at the top of the steep, banked road that leads away from the stadium. My journey from home was exactly the route I used to take to the ground when I was manager of Huddersfield. So when I climbed into the car, I pretended that I was going back to my office at the ground rather than up to Dalton to change a few catheter bags and incontinence pads.

Only this time I wasn't driving my Range Rover or Mercedes but a second-hand Renault Clio with Caremark written on the side. And instead of turning right into the ground when I came to the roundabout in front of the Odeon cinema, it was time to take a deep breath, get back into the real world, change gear and set off up Dalton Bank.

I never knew what might be waiting for me. It might be just a wake-up call, making breakfast and a cup of tea, helping an old person get dressed and set up for the day. Usually there was more: changing an incontinence pad or a catheter bag, changing soiled sheets, giving medication. Maybe a client had fallen out of bed, wet or soiled themselves. Or perhaps the electricity had blown or a room flooded because a tap had been left on. It's the carer's job to make the necessary calls for help.

Once I called into a house to make a gentleman's breakfast and found him sitting on the stairs covered in faeces from head to toe. I should have been there for 15 minutes to see if he was OK, make his breakfast and give him his medication. I showered him and cleaned everything up but obviously the call lasted a bit longer than it should. But it wasn't his fault, was it? These things happen and it's a carer's job to help. Sometimes I work with another carer, using a hoist to help an elderly person into the bath, and I've turned my hand to more or less anything that involves bodily functions.

One day, I suppose, I will arrive to discover that a client has died in the night. It's happened to other carers and it will happen to me and it will be difficult and upsetting, particularly if it's a client I've been looking after for a couple of years.

But I've come a long way since the first catheter bag. I suspected it would be horrendous and it was. But now it's become just another part of the job… and I've even learned how to cook scrambled eggs! I never thought that I would end up doing something like this but the longer I've been here, the more I've felt at home. It's hugely rewarding and as it stands now, it won't be the end of the world if I don't go back into football. I never thought the day would dawn when I'd say that.

I have some really good relationships with my clients and that's so important because they see us as part of the family. They are reliant on Caremark. We could be the only people they see in a week if their relatives live away. Neighbours or friends may pop in once in a while but we are their regular visitors, their lifeline in some ways. The only people who walk through their door and say good morning on a regular basis.

Care is about going into people's houses and treating them as you would want a parent to be cared for. There's a lot of pressure and carers don't receive the credit they deserve. They aren't paid a lot of money but they are happy to get up at six o'clock in the morning and be on the road by seven with no idea what they might have to face in their working day. There isn't much in the way of praise or thanks when they do the job properly. But it's a different story if a carer is late or if the job doesn't go smoothly. We might do 1,500 calls in a week and if 1,499 go smoothly we never hear a word. But just wait until something goes wrong on the 1,500th!

One of my clients is Dean. He's wheelchair-bound and we take him out on respite care for five hours a day, three times a week.. It's a pleasure being with him. He was badly injured in an accident 17 years ago and has a memory span of about ten minutes. I'll say, "Hello, I'm Peter," when I arrive and ten minutes later he's forgotten who I am. We go all over. He has three separate carers and if it's me, I might take him to Hollingworth Lake, a big freshwater lake near Milnrow close to the M62, or maybe the butterfly garden at Manor Heath Park in Halifax. Or even somewhere like the White Rose shopping centre near Leeds. We have a converted Renault Kangoo and I have to hoist him into the back with the ramp, fasten him in and then set off. It's a big responsibility and I sometimes have visions of driving down the road, looking in the rear view mirror and seeing Dean wheeling off in the opposite direction!

Quite a lot of the people I've cared for have known who I am and at first, I could see they were shocked by what I was doing. I suppose it must have been difficult for them as well. After all, it isn't every Huddersfield Town fan who has his catheter bag changed or his breakfast cooked by a former manager of the club!

Most of my ex-teammates or other managers and people who are still in the game can't get a handle on what I actually do either. Fair enough, I suppose. If, when I was in football, I'd been told that a former player or manager was now a care worker, it would have taken some believing. Mainly, they seem to think Alison and I run a care home, rather than a domiciliary (there was a time when I couldn't pronounce that!) care service. When Alison launched the business there was some publicity locally about my involvement and people probably saw the word 'care', put two and two together and made five.

So these days, when I'm asked how the care home is going, I have a script ready: "No, we're not a care home, we're a care provider. We cover wake-up calls, medication calls, lunchtime, teatime, bedtime and so on." They always say, "Good on you, that's brilliant."

Alison has been amazing. When we first started, she was leaving home at six in the morning and sometimes not getting in until ten at night. Ridiculous hours, really, but it had to be done if the business was going to be successful. It was tough at first but she's turned it round now. She's an incredible businesswoman and working alongside her, I've seen what an incredible person she is, too. I'm there to help and support her in any way I can. Just like she helped and supported me through the good and bad times in my life.

And now?

July 31, 2013. Deadline day minus one...Living with Jacko goes to print tomorrow. What better time for Alison and Peter to start looking forward to the good times ahead...

Alison: We've got a big map of the world at home with stickers showing every single place we've visited. We sometimes look at it and think it's a big, big world and there's a hell of a lot of it we haven't seen yet. We've been lucky. We've been to places a lot of people can only dream about. But we have new dreams, too.

Peter: And two more of those dreams will have come true by the end of 2013. Oliver and Stacey were married in May and Charlotte and Stephen will be married in October. I suppose when I was ill, there were times when perhaps we all wondered whether I'd be around to see those weddings happen.

Alison: So soon the kids will both have moved on to the next stage of their lives...and fingers crossed, we can look forward to the next stage of ours as grandparents. We can't wait for that and we'll be very hands-on! Peter will be an absolutely fantastic granddad. His role as a carer is a very serious and responsible position and after football, he's found himself living in the real world. But having a grandchild will mean he could go back to being a big kid again. He'll love that. But over our time together, we've both learned never ever to take anything for granted. When you are living the good times, enjoy them and be ready to relish every minute. You never know when they will be whipped away from you.

Peter: That's right. I care for some clients who are really, really ill and the one thing so many of them say is that these things can happen overnight, literally. Some of them have had marvellous lives, been successful in their work and some have travelled the world. One day they are fit and healthy and then in no time they find themselves bed bound and desperately ill. Their life has changed completely and they will never be the same again. I've had two life-changing experiences, first the throat cancer and now seeing life from a carer's point of view. Who knows whether there will be another one somewhere down the road. Or what the future may hold. We've had our ups and downs like all families but to do all we've done and to have had a great lifestyle is everything we could have asked for.

Alison: Above all, we've had a happy marriage for 32 years. We've survived everything that's been thrown at us.

Peter: Yes, there might have been a few bad times but don't we always say there's no point in looking back?

Alison: Exactly. We've always, always been positive and that's so important. Concentrate on looking forward but when you do look back, reflect on the good times.

Peter: That's something I took into football management. Always show people your positive side.

Alison: And be optimistic. I know that especially well from the time I spent looking after Peter during his treatment and recovery from cancer. There were some dreadful times for us all but however bad one day might have been, I went to bed determined that tomorrow would be better. And that I'd make the best out of a bad situation.

Peter: I'm trying to put that across now to the people I'm caring for. After being in the limelight as footballer and manager to go into care has been humbling. And I feel I am a better person for it. I've learned so much over the last couple of years.

Alison: When Peter was in football, both as a player and manager, we never knew almost from one week to the next what might be waiting round the corner. We were ready to face whatever challenges there may be. Now the business comes first and that's the big challenge facing us. But as I've said before, every business has a lifespan and the time will come when we'll start looking at something else.

Peter: We'd both like to do more travelling at some point. Maybe South America or Vietnam. In some ways you could say we've cracked it after 32 years and these days, even being married for as long as we have is an achievement in itself. But we're not past it yet...although before long I suppose we'll have to start thinking about moving house and looking at places with built-in stairlifts and ramps...

Alison: What? You must be joking...and there was me talking about positive thinking! There's still another 20 holidays in us. In fact I don't feel as if we've really changed at all since that night we met in the Time & Place nightclub all those years ago. Same dress size for me? If only....

Peter: Same waist measurement for me? Well, sort of! But I don't think either of us would have changed a thing, would we? It's been fantastic.

Peter Jackson.

Born Bradford, West Yorkshire, April 6, 1961

Career as a player

Football League

	League	FA Cup	League Cup	Other
Bradford City (7-4-79 – 23-10-86)	267(11)	10(1)	27(0)	4(0)
Newcastle Utd (23-10-86) – 15-9-88)	60(0)	6(0)	3(0)	3(0)
Bradford City (15-9-88 – 6-9-90)	55(3)	4(0)	7(0)	2(0)
Huddersfield Town (6-9-90 – 29-9-94)	152(3)	13(0)	11(0)	18(0)
Chester (29-9-94) – 31-5-97)	99(0)	2(0)	5(0)	2(0)
Totals	633(17)	35(1)	53(0)	29(0)

Football Conference

Halifax Town (1-8-97 – 7-10-97)	8(0)			

As a manager

Huddersfield Town October 1997 – May 1993

Huddersfield Town July 2003 – March 2007

Lincoln City October 2007 – September 2009

Bradford City February 2011 – August 2011

Five Manager of the Month awards, three with Huddersfield Town and two with Lincoln City